D1562917

Communication Programming
for the Severely Handicapped:
Vocal and Non-vocal Strategies

Caroline R. Musselwhite, Ed.D., C.C.C.

and

Karen W. St. Louis, M.S., C.C.C.

COLLEGE-HILL
PRESS

This book is dedicated to women who are pursuing their professional goals while juggling families, homes, jobs, continuing education, and other personal responsibilities.

College-Hill Press
4284 41st. Street
San Diego, California 92105

© 1982 by College-Hill Press

Library of Congress Cataloging in Publication Data

Musselwhite, Caroline Ramsey.
    Communication programming for the severely handicapped.
    Bibliography.
    1. Communicative disorders. 2. Handicapped—
Language. I St. Louis, Karen Waterman.
II. Title

RC423.M76   6.6.85′5   81-2111

ISBN 0-933014-64-3   AACR2

Contents

83-- 1973

Dedication

This book is dedicated to women who are pursuing their professional goals while juggling families, homes, jobs, continuing education, and other personal responsibilities.

Preface

This book was not originally intended as a book. Several years ago we started from different directions: Karen was collecting information on communication programming for the severely and profoundly retarded for a curriculum she was developing, and Caroline was doing research for a doctoral project. In comparing notes, we realized that both of us were frustrated by the inadequate information available and the degree to which it was scattered among numerous sources, many of which were not published. We decided to collaborate on an annotated bibliography of sources of information on communication for the severely handicapped. That project became a working paper which is distributed through the University Affiliated Center for Developmental Disabilities at West Virginia University in Morgantown. We then decided to expand a paper written previously by Caroline on communication for the severely handicapped. By the time this work was expanded sufficiently, it became clear that it was more than a paper in both length and depth. Since the paper and the bibliography complemented each other, we decided to update and expand both into a book. The book has since mushroomed, as we have attempted to address issues in sufficient detail. For example, coverage of the various gestural and symbolic communication systems was enlarged greatly from our original plan, as we believed it necessary to provide enough detail to give communication specialists a rationale for selecting a communication mode and implementing a training program. In so doing we have not only reviewed the appropriate literature, but have also drawn from our own clinical experiences with severely handicapped clients and those of our colleagues.

This project began and ended without institutional support, and we endured the many interruptions and absorbed travel and other costs on our own. However, the moral and technical support we received from our families, colleagues, friends, and new acquaintances was both encouraging and sustaining. We would like to acknowledge and thank the many people who have provided this support.

First, our immediate and extended families have given all types of assistance. Our preschool children, Matt, Katie, and Melinda, have enjoyed new experiences as a result of this project. They have learned the value of quiet play and have acquired some new skills, such as saying "See you later, alligator" in sign language, and have been introduced to Blissymbols, rebuses, and lexigrams. They have been patient with us through many interruptions of their daily routines. Our husbands, Robert and Ken, have been supportive throughout this endeavor by increased sharing in child care as we traded visits to each other's homes. They have also served as sounding boards for ideas and have proofed various sections of the book. Our mothers, Julia and Louise, and mother-in-law, Sallie, have shared in child care whenever possible, although many miles separate us. Our fathers, Gene and Ed, have also been very supportive. Other family members, including Ruth Johnson Tompkins (Caroline's grandmother) and Diane Fletcher (Caroline's cousin) have searched through newspapers and personal files to find additional information for this book.

Numerous professionals from all over this country provided us with current information and technical support. Chief among these are Diane DeHaven, Judy Montgomery, Orin Cornett, Howard Shane, and the staff at the Blissymbolics Communication Institute in Toronto.

Special appreciation goes to Ronjit Majumder and Katherine Greever for their encouragement during this project.

Several colleagues in speech-language pathology and special education have also provided assistance. Gerry Killarney and Louise Kaczmarek read portions of the manuscript and gave both suggestions and materials. Fred Orelove and Linda Luther gave general assistance and moral support. Barbara Ludlow served as a pony express, carrying materials between Buckhannon and Morgantown, West Virginia.

The students, teachers, and directors of the School of Movement Theatre in Elkins, West Virginia, were most helpful in contributing information and ideas for the section on mime.

Ricky Creech shared insights and information from the perspective of a non-vocal person and offered ideas for preparing professionals to work with non-vocal clients.

We would also like to acknowledge the many severely handicapped clients and their families with whom we have worked.

People from local service agencies have also been extremely helpful in our attempts to gather information. We are especially grateful to the staff at the Stonewall Jackson Regional Library in Buckhannon, who managed to locate numerous hard to find sources for us, and to Jay Newman of the Buckhannon radio station.

Our close friends, Tammy Murray, Patty McCartney, Suzanne Smart, and Tammy Wilson, encouraged us when we were discouraged and helped care for our children.

Preparing this manuscript has been a logistical nightmare. Typing assistance has been begged, borrowed, and bought. Special thanks go to Cathy Samargo and the other typists who have contributed their time and skill to this project. Caroline deserves a special acknowledgement for typing some sections herself amid the frenzy of meeting our deadlines.

Part One: Preliminary Issues

Chapter 1: Introduction

"The closest simile as to how people treat nonspeech people is how they treat pet dogs. . . . think about that for a minute. How much difference is there? People take good care of pet dogs. They give them love, food, warm homes, attention when they are not busy. And people don't expect much out of their pet dogs. Just affection and obedience. This is the sad part. People just don't expect much from nonspeech people."

> *Personal communication via voice synthesizer,*
> Ricky Creech, *non-vocal person*

Focus

This book covers both vocal and non-vocal communication strategies, as well as related topics such as preliminary skills and support systems. We chose not to limit the scope of this book to non-vocal strategies because we believe strongly that vocal communication, being the primary and normative mode, must always be considered. Including vocal language programming in conjunction with a more in-depth coverage of non-vocal programming will, we hope, help keep these communication modes in perspective. Throughout this book we will stress the potential usefulness of non-vocal modes to facilitate or supplement vocal language. It is important to recognize that for some individuals non-vocal modes will serve as an alternative to speech, at least for a portion of their lives.

The emphasis in the various chapters of this book reflects our varied purposes in covering different topics. Chapters in Part I are designed to acquaint the reader with background information and considerations that apply to all modes of communication programming. Therefore, these chapters explore important topics and provide directions and resources for further study. Part II presents an overview of selected vocal language programs and issues in vocal language training. Because of the large number of available programs, this is not intended to be a comprehensive literature review. Its purpose is to provide the reader with a basis for comparing various programs in relation to specific issues about developing communication strategies. Part III receives the greatest emphasis, as information concerning non-vocal communication is less available and less integrated. In addition, this part covers a wide variety of communication systems rather than focusing only on specific programs. We think it is important to provide sufficiently detailed descriptions of each system to allow the communication specialist to make informed decisions. Part IV consists of four appendices designed to supplement, through various types of resources, the information presented in the first three parts.

Overview of Chapters

Chapter 2 presents a decision process model which can be used for structuring the increasingly detailed decisions that must be made regarding communication programming. Recent theoretical approaches to selecting communication modes for primary emphasis in training are described, and a visual continuum is presented as a means of following client progress.

Chapter 3 presents selected issues that relate to general communication programming. These issues, such as methodology selection, the content to be trained, and the context in which the training will take place, are described and then presented in later chapters as they relate to each communication mode (vocal, gestural, or symbolic).

Chapter 4 presents preliminary training strategies for skills usually considered prerequisites to language training. We have stressed the idea and trend apparent in recent literature that these preliminary skills, such as attending, can often be taught concurrently with language oriented tasks.

Support services are described in Chapter 5. The need for a team of professionals, including occupational, physical, and speech-language therapists along with the classroom personnel and parents, is emphasized in planning and implementing communication programming. Sources of funding at the local, state, and national levels are discussed.

Vocal communication strategies are presented in Chapter 6. Twenty-four language programs are reviewed as they relate to the general issues in communication programming raised in Chapter 3. Both general and prescriptive assessment strategies are presented. Involvement of parents in their child's programming is also discussed.

Chapters 7, 8, and 9 deal with non-vocal communication strategies. Chapter 7 describes the functions of non-vocal systems and the implications for their use. Factors to consider in choosing between gestural or symbolic modes are briefly discussed. Chapters 8 and 9 deal specifically with gestural and symbolic modes, respectively. An in-depth description of the communication systems that can be utilized with each of these modes is presented.

Populations for Whom This Book is Intended

This book is intended for a wide variety of client populations. They may be divided into five categories according to the basic impairment which influences the communication disorder. Table 1-1 lists those five categories and indicates client populations that may fall within each. These lists are meant to indicate clients that might fall under a specific category, but they do not include all possible client populations. The five categories are not mutually exclusive; clients often have more than one impairment contributing to the communication disorder. For example, mental retardation may accompany autism or cerebral palsy. Our opinion is that considering the impairment leading to the communication disorder will often be more helpful than looking at population labels. The wide range of capabilities and limitations existing within a client population requires that decisions ultimately be made on a case-by-case basis.

Table 1-1.
Categories of impairment frequently accompanied by severe communication disorder.

Cognitive Impairment	Sensory Impairment	Neurological Impairment	Emotional Impairment	Structural Impairment
Mental Retardation	Deafness Blindness Deaf-Blind	Cerebral Palsy Aphasia Apraxia Dysarthria Progressive Disorders (e.g., Myasthenia Gravis, Multiple Sclerosis, Parkinson's Disease) Dysphonia from vocal fold paralysis	Autism Elective Mutism Childhood Psychosis	Glossectomy Laryngectomy

This book is also intended for a wide range of persons involved in working with severely handicapped clients. It will be primarily useful for professionals designing and implementing communication programs for the severely handicapped. The major professional groups involved in these activities are speech-language pathologists and special educators. Physical therapists, occupational therapists, and developmental psychologists, too, may find this information useful in their overall program planning. Portions of this book could serve as background information for others working with the severely handicapped, such as social workers and rehabilitation specialists.

Terminology

Terminology is always a controversial issue. Newsletters in the field of non-vocal communication frequently print articles or letters concerning terminology, especially as it relates to labeling individuals or populations. At this point we will offer our definitions of some of the key terms we have selected. We have chosen to use the term *non-vocal* to describe persons who do not communicate through oral language. There were many terms to choose from, including *nonspeech*, *nonoral*, and *non-verbal*. We decided on *non-vocal* because it is widely used in the literature and because it provides a clear opposite to *vocal* communication, which is a descriptive term. We have divided non-vocal communication into two categories, gestural and symbolic. *Gestural communication* includes systems which require movement of the body, typically the arms and hands, but do not require access to equipment or devices separate from the body. Examples are sign languages, sign systems, and mime. *Symbolic communication* comprises systems which require access to a symbol system separate from the body, such as Blissymbols, rebuses, or words. We have used the word *mode* as a broad term to indicate overall categories such as vocal and non-vocal modes of communication. The term *systems* is used to refer to specific subcategories within these modes. For example, Amer-Ind is considered a gestural system and Blissymbolics is listed as a symbolic system.

We have chosen to use the terms *client, trainer,* and *communication specialist.* Although we believe that *client* is somewhat sterile, it is clearer than *person* or *individual* and is less restrictive than terms such as *child, patient,* or *student.* *Trainer* is also a rather cold term; however, it is not as restrictive as *teacher, professional,* or *speech-language pathologist.* Our view is that any of these professionals as well as parents, paraprofessionals, and others, may serve as trainers for some activities. The term *communication specialist* refers to the professional who coordinates communication programming; this will often be a speech-language pathologist but may be another person who has extensive training in communication.

The most difficult terminology problem was choosing descriptive terms for training approaches. After several hours of discussion with colleagues, we decided on *artificially-structured techniques* and *naturally-structured techniques.* We are not completely satisfied with these terms, as we recognize that they are not sufficiently exact. However, we think that their meanings will be immediately clear to readers, unlike some of the terms we considered as substitutes. *Artificially-structured techniques* refer to techniques which utilize rote instruction apart from context. An example is presenting pictures, one after the other, and asking, "What is this?" In that example the activity presumably lacks contextual support and communicative intent. *Naturally-structured techniques* refer to techniques focusing on events which are, or at least appear to be, naturally-occurring. An example is training the motor imitation of waving good-bye as staff members or peers leave the area. In this example contextual support and, possibly, communicative intent may be present. The inclusion of the word *structured* in each term indicates that neither approach is haphazard. Both can be carefully planned and monitored.

As to our opening quote from Ricky Creech, it is our hope that this book will help professionals to better serve the needs of nonspeaking clients so that we may expect more of them and they may experience greater self-fulfillment in the future. It must also be a goal of professionals and clients alike to educate the public to recognize the communication capabilities of severely handicapped people, even though they may not be expressed through traditional modes.

Chapter 2: The Decision Process

Introduction

Developing and implementing a communication program for the severely handicapped client involves making a series of decisions. Ordinarily, this initial decision involves a number of related, increasingly fine decisions. Even if very little time and thought go into the decision process, the resulting communication plan reflects a number of crucial decisions. It is most important that this process be brought to a high level of awareness so that decisions for an individual are based on the best information available about that individual and about severely handicapped persons in general.

A four-stage decision process model is presented as a framework for making the major decisions. Figure 2-1 illustrates this model, which will be followed throughout this book. The first stage involves determining whether a vocal or non-vocal mode will be used as the primary communication mode. Stage two involves selecting a gestural or symbolic mode as the primary mode for a non-vocal client. The third stage covers system selection decisions, such as use of Blissymbols, and the fourth stage considers implementation features such as content and method of training. The following discussion focuses on a number of considerations and procedures for use at each point of the decision process.

Stage I: Vocal/Non-vocal Modes of Communication

This stage of the decision process involves determining how much emphasis to place on vocal or non-vocal modes of communication. This decision concerns both input and output. For example, a severely physically handicapped client may receive messages primarily through the vocal mode but may transmit primarily through a non-vocal mode, such as an electronic device utilizing printed words. It should be noted that pure examples of either vocal or non-vocal modes are rare. Obviously, vocal communicators transmit a proportion of their message non-vocally, through facial expressions, gestures, and so forth. Likewise, non-vocal communicators may support their messages by vocal expressions such as laughter or grunts. Selecting a communication mode may be viewed as a continuum, with non-vocal at one end and vocal at the other, as illustrated:

Non-vocal ———————————————————————————————— Vocal

The decision would then change from an either/or issue to a question of which communication mode should receive primary emphasis in training.

It is generally agreed that vocal communication should be given priority since it is more normative. However, it may be necessary to train even a primarily vocal client in non-vocal techniques for use when there is a communication breakdown. For example, a dysarthric client might be intelligible only when the context is known. This person might use a non-vocal mode, such as a communication board with rebus symbols, to establish context when necessary. Such an instance is visualized on the continuum as follows:

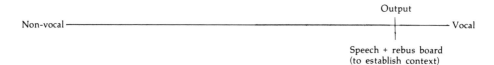

For some clients it may be desirable, at least initially, to place equal emphasis on vocal and non-vocal components. In this case the word would be spoken simultaneously with a symbol or sign for the word. This pairing is often used for input to severely handicapped clients, as in trainers' use of Total Communication (speech plus signs). The client may also use simultaneous production for output, such as signed speech, Cued Speech, or Blissymbols plus speech. An example of one equally emphasizing vocal and non-vocal modes is the severely dysarthric client who uses a letter board to indicate the first letter of each word as it is spoken (Beukelman and Yorkston 1977). This would be represented on the continuum as follows:

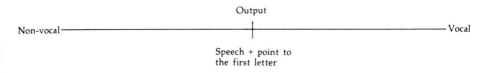

In many cases the equal emphasis would change as the client progressed, with emphasis shifting toward the vocal end of the continuum. In the

Figure 2-1

The Decision Process Model

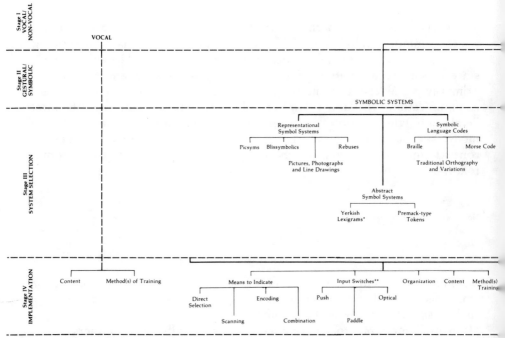

*Indicates communication systems which are not covered in depth in this book.
**Indicates that entries are merely examples of possible entries.

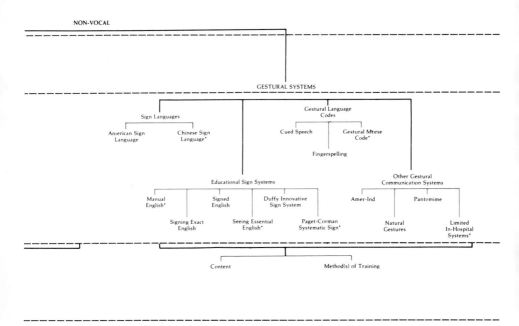

NON-VOCAL

GESTURAL SYSTEMS

Sign Languages

American Sign Language

Chinese Sign Language*

Gestural Language Codes

Cued Speech

Gestural Morse Code*

Fingerspelling

Educational Sign Systems

Manual English*

Signed English

Duffy Innovative Sign System

Signing Exact English

Seeing Essential English*

Paget-Corman Systematic Sign*

Other Gestural Communication Systems

Amer-Ind

Pantomime

Natural Gestures

Limited In-Hospital Systems*

Content

Method(s) of Training

example above, the client could begin pointing to first letters for only those words not understood by the listener. This was the approach taken by Schaeffer (1980), with four autistic clients; gradually, the signs were faded from both input and output so that the clients ultimately listened to and produced spoken utterances.

Some clients may need initial emphasis on non-vocal communication. For example, a client who demonstrates persistent (abnormal) oral reflexes such as biting or rooting may be considered a poor candidate for early development of functional speech. Here a non-vocal system such as a Blissymbol board might serve the child's immediate communication needs while therapy focuses on inhibiting the abnormal reflexes and developing functional speech. Useful vocalizations (e.g., appropriate laughter) would also be encouraged. This situation would be represented on the continuum as seen below:

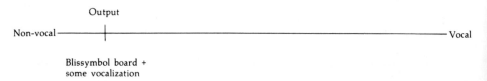

The input to the client may also emphasize vocal or non-vocal approaches. Typically, the trainer will provide input that is primarily vocal (speech) or a combination of vocal plus non-vocal (Total Communication or speech plus symbols). Primary emphasis on non-vocal modes is less common for input than for output. A variety of possible input modes may be represented on our non-vocal/vocal continuum:

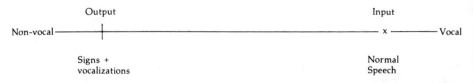

It would also be possible to represent both input and output on the same line. An example of a sketch for a client who receives normal speech as input and produces signs plus vocalizations as output is shown below:

There are several reasons why it could be useful to chart the input and output emphasis on a non-vocal/vocal line. First, and most important, such a visual device could help bring the decision to a higher level of consciousness and possibly result in greater individualization. Second, such a device helps indicate the client's present distance from normalization. A rule of thumb would be that the closer the input and output marks are toward the vocal end of the continuum, the more normalized the client is. Finally, this visual aid could be used to follow progress across time, with the sketch redrawn each time the mode is changed significantly (e.g., when signs are faded from either input or output). Progress toward the vocal end would, one hopes, be seen. Change toward the non-vocal end might also be noted across time, especially in clients with progressive disorders. For example, a client with Parkinson's Disease might initially use primarily vocal output, but at a slower rate; gradually, it might be necessary to introduce a communication board for establishing context and, finally, to use a communication board as the primary mode, accompanied by vocalizations. Dates of charting would be noted as follows:

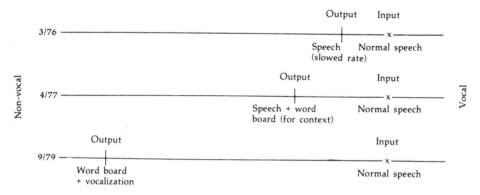

In summary, this continuum emphasizes the normalization part of the vocal/non-vocal decision and provides a method of visualizing that decision. Obviously, several factors other than normalization must influence the initial decision. Several authors (e.g., Harris and Vanderheiden 1980; Harris-Vanderheiden and Vanderheiden 1977; Kladde 1974; Kohl et al. 1977; Shane and Bashir 1980) have suggested a number of such factors. Shane and Bashir (1980) have operationalized this process by using a branching type decision matrix intended for use with clients having congenital disorders. Their matrix includes ten categories (see table 2-1). Answers to questions in each of the ten categories lead to a decision to elect, delay, or reject a non-vocal communication system. They discuss each of the categories and provide several case examples demonstrating use of the decision matrix.

A formalized system such as Shane's and Bashir's has several advantages. First, it is a comprehensive system. Use of the matrix helps ensure that decisions will not be based on limited information. This system requires considering ten clusters of factors. Second, the system is efficient because the branching allows the evaluator to eliminate some clusters for specific clients. For example, evidence of oral system persistent reflexes which interfere with control of the oral mechanism yields a decision to elect a non-vocal system, without requiring completion of the entire decision matrix. Third, this system provides documentation of this important decision, an increasingly

Table 2-1. Election Decision Matrix (Shane and Bashir 1980).

LEVEL I COGNITIVE FACTORS
At least Stage V sensori-motor intelligence?
At least 18 months mental age; or ability to recognize at least at photograph level?
    YES → Go to II
    NO → Delay

LEVEL II ORAL REFLEX FACTORS
Persistent (1) Rooting; (2) Gag; (3) Bite; (4) Suckle/Swallow; or (5) Jaw Extension Reflex?
    YES → ELECT → Go to X
    NO → Continue to III

LEVEL III LANGUAGE AND MOTOR SPEECH PRODUCTION FACTORS
A. Is there a discrepancy between receptive and expressive skills?
    YES → Go to III B
    NO → Go to V

B. Is the discrepancy explained predominantly on the basis of a motor speech disorder?
    YES → Go to V
    NO → Go to III C
    UNCERTAIN → Go to IV

C. Is the discrepancy explained predominantly on the basis of an expressive language disorder?
    YES → Go to VII
    NO → Go to VI
    UNCERTAIN → Go to V

LEVEL IV MOTOR SPEECH—SOME CONTRIBUTING FACTORS
Presence of neuromuscular involvement affecting postural tone and/or postural stability?
Presence of praxic disturbance?
Vocal production consists primarily of vowel production?
Vocal production consists primarily of undifferentiated sounds?
History of eating problems? Excessive drooling?
    YES → Evidence to support motor speech involvement (Go to V)
    NO → Evidence against motor speech involvement (Go to V)

LEVEL V PRODUCTION—SOME CONTRIBUTING FACTORS
Speech unintelligible except to family and immediate friends?
Predominant mode of communication is through pointing, gesture, facial-body affect?
Predominance of single word utterances?
Frustration associated with inability to speak?
    YES → (Evidence to ELECT) Go to VII
    NO → (Evidence to DELAY or REJECT) Go to VII

LEVEL VI EMOTIONAL FACTORS
A. History of precipitous loss of expressive speech?
    YES → Go to VIII
    NO → Go to VI B

B. Speaks to selected persons or refuses to speak?
    YES → Go to VIII
    NO → Go to V

LEVEL VII CHRONOLOGICAL AGE FACTORS
A. Chronological age less than 3 years?
    YES → Go to VIII A

B. Chronological age between 3 and 5 years?
    YES → Go to VIII A

C. Chronological age greater than 5 years?
    YES → Go to VIII A

LEVEL VIII PREVIOUS THERAPY FACTORS
A. Has had previous therapy?
    YES → Go to VIII B
    NO → Go to IX, weigh evidence (DELAY with Trial Therapy or ELECT) Go to X

B. Previous therapy appropriate?
    YES → Go to VIII C
    NO → DELAY with Trial Therapy

C. Therapy progress too slow to enable effective communication?
    YES → ELECT → Go to X
    NO → DELAY → continue therapy

D. Therapy appropriately withheld?
    YES → ELECT → Go to X
    NO → DELAY with trial therapy

LEVEL IX PREVIOUS THERAPY—SOME CONTRIBUTING FACTORS
Able to imitate (with accuracy) speech sounds or words; gross motor or oral motor movements?
    YES → (Evidence to DELAY) Go to VIII
    NO → (Evidence to ELECT) Go to VIII

LEVEL X IMPLEMENTATION FACTORS—ENVIRONMENT
Family willing to implement (use, allow to be introduced) Augmentative Communication System recommendation?
    YES → IMPLEMENT
    NO → COUNSEL

important matter in this "age of accountability." In addition, it may be helpful in supporting an intuitive clinical decision and helping to demonstrate to parents, teachers, administrators, and clients the rationale behind the output mode selected. Finally, using a decision matrix may help evaluators and trainers avoid employing non-vocal systems as a panacea for all new clients. Shane and Bashir (1978) suggest that their system may result in fewer individuals being inappropriately assigned to non-vocal communication individuals being inappropriately assigned to non-vocal systems.

For some clients, results of the decision matrix in Stage I will point clearly toward either a vocal or non-vocal output mode. For clients in the vocal track, content and method of training will be determined next in Stage IV of the matrix. For clients in the non-vocal track, the next decision will involve the general type of output mode selected (gestural or symbolic), proceeding to Stage II of the decision process model.

For many clients, however, even this clearly delineated decision matrix may not yield a definitive choice. Failure to clearly "reject" or "elect" a non-vocal system could be due to one of two reasons. First, the evaluator might be forced to "delay," due either to lack of cognitive readiness in the client or to inadequate therapy. A number of very young and/or severely retarded individuals will "fail" Level 1 of the decision matrix. That is, they will not demonstrate at least Stage V sensorimotor intelligence,[1] 18 months mental age, or the ability to recognize at least at the photograph level. Rather than stopping at Level I in such cases, however, we have found it helpful to proceed as far as possible through the decision matrix in order to identify those clients who may have future difficulty in learning to produce speech. McDonald (1980) addresses this issue of the child who is "at risk for speech development," recommending early identification through studying the child's history, developmental lags, and examination findings. Most areas of concern noted by McDonald are covered in Shane and Bashir's (1980) decision matrix. For example, Shane and Bashir note that ". . . persistent oral reflexes suggest an extremely poor prognosis for oral speech development. We view these factors as an early predictor of failure to develop speech and one which leads to election of an augmentative communication system" (1980).

Clustering of factors included in Level IV of the matrix (such as neuro-muscular status, eating skills, and vocal repertoire) may also help identify high-risk clients. Thus, although the client may not presently have the cognitive skills necessary to use a non-vocal system, the evaluator will know that the client has a poor prognosis for early vocal language development. The trainer may use this additional evidence in designing a pre-symbolic program for the client. For example, the trainer might focus on skills such as head-control, tracking, scanning, and motor imitation if necessary, to prepare the client for later learning of a non-vocal output mode. This seems to be a safe approach which in no way rules out the eventual development of vocal

---

1. Stages of sensorimotor intelligence are described in Chapter 4 under cognitive skills.

language. Chapter 6 in this book includes further discussion of prognostic factors related to vocal language development.

There is also a possibility that non-vocal systems may be helpful in facilitating cognitive representational skills; thus they might be introduced even before the client reaches the "pass" level for cognitive development on the Shane and Bashir matrix. Chapman and Miller (1980) note that we currently have no answer to the basic question about non-vocal systems used as facilitators: "Are nonvocal systems a means to teach representational skills, or do they themselves require representational skills in order to be learned?" (p. 180). Since the possibility still exists that non-vocal systems may foster cognitive/linguistic development, perhaps trial therapy is justified even for clients who do not meet the minimum requirements for candidacy in a non-vocal system. This is consistent with current thought on concurrent teaching of skills previously considered to be "prerequisites" to language training. This issue is discussed further in Chapter 4.

There is a second reason why the Shane and Bashir matrix may not yield a definitive decision regarding output mode. For some clients, answers to several of the questions within the ten levels may not be a clear "yes" or "no." In this case the evaluator may find it difficult to make the final decision. Shane and Bashir note that "intuitive good sense" will be a part of this process. When neither a vocal nor a non-vocal mode is clearly "right," the most appropriate choice is probably a combination of output modes falling more toward the center of the non-vocal/vocal continuum presented earlier.

Chapman and Miller (1980) present another scheme for making the vocal/non-vocal decision. Their scheme involves gathering information on several dimensions of client behavior. The client's chronological age is compared with behavior in five areas:

1. Cognition (informal and formal);
2. Comprehension (syntax and vocabulary);
3. Production (Brown's stages [1973]: syntax, semantics, and phonology);
4. Communication function (functions and interactions);
5. Motor skills (gross, fine, and visual-motor).

The decision regarding emphasis is based on the presence or absence of discrepancies among the developmental areas as compared with chronological age. Chapman and Miller suggest that ". . . when development is equal across these four dimensions [cognitive development, comprehension, production, and communication function] (and the speech production mechanism is normal), the child is not a candidate for nonvocal systems" (p. 183). While such a client may not be a candidate for a primary non-vocal system, he or she might be helped by a non-vocal system used as a speech or language facilitator, as discussed earlier.

The issue of whether non-vocal systems facilitate speech and/or language development is an important one with regard to choosing an output mode. Silverman (1980) reviewed a number of published and unpublished reports to determine the impact on speech of non-vocal output modes. He concludes that ". . . intervention with nonspeech communication modes can be rationalized for the purpose of speech facilitation as well as improving

Table 2-2
Advantages and disadvantages of non-vocal systems
(as compared to vocal systems)**

Advantages	Disadvantages
1. Non-vocal systems provide two simultaneous inputs (e.g., auditory and visual).*	1. Non-vocal systems are not typical systems of communication and may not be as readily reinforced by vocal language users.
2. Non-vocal systems have not been found to inhibit development of vocal language; in fact, a number of studies suggest that non-vocal system may enhance speech and/or language development (see Silverman 1980).	2. Persons in the environment may be hesitant to accept use of a non-vocal system, as they may feel it represents giving up on vocal language.
3. Non-vocal systems may serve various purposes relative to vocal language: a. Interim communication system (thus may reduce frustration level); b. Speech and/or language facilitation; c. Supplement to vocal language; d. Ultimate communication system.	3. Persons in the environment may be unable to receive the message (e.g., may not know sign or Blissymbols).
4. Non-vocal systems are typically more static, which should help in learning (that is, each entry is available longer).	4. Persons in the environment may not be willing to take the time necessary to receive messages.
5. Non-vocal systems are often more amenable to physical prompting (e.g., the client can be taken through a sign or the gesture of pointing to a symbol).	5. Non-vocal systems may be more expensive due to the need to buy equipment and/or to train persons to teach and receive the message.
6. Non-vocal systems may be slowed down more than vocal language, with less distortion.	

*Although there is some visual input in vocal language, it is not as intense or lasting as in non-vocal language.
**Taken in part from Beukelman and Yorkston (1977); Harris and Vanderheiden (1980); Vicker (1974b); Wilson, Goodman, and Wood (1975).

message transmission" (p. 45). Silverman's reports covered children and adults having a wide variety of diagnoses and using a number of non-vocal communication modes. This may support augmentative use of a non-vocal mode, possibly on a trial therapy basis, at least for those clients for whom the vocal/non-vocal decision is not clear-cut. Table 2-2 presents a list of advantages and disadvantages of non-vocal output modes, as compared to vocal output modes. For the client who could potentially use either mode, this list may facilitate the decision concerning primary emphasis.

The program planner must also follow a thorough decision process in determining the appropriate input mode for a client. The relevant considerations here may be quite different from those involved in the decision regarding output mode. Sensory deficiencies, especially those involving vision and hearing, assume a greater importance, while motor impairments, such as cerebral palsy, will be of less concern. Cognitive and emotional status of the client should also be considered. Numerous researchers have been successful in using various non-vocal systems as primary or supplemental input modes. This research is discussed in Chapters 8 and 9. As illustrated earlier, input can extend on the non-vocal/vocal continuum from normal speech to a combination (such as speech plus sign or symbols) to primarily non-vocal input (such as sign or symbols alone). Even in clients labeled "non-vocal," input will often be primarily vocal or simultaneously vocal and non-vocal.

To summarize, Stage I of the decision process involves determining whether primary emphasis will be placed on vocal and/or non-vocal modes, a decision regarding both input and output. It may be represented visually on a non-vocal/vocal continuum. The output decision may be based, at least in part, on use of Shane's and Bashir's (1980) decision matrix and/or Chapman's and Miller's (1980) decision scheme. The input decision may be based on some or all of the factors described above. In any case, it is recommended that "clinical intuition" be supplemented by methodological procedures.

Stage II: Gestural/Symbolic Systems

The second stage of the decision process relates to those clients who are candidates for a non-vocal output mode as a primary or supplementary system. The program planner must next decide whether to use a gestural or a symbolic system as the primary non-vocal system. Several authors (e.g., Harris and Vanderheiden 1980; Hamre-Nietupski et al. 1977) suggest teaching more than one non-vocal system to reduce limitations placed on the client. For example, a client who uses a sign language with family and close friends might use a word board with people who do not know sign.

Harris and Vanderheiden (1980) caution that use of such generic terms as "nonvocal" or "nonspeaking" to describe all persons who have not developed functional oral communication skills may be confusing. They assert that "Individuals may be nonvocal for a variety of reasons, each of which might require a different intervention program" (p. 230). They note the need to clearly differentiate the primary cause of a non-vocal condition. Thus, they recommend examining a variety of behavior, as suggested by Chapman and Miller (1980). The data included on a profile developed from their assessment system should be helpful in determining whether to use a gestural or symbolic output system; for example, the client who demonstrates poor fine and gross motor skills would be a poor candidate for most gestural systems. The specific capabilities and limitations of each client should be considered in matching that client to a general mode (gestural or symbolic) and a specific system (e.g., American Sign Language, Blissymbols). While there may be systems which are particularly appropriate for different handicapped populations, the wide range of individual differences and the overlapping of categories require that decisions be made on a case-by-case basis. In addition to the areas of behavior included by Chapman's and Miller's (1980) assessment profile (e.g., cognition, production), a number of considerations related to the general systems should help in making the Stage II decision. Several primary considerations are presented in Chapter 7 and listed in table 7-1. These should be compared to the needs and capabilities of the client. For some clients, notably the severely physically handicapped, use of one mode (e.g., gestural) may be ruled out at this stage. For many clients, however, it may be impossible to reject either gestural or symbolic systems. In either case the planner should proceed to the next stage.

Stage III: System Selection

This stage involves choosing a specific system for primary emphasis. Increasingly detailed information about the system and the client will be required to make the optimal match.

Table 2-3 presents a number of crucial considerations in selecting a non-vocal system for input and/or output. This table may also be modified for use as a worksheet at this stage in the decision process. Client-related factors are listed in the first column. Information regarding many of these criteria will have been gathered during Stage I through use of the decision schemes. Client-related factors are matched in the second column by corresponding system features. The third column provides an example of how the client and system information would be combined in decision-making. For example, some systems require trainers with special skills or training. Thus the systems which require specific training, such as Blissymbols or any of the sign systems, would be less desirable options in situations where trained teachers are not readily available. Word or picture systems might be more realistic choices in these situations. The two chapters covering non-vocal systems (Chapter 8 and 9) present a number of systems in some detail. Information will be provided on the features of each system and their relationship to the client factors listed in Table 2-3. The reader is also referred to Appendices A and B of this book for specific annotations regarding non-vocal systems.

Silverman (1980) recommends that the planner first determine which systems would be possible for the client to use. The optimal system would then be selected from this narrowed list. Alpert (1980) suggests that for clients who are candidates for several systems, two non-vocal systems should be selected for trial therapy. Her training-assessment model involved a pilot study of approximately seven weeks of trial therapy. Three "indicators" were used to determine which of the two non-vocal systems was optimal for the client:

1. Learning of nonspeech responses taught in each training condition;
2. Percentage of correct vocalizations produced during each training condition;
3. Performance on the probes [10 probes, including production, comprehension, association, and cross-modal transfer/probes] (p.412–13).

Several additional or alternate indicators might help in choosing the preferred system. Measuring trials to criteria would help determine the efficiency of each system. It would also be helpful to consider generalization with respect to untrained items; for example, Blissymbolics makes use of a number of different strategies and basic elements which may reduce teaching time through client generalization. The client's spontaneous use of entries in

Table 2-3

Considerations in selecting non-vocal input or output systems.

Client-Related Features	System Features	Implications for Non-Vocal Systems
Client's abilities/ limitations		
Cognitive level	There is a wide range in the cognitive level needed to use various systems.	Stage 4 or 5 sensorimotor level: natural gestures, photographs Late preoperations to early concrete operations: traditional orthography, fingerspelling
Gross motor skills	Positioning and gross pointing abilities are needed with many systems.	Many symbolic communication aids require head control and adequate posture. All gestural systems require adequate positioning and some control over gross motor skills.
Fine motor skills	High degree of coordination is needed for one or both hands with many gestural systems.	Sign systems, except for Duffy's System and mime, require moderate to good control of at least one hand. Symbolic systems can be adapted for clients with poor fine motor skills.
Sensory or processing problems		
Vision	Most systems require adequate visual acuity. A range of visual discrimination skills is needed.	Exception: Braille High level: traditional orthography Moderate level: Amer-Ind
Hearing	Most systems do not require hearing but it makes learning easier; some systems are designed for hearing impaired.	Example: Cued Speech, most sign systems
Touch	Several systems are based on tactile information.	Example: Braille, Tadoma
Memory	Memory may be more important for systems which do not use visible symbols. Some symbols or gestures may be easier to remember.	Gestural systems may be more difficult for clients with memory problems. Example: Picsyms, Amer-Ind

Client's needs

Present communication "system"	Some systems build on specific skills the client already uses.	Example: natural gestures and pantomime may be developed into a sign language; pointing may be adapted to use of a communication board.
Current communication needs	Some systems are most appropriate for basic needs, while others can code abstract meanings and complex grammatical structures.	Basic needs: natural gestures, pictures. Complex needs: Signing Exact English, Blissymbolics
Anticipated future communication needs	Those systems which parallel English should build a better base for clients expected to learn to read or speak English.	Parallel to English: Cued speech, traditional orthography. Structure typically different from English: Amer-Ind, American Sign Language, Blissymbolics

Implementation

Audience	Some systems are more transparent than others to untrained audiences.	Transparent: Amer-Ind, mime, pictures. Translucent: Blissymbolics. Opaque: Cued Speech, Premack-type, symbols
Willingness to implement	Systems which appear highly non-normative or are difficult to learn may not be implemented.	Example: Premack-type symbols.
Funding	Systems requiring extensive equipment or training will generally cost more.	Symbolic systems will cost more if they must be displayed on complex electronic prostheses.
Availability of trainers	Some systems may be readily learned from a book or may already be in trainer's repertoire, while others require more direct training.	Systems already in repertoire: natural gestures, traditional orthography. Systems which may be self-learned: Signed English, rebus, Picsyms. Systems which require direct training: Blissymbolics, American Sign Language

a system would be another positive indicator for future use of that system. Finally, the reaction of others in the environment (parents, teachers, students) might be noted formally (e.g., number of times others attempt to use each system) or informally (through soliciting opinions).

After the primary system has been selected, the evaluator must determine whether a secondary system will be chosen at this time. This will be especially important if the system chosen is one which limits the client's available audience, such as Signing Exact English. In this case a supplementary non-vocal system may be provided. The client-related factors listed in table 2-3 should be considered in determining the need for and type of second system.

The Stage III decision, system selection, necessitates making a number of further decisions based on the system chosen. The program planner should now move to Stage IV. The client for whom a vocal system was selected in Stage I will re-enter the decision process at Stage IV.

Stage IV: Implementation

This stage covers a variety of implementation factors. Some of these factors (content, method of training) are relevant to all systems, while others (e.g., means of indicating, output mode) are specific to individual systems. These issues are discussed within the four chapters covering vocal and non-vocal systems (Chapters 6, 7, 8, and 9).

Summary

This chapter presents a process for making the decisions necessary to develop a communication plan for a severely handicapped client. Four stages are described and at each stage strategies are discussed. We stress that a decision will often not determine an "either/or" strategy, but rather a primary emphasis for training. Finally, it should be noted that this decision process is not a one-time undertaking. The client's needs and capabilities must be constantly re-assessed in order to make the system and its implementation optimal for the client.

Chapter 3: Issues in Communication Training

Introduction

Some issues appear with considerable frequency in the literature related to language training of the severely handicapped. The following issues will be presented generally in this chapter and then related to specific types of communication modes (vocal, gestural, and symbolic) in the appropriate chapters:

1. Model of language training;
2. Theory of intervention approach;
3. Content and context of training;
4. Methodology;
5. Generalization of skills;
6. Self-initiation/self-regulation;
7. Role of imitation in training;
8. Relationship between comprehension and production.

These issues are important regardless of whether the trainer selects a vocal or a non-vocal mode of communication.

Models of Language Acquisition and Training

The two models used most often in language training of the severely handicapped are the developmental and the remedial. The developmental model follows the sequence of normal language acquisition. Most authors (e.g., Bloom and Lahey 1978; Bricker and Bricker 1974; Miller 1977; Ruder and Smith 1974; Tilton, Liska, and Bourland 1977; Yule and Berger 1975) have accepted the developmental model in planning language intervention, thus assuming that the acquisition process should follow the same sequence for severely handicapped children as for normal children. A number of sources of developmental data are available. Trantham and Pedersen (1976) have collected data on eight children who acquired language normally. Bloom and Lahey (1978) present plans for language development goals based on normal development. Cohen, Gross, and Haring (1976) have compiled sets of "developmental pinpoints," or measurable behavior, in a variety of areas, including receptive and expressive language. Their pinpoints are drawn from studies of large numbers of subjects, screening batteries, and developmental checklists, and cover ages from 0.1 months to 72 months. Barrie-Blackley, Musselwhite, and Rogister (1978) have prepared an annotated bibliography of selected sources of developmental data. Ruder and Smith (1974) summarize the justification for using a developmental model in saying, "It might be that little is to be lost and perhaps a great deal is to be gained from structuring training programs on such developmental data" (p. 566). Thus it seems that the primary reasons for using developmental data from normal children may be their availability and the lack of extensive and accurate information with regard to language acquisition in various severely handicapped populations.

Bloom and Lahey (1978) note that a typical objection to the developmental model is that this approach merely provides the child with more of the same experience, while the child may really need something different from the normal model. They contend, moreover, that children with disordered or delayed language do not continue to receive simple language models. For the severely handicapped, the language models may never have been "normal."

The remedial model follows sequences other than those involved in normal development, the rationale being that the normal sequence is not appropriate for these populations or is no longer appropriate to the client's age (Hogg 1975; Switsky et al. 1979). That is, the client with a measured mental age of 18 months will likely not parallel the normal 18-month-old infant in terms of knowledge and abilities. The client may display behavior that is significantly above or below that of a normal 18-month-old infant.

Although the remedial model is typically discussed as a single entity, it appears that several types of remedial sequences exist. Remedial sequences may be data-based, utilizing language acquisition data from children with learning problems similar to those of the target population, just as the developmental model uses normal acquisition data. The assumption behind a data-based remedial model is that persons with the same problem tend to learn language in the same way. Remedial sequences may, instead, be teacher-devised, based on "adult intuition" and/or analysis of the learning environment. An example of an intuitive approach is an additive sequence in which the language segments taught increase in length as the client progresses. An example of an approach based on an analysis of the learning environment is a task analysis which teaches all necessary skills, beginning with the first step not already in the client's repertoire and adding steps until the goal is met. Both of these teacher-devised sequences share the assumption that steps can be programmed more "logically" than the "normal" sequences and thus result in more efficient learning. Bloom and Lahey (1978) caution that intervention programs using a remedial model based on adult intuition may result in "clichés." For example, such programs typically teach labeling of objects first, followed by word combination; however, developmental data show that, even at the single-word level, children talk about relations between objects and events rather than merely labeling objects.

Leonard (1975) experimented with a developmental and a remedial hierarchy (in this case an intuitive sequence of increasing response length) in designing a model procedure for language intervention. He found that use of the developmental sequence enabled the children to reach objectives with significantly fewer responses and to achieve a significantly higher percentage of correct responses than did the remedial (intuitive) sequence. Although his subjects were not severely handicapped persons, they were having difficulty acquiring language normally; therefore, it seems reasonable to speculate whether his findings might relate to severely handicapped persons as well.

As noted, most authors have chosen to follow the developmental model in planning language programs. Primary advocates of the remedial model using data from severely mentally retarded persons are Guess, Sailor, and Baer (1974, 1976, 1977, 1978). Their rationale for using this remedial model is that severely mentally retarded children undergoing training in the authors' program seem to make faster progress when using sequences established by severely mentally retarded children who have completed those phases of the program. Thus the authors used developmental data as a place to start and are currently modifying the program on the basis of acquisition data from severely mentally retarded children involved in the program.

Many other authors have also combined the developmental and remedial models to some extent, so that few, if any, pure examples of either model are available. Even those authors advocating a remedial model (e.g., Guess et al. 1974, 1976, 1977, 1978; Hogg 1975; Switsky et al. 1979) use developmental data as a starting point. Conversely, authors using the developmental model will usually fill in the gaps with intuitive or task-analyzed steps (e.g., Struck 1977, St. Louis et al. 1980). Special applications of the remedial and developmental models to vocal and non-vocal language systems will be discussed in appropriate chapters.

Theories of Intervention Approaches

In addition to the model of language acquisition, the program or approach chosen may follow a specific theory of language acquisition (e.g., cognitive, operant). However, it should be noted that disciplines such as speech pathology, special education, and psychology may interpret various theories differently. In addition, programs may not be based on a single theory but, instead, may incorporate features from several theories. As with the question of model, it may be concluded that these clients have not acquired language in the "normal" manner; therefore, intervention approached need not follow theories of normal acquisition. Siegel and Spradlin (1978) assert that ". . . behavior modification is now seen as a form of behavioral engineering rather than a theoretical system" (p. 371). This may help explain, for example, the widespread use of behavior management techniques in a number of different approaches, not all of which are based on behavioral theory (e.g., Bricker and Bricker 1974; Bricker and Dennison 1978; Bricker, Dennison, and Bricker 1975; Bricker et al. 1973; Bricker, Ruder, and Vincent 1976).

Content and Context

Two primary areas of concern in developing a language program for the severely handicapped are the content and context of that program. The following discussion uses Holland's (1975) definitions. She defines content as the words focused on in therapy, while context refers to the interrelated environmental conditions in which therapy exists. To a great extent the content and context of language therapy for the severely handicapped are determined by the model and theory chosen by the trainer. Thus the trainer using a developmental model and a cognitive theory would be likely to select items based on a sequence described by normal acquisition and would choose only those lexical items and relations over which the client has demonstrated cognitive control. For example, "wash dolly" would be introduced in a normal developmental sequence after the client has demonstrated, through symbolic play, that the concept is in his or her repertoire.

Increasingly, researchers have stressed that communication intervention must be a part of the total environment, rather than being concentrated into therapy sessions with one trainer and one client (e.g., Hamre-Nietupski et al. 1977; Hart and Rogers-Warren 1978; Kopchick and Lloyd 1976; Williams and Fox 1977). This focus on an environmental context also supports a greater role for parents as intervention agents (e.g., Bloom and Lahey 1978; Harris 1976; Horstmeier and MacDonald 1978a,b; Schumaker and Sherman 1978).

This discussion will focus on strategies for selecting initial content and context for the client with no or limited language. Included are general strategies appropriate to vocal or non-vocal systems. Strategies suited to specific systems or populations are presented where appropriate.

The first strategy is to *develop a core lexicon,* or a small, functional vocabulary which can be adapted to the needs of the individual client (Holland 1975; Lahey and Bloom 1977). Holland suggests a 35-entry core lexicon which fits a psycholinguistically based therapy model such as the one developed by MacDonald and Blott (1974). This model includes eight semantic-grammatical formations, such as the following: agent plus action (e.g., car go); action plus object (e.g., gimme ball). All but two of the words in Holland's lexicon can be combined to produce at least five phrases that can be related to at least two of the semantic-grammatical formations. Thus, although the lexicon includes only 35 entries, the client has considerable flexibility. Examples of the items in Holland's lexicon are the following: specific words such as "you," "hate," "no," "go," and word categories such as "the names of specific others in a given child's life." Lahey and Bloom also suggest using a core lexicon but disagree with some of Holland's lexical items; for example, they do not recommend inclusion of "hate" and "yes." Lahey and Bloom organize their lexicon according to content and form. Form is sub-divided into substantive and relational words. Substantive words refer to specific objects of categories, and relational words refer to connections between objects or events. Content categories such as "rejection" and "actions on objects" provide the second level of organization. Lahey's and Bloom's lexicon is presented in table 3-1. The remaining strategies discussed here will center on use of a lexicon such as the ones discussed above.

Table 3-1
Organization of a first lexicon by content and form
(Lahey and Bloom 1977, p. 350).

Content Category	Relational Words		Substantive Words
	Relational words that are not object specific	Relational words that are more specific to objects but still relate to many objects	
Rejection	no		
Nonexistence or disappearance	no, all gone, away		
Cessation of action	stop, no		
Prohibition of action	no		
Recurrence of objects and actions on objects	more, again, another		
Noting the existence of or identifying objects	this, there, that		
Actions on objects		give, do, make, get, throw, eat, wash, kiss	
Actions involved in locating objects or self		put, up, down, sit, fall, go	
Attributes or descriptions of objects		big, hot, dirty, heavy	
Persons associated with objects (as in possession)			person names

The initial strategy in selecting a lexicon will often be to *use the principles of normal verbal language acquisition* (Hamre-Nietupski et al. 1977; Holland 1975; Lahey and Bloom 1977). This will help yield a list of entries[1] to use as a starting point. The entries presented in both the Holland and the Lahey and Bloom lexicons are words common to early verbal language. Strategies could then be used to expand or delete this preliminary list to include entries which will meet the client's current and future communication needs.

Many strategies involved in selecting an initial lexicon relate to the client's current communication needs. *Client preference* is a primary factor in selecting initial vocabulary, whether signs, symbols, or spoken words. Hamre-Nietupski et al. (1977) have operationalized this strategy through use of student preference checklists for objects, actions, places, and persons. For each category the observer notes those entries which the client appears to prefer or dislike, on the basis of attention to and interaction with the object. This record is kept for several settings, such as home and school. The authors caution therapists not to rely solely on this strategy, as exclusive use of entries the client already attends to might inhibit his or her future growth in knowledge about the world.

Frequency of occurrence is also useful in developing a core lexicon because this indicates those entries to which the client has repeated exposure. This procedure would suggest entries which might be important for the client to learn; in addition, practice would be available throughout the day. Hamre-Nietupski et al. also suggest a frequency of occurrence checklist to determine various entry categories (e.g., "nouns," "pronouns," "verbs," "adverbs"). These categories could be modified to represent the content categories included in the Lahey and Bloom lexicon. Both Holland and Lahey and Bloom recommend that an initial lexicon should code the *here-and-now*, or objects that are present and events that are occurring in the milieu of training. Related to this issue, Holland suggests attention to Ashton-Warner's (1971) concept of *organicity*. Organicity refers to the essential interrelatedness of the word, the activity, and the child. As Holland stresses, "Wants and the centrality of *me* are the fabric of talk, not *blue* or *cup*" (p. 517). Developing a lexicon based in part on client *preference, frequency of occurrence,* and the *here-and-now* should help ensure *organicity*.

Another strategy useful in matching the lexicon to the client's needs is to provide entries that code a *variety of communicative functions*. For example, Holland (1975) and Yule and Berger (1975) note the importance of teaching the use of one-word utterances in a variety of ways, depending on function. For example, the word "eat" may be used as a comment (e.g., "The dog is eating"), a demand regulating the behavior of another (e.g., "Mommy, fix me something to eat"), or a request (e.g., "May I have something to eat?"). This strategy may remain useful for the client who is cognitively and linguistically beyond the one-word stage but has a limited rate of output due to motoric problems.

Another strategy relating to the client's immediate needs involves the

---

1. In the discussion that follows, "entries" refers to words, signs, or symbols.

ease with which the concept can be demonstrated in context (Lahey and Bloom, 1977). This will be especially important for the client with a low receptive language level. Some concepts (e.g., "hate") may be difficult to demonstrate, regardless of the input mode, while others may greatly depend on the mode. For example, the concept "want" may be difficult to picture on a symbol communication board; however, the sign for that concept may be transparent or easy for the decoder to guess (Fristoe and Lloyd, 1980). Thus selection of entries for linguistic input will depend in part on the mode of input.

A final strategy relating to the client's current communication needs concerns the *ease of production and discrimination*. Again, this must be based in part on the client's output mode. Bloom and Lahey (1978) stress the importance of the signal configuration (e.g., sounds in entry, number of syllables) in selecting spoken words. The motoric configuration is an important consideration in choosing an initial sign lexicon. With regard to symbol systems, the number of movements necessary to indicate the entry would be important. This would probably not be a major factor, as it is unlikely that early symbols would require spelling or otherwise combining symbols. Therefore, the number of movements would not be based on the symbols, but rather on their positions on the display. Considerations in determining ease of production will be discussed relative to each major system (vocal, gestural, and symbolic) in the appropriate chapters.

Primary emphasis in selecting an initial lexicon should focus on the client's *future* as well as current communicative needs. Bloom and Lahey (1978) refer to this strategy as the *efficiency of a lexical item*. For example, both Holland (1975) and Lahey and Bloom (1977) include entries that combine with others to code a wide range of ideas about the environment. This efficiency is important in measuring the client's development from using a predominance of one-word utterances to employing longer utterances. It is also an important consideration for the client who will be limited in the ultimate number of lexical entries available to him or her because of motoric or cognitive limitations.

In conclusion, a number of strategies have been offered which merge content and context in determining an initial lexicon for a severely handicapped client. These strategies and others will be discussed further as they relate to specific systems. It should be recognized that no one strategy will be sufficient in choosing a lexicon. Emphasis on the various strategies will depend on the needs and limitations of the individual client.

Methodology of Language Training for the Severely Handicapped

As with content, methodology is greatly dependent on the theory underlying the approach chosen. An approach based on operant technology would be expected to use operant procedures; as noted, however, many approaches based on other theories use operant techniques to some degree. Guess et al.

(1974) in a review of the literature on language acquisition and training in the severely mentally retarded, noted the widespread use of operant techniques. They assert that "It seems appropriate to conclude that an operant technology presently exists for the establishment and maintenance of imitative and expressive speech" (p. 540). Obviously, not all approaches are based on operant theory or techniques. Some approaches (e.g., those based on cognitive theory) may make more use of a discovery approach, presumably structured to some degree but more closely representing natural language learning. As noted in the section on content and context, many authors are shifting to a more environmental approach (e.g., Hart and Rogers-Warren 1978; Horstmeier and MacDonald 1978a,b; Kopchick and Lloyd 1976; MacDonald and Blott 1974). Such a change would affect methodology somewhat by, for example, spreading trials across a wider time span, making use of more than one trainer, and providing "natural" trials and consequences. Thus the methodology of communication intervention approaches may differ as much as, and in conjunction with, the variety of models and theories of language.

Generalization

Guess et al. (1977) assert that "the issue of generalization is certainly the most current and pressing problem re: language training" (p. 363). Two types of generalization are important to the ultimate language learning of the severely handicapped child: (1) generalization of response classes (e.g., morphological inflections such as markers) across items and across modalities (e.g., comprehension and production, or non-vocal and vocal imitation); and (2) generalization of language learned in the training situation to other communicative situations and in response to other antecedent events (traditionally referred to as "carryover"). Guess, Keogh, and Sailor (1978) have termed the former "response differentiation" and the latter "stimulus generalization."

The concept of a zero inference strategy (Brown, Nietupski, and Hamre-Nietupski 1976) has been suggested to account for a lack of generalization across cues, modalities, persons, and so forth. The implication is that some severely handicapped persons (particularly the severely mentally retarded) do not infer from one instance or one situation to another. Therefore, it would be necessary to teach directly all desired behavior in all desired settings. Obviously, this would be a formidable task even for relatively discrete goals. A number of strategies might be helpful in increasing the level of inference, thus promoting generalization. One way to attack this problem is to *train generalized learning strategies*. Two examples of this are training in generalized instruction-following (e.g., Streifel, Wetherby, and Karlan 1976, 1978; Whitman, Zakaras, and Chardos 1971) and generalized imitation skills (e.g., Baer 1978; Bricker and Dennison 1978). In each case the client is presumably "learning-to-learn" rather than merely learning a small set of responses. In generalized instruction-following the client learns to "Do what I say," while in generalized imitation the client learns to "Do what I do."[2] Either of these skills may enable the client to learn incidentally rather than to depend solely on direct teaching. In addition, generalized learning skills will increase the number of people the client can learn from, even though these people may not realize that they are serving as models.

Some evidence indicates the possibility of producing a response class which will generalize across items; for example, teaching plural markers to one set of nouns increases the probability that the markers will be used with other similar nouns (Garcia and DeHaven 1974; Guess et al. 1968). Several authors (Garcia and DeHaven 1974; Harris 1975) have noted, however, that many severely handicapped children do not automatically generalize from comprehension to production, or vice versa, although some studies suggest that training in one modality may facilitate learning in the other. Therefore, Guess et al. (1977) recommend that the trainer "train both modalities simultaneously or in rapid succession, but do not necessarily expect that the development of one, through training, will automatically enhance the development of the other, without direct training" (p. 363).

The second aspect of this issue, generalization from training to other communicative situations, seems even more crucial than generalizing across response classes. However, in her review of problems with generalization, Harris (1975) notes that many of the better designed studies of teaching language to non-verbal persons failed to extend functional speech from the training situation to other people. She suggests that two ways of overcoming this problem are (1) to train subjects to respond to more than one person (perhaps from the outset of therapy), and (2) to train in more than one setting, with some training taking place in a group setting. Brown et al. (1976) also recommend using a variety of instructional arrangements in addition to the traditional one trainer-one student arrangement. They suggest considering each of the following for a portion of the day:

1. Group instruction;
2. Clustered individualized instruction in which one teacher engages in individualized interactions with a cluster of three, four, or five students;
3. Instruction that generates adaptive student interactions without the direct involvement of persons in authority.

Recent studies (e.g., Flavell, Flavell, and McGimsey 1978; Storm and Willis 1978) have demonstrated that small-group instruction is as effective as individualized training and employs staff time more efficiently. This finding was demonstrated in an imitative training program with profoundly retarded men (Storm and Willis 1978) and through a word-recognition task with

---

2. Baer (1978) presents an 18-step program for training generalized imitation. Wetherby and Striefel (1978) and Whitman et al. (1971) present strategies for training generalized instuction-following.

severely retarded[3] persons across a wide age range (CA = 9 to 25 years) [Flavell et al. 1978]. Thus, at least for some tasks, use of small groups appears preferable.

Brown et al. (1976) assert that utilizing a variety of instructional arrangements may help to reduce the stimulus-bound nature of clients, thus increasing self-initiating behavior. In addition, clients will have more opportunities to learn from each other and will rely less on the trainer.

Stokes and Baer (1977), having reviewed 200 studies involving generalization, suggest several tactics for producing generalization. These strategies relate to both response differentiation and stimulus generalization. Each of the seven tactics is described and illustrated. These seven hypothetical tactics for generalization are as follows:

1. "Loose training"—assumes that using a wide variety of nonrepeated stimulus items rather than using "structured repetitive lists" for training drills will aid in generalization;
2. "Indiscriminable contingencies"—assumes that the use of an intermittent reinforcement schedule will increase generalization by making the reinforcement contingency less discriminable to the subject;
3. "Training sufficient exemplars"—assumes that increasing the number of examples of new items or settings will increase generalization;
4. "Programming common stimuli"—assumes that the use of sufficient common stimuli in both the training and generalization settings will enhance carryover;
5. "Mediated generalization"—assumes that establishing a response with some similarity between the original response and the new response to be learned will increase generalization;
6. "Training to generalize"—assumes that the occurrence of any novel response which demonstrates generalization requires immediate reinforcement of that generalization;
7. "Introduction to natural maintaining contingencies"—assumes that there must be a transfer of control from the trainer to the student's natural environment, stressing functionality and therefore being potentially naturally reinforcing.

A few authors have included specific procedures for generalization in their programs (e.g., Guess et al. 1976; Gray and Ryan 1973; Kent 1974). Many authors recommend that new skills be performed under varying conditions (e.g., different settings, response cues, etc.) to increase the probability of generalization. Williams and Fox (1977) have operationalized this procedure by stipulating a strict definition of mastery. To achieve mastery the client "must perform the skill in the 'normal' manner, or a functional alternative, across functional tasks which frequently occur throughout the day, people, cues to respond (verbal cues and the task itself cuing the behavior), materials and time" (Introduction, p. 24). These authors have chosen a time span of two months and a minimum of three instances of each

---

3. Though subjects in the Flavell et al. (1978) study are referred to as "severely retarded," their Stanford-Binet Intelligence Scale IQ's ranged from 36 to 59 with a mean of 45.7.

other condition (e.g., people, response cues) across which the skill must be demonstrated. A mastery assessment sheet (see table 3-2) is provided to help the trainer ensure that all five conditions are met the minimum number of times for each skill.

Much attention has been given to the problem of generalization, including response differentiation and stimulus generalization. However, this area remains a significant problem to the professional or parent working with the severely handicapped. Several strategies for enhancing generalization have been presented. In addition, generalization procedures are specifically considered for each of the vocal and non-vocal language programs reviewed in Appendix B.

Self-Initiation/Self-Regulation

Self-initiation and self-regulation are another crucial issue with regard to training of the severely handicapped. Several authors (e.g., Brown et al. 1976; Williams, Brown, and Certo 1975) have noted that many severely handicapped clients lack these skills. This problem, which is closely related to the generalization issue, must be considered relative to communication training, whether vocal or non-vocal. Williams et al. (1975) state that those labeled severely handicapped are often referred to as externally controlled, relying on prompts and cues from caregivers. They note that there are situations when it is appropriate to make a specific response to a specific cue (e.g., "What is your name?"); instances when a series of responses should be provided to a single cue (e.g., "Tell me about your family."); and still other situations when one or a series of responses is required to nonspecific cues, such as environmental cues (e.g., client is lost and must ask for help). In addition, it may be necessary to engage in a series of responses, evaluate their correctness, and correct them if necessary. All of this should be possible without direct cues from persons in authority. The authors recommend that the trainer include self-regulation training within a curriculum. Nietupski and Williams (1974) developed a training sequence for redimentary self-regulation skills, consisting of the following steps:

1. Detecting or defining the task;
2. Arriving at alternative ways to complete the task;
3. Implementing an alternative;
4. Assessing the outcome of the alternative;
   a) if the task is not correctly completed
   b) if task is correctly completed, end of task.

The first step covers the client's self-initiation skills, while later steps cover abilities to make, implement, assess, and, if necessary, revise decisions regarding appropriate action. Application of such a self-regulation model could serve as the final step in generalization. The use of self-regulation techniques will be discussed in the chapters on vocal and non-vocal communication systems.

Table 3-2
Mastery Assessment Score Sheet (Williams and Foxx 1977, p. 26).

Mastery Assessment Score Sheet

TARGET MO	School			Home			Other
	Functional Task 1	Functional Task 2	Functional Task 3	Functional Task 1	Functional Task 2	Functional Task 3	Functional Task 1
Gross Motor: supported sitting with head control	Head control while eating	Head control while sitting and playing w/ busybox		Head control while washing after meal			
Response Cue	"head up"	No cue provided by teacher; self-initiated		"Sit up"			
Person	Milly	Tutor - Ann		Mother			
How data obtained: a. Observed by evaluator	Yes	No		No			
b. Observed and reported to evaluator by	Tutor-Ann	Tutor-Ann Tutor-Carol		Mother and sister			
Date	9/10/76	10/20/76		11/1/76			

Imitation, Comprehension, and Production

Historically, researchers have been interested in the roles of relationships among imitation, comprehension, and production in language acquisition and training.

Imitation

The role of imitation is a major issue, in terms of both language acquisition and language training. With regard to acquisition, Bloom and Lahey (1978) conclude that ". . . there has not been a consensus in the literature as to whether imitation contributes to language learning" (p. 272). Risley, Hart, and Doke (1972) assert that "Whether or not imitation is crucial to the normal development of language, it is a crucial part of all procedures for remediating language deficits" (p. 110). While such a blanket assertion may be an overstatement, a casual review of both vocal and non-vocal language programs reveals that imitation is indeed widely used in training. This is perhaps not surprising in view of the potential increase in efficiency possible with imitative procedures, especially when the child learns generalized imitation skills. However, several authors (Bloom and Lahey 1978; Siegel and Spradlin 1978; Rees 1975) have expressed cautions regarding extensive use of imitation as a training technique. First, imitation may be defined differently by different disciplines or even by different workers within a single discipline. For example, for an instance of imitation to be counted, the following conditions might be considered:

1. Must the two behaviors be exactly alike? (For example, if the trainer says "eat cookie" and the client says "cookie," will an instance be counted?);
2. Must the model and the response have a specific temporal relationship? (If the trainer says "eat cookie" and the client says "eat cookie" in one second or one minute or one hour, would all be counted as instances of imitation?).

These examples may give some indication of why there is currently so much confusion over the issue of imitation.

A second concern regarding imitation relates to its functionality. Bloom and Lahey (1978) caution that imitation not supported by context or intention may not yield desired results. That is, if the child does not see a cookie, and does not desire a cookie, his merely repeating "eat cookie," whether verbally, gesturally, or symbolically, may not be meaningful. Guess et al. (1978) also stress the need for functional imitative responses. They define imitative responses as ones that:

1. produce an immediate consequence for the child;
2. produce a consequence which is potentially reinforcing;
3. produce a consequence which is specific to the response;
4. produce a response which is natural to the child's interaction with the environment.

A theory expressed by Kuhn (1973) also seems to have important implications for the use of imitation in language intervention. Kuhn suggests

33

that children imitate only those behaviors already in their repertoires. Thus Siegel and Spradlin (1978) question, "Is it possible that generalized imitation does not really involve imitation of novel behavior but simply the rearrangement of components already learned?" (p. 382). This component recombinations notion suggests that training should focus on recombinations of components already established. Although still in the theory stage, it is yet one more aspect to consider when using generalized imitation as a strategy.

Two major types of imitation are traditionally described, non-verbal and verbal (Harris 1975). Non-verbal imitation may include gross and fine motor imitation, while verbal imitation may cover vocal imitation (i.e., imitation of non-meaningful sounds and sequences) and imitation of words or larger linguistic units. Non-verbal imitation is often initiated first because researchers have reasoned that gross motor movements are topographically less difficult and can be physically prompted more readily than verbal responses (Baer, Peterson, and Sherman 1967; Kent 1974; Harris 1976; Sloane, Johnston, and Harris 1968). However, as Harris (1975) notes, " . . the value of nonverbal imitation training has been more a clinical assumption than an empirical fact" (p. 566). Siegel and Spradlin (1978) assert that if their theory of component recombinations is correct, there would be little reason to expect generalization from non-verbal to verbal imitation. Finally, Guess et al. (1978) suggest that the important factors regarding type of imitative response do not hinge on verbal/non-verbal but on whether the response is in the client's repertoire and how functional the response is to the client, as discussed earlier.

Thus, the role of imitation in language training is not entirely clear, although it is certainly a widely used strategy. The role of imitation will be discussed further in conjunction with preliminary training strategies and vocal and non-vocal systems.

Comprehension and Production

Although traditionally it has been taught that in language acquisition comprehension precedes production, some recent studies (Chapman and Miller 1975; Keeney and Wolfe 1972; Lahey 1974) have suggested that in certain cases the reverse may be true. Following an extensive literature review, Bloom and Lahey (1978) propose the following hypothesis:

> . . . [comprehension and production] represent mutually dependent but different underlying processes . . . [and] . . . the developmental gap between comprehension and speaking probably varies among different children and at different times, and that the gap may be more apparent than real. (p. 238)

Many researchers (Reike, Lynch, and Soltman 1977; Schumaker and Sherman 1978) have continued to use the traditional approach of training comprehension first, for reasons which appear much the same as those cited in choosing the developmental model, mainly that it appears to be a "safe" choice. For example, Schumaker and Sherman (1978), in an extensive literature review, found no studies in which receptive speech skills adversely affected production. Therefore, they concluded that " . . . it seems safe to say that providing children with opportunities to discriminate differences in words and sentence forms can not hurt and, in some cases, may well foster productive language acquisition" (p. 248).

The opposite strategy, training production before comprehension, has been selected by some researchers (e.g., Bloom and Lahey 1978; Guess et al., 1976; 1978). Bloom and Lahey (1978) focus primarily on production goals "... simply because more is known about the development of children's production of content/form/use interactions than is known about the development of children's comprehension of these interactions" (p. 377). However, they stress that comprehension is also facilitated since content/form interactions are always presented in a context which represents the meaning relation being coded. For example, context would help define whether the word "milk" is intended as a comment ("You have milk") or a request ("May I have milk?"). Guess et al. (1978) note that production skills allow the client greater opportunity to manipulate and control the environment than do comprehension skills. The client may thus receive immediate reinforcement. A study by Miller, Cuvo, and Borakove (1977) reported almost complete transfer from production to comprehension in clients describing the number of cents in various coins, while teaching comprehension did not affect production.

A third alternative is to train comprehension and production concurrently (Bloom and Lahey 1978; Siegel and Spradlin 1978). This is consistent with current practices of concurrent training, where appropriate, the aim being to avoid long delays while waiting for the learning of prerequisites.

To summarize, the production/comprehension question is yet another issue which must await further research before a definitive answer may be given.

Chapter 4: Preliminary Training Strategies

Introduction

During the evaluation and information gathering stage of planning an educational program for a severely handicapped person, certain behavior (e.g., lack of cooperation during testing, limited motor control, poor attention) may suggest that the client needs to learn other skills before language training can be initiated. These may be termed preliminary, prerequisite, precursory, or prelanguage skills. Throughout this chapter the term preliminary skills will be used to discuss initial training strategies that will lead to training in higher level language tasks. Although these preliminary behaviors have traditionally been taught *prior to* beginning a language training program (Horstmeier and MacDonald 1978b; Kent 1974), a current trend advocates teaching them concurrently with language training (Hamre-Nietupski et al. 1977; Miller et al. 1980; Sapon et al. 1976). The concurrent training approach may be described as a horizontally arranged training model in which, for example, tracking, scanning, and imitation skills are taught as a part of language training (Hamre-Nietupski et al. 1977). This contrasts with a vertically arranged training model, in which skills such as on-task behavior or imitation are taught prior to beginning direct language training (Bricker and Dennison 1978; Kent 1974). The decision to use a horizontal or vertical training model must be based on a number of factors, such as the client's desire to communicate and his or her current level of functioning on non-language tasks.

Our view that language is an integral part of every activity or interaction throughout the client's waking hours at home, school, and in other situations (e.g., shopping, traveling, visiting neighbors) will be evident throughout this chapter. Realistically, concurrent training in preliminary skills can quite naturally take place within language training sessions and general daily activities. For example, when training attention, the trainer usually creates a situation in which he or she rewards attention by an interesting consequence, such as allowing the client to play with a desired toy. The client may be learning to use the object or to associate a word label with the object as well as learning to attend to a particular task.

The preliminary behavior to be discussed in this chapter is as follows: (1) Establishing the desire to communicate; (2) Eliminating interfering behavior (e.g., self-stimulating and self-injurious behavior); (3) Improving attention; (4) Increasing cognitive skills; (5) Establishing motor imitation; and (6) Developing oral-motor control. This is not intended to be an exhaustive review of these areas, as such a review would be beyond the scope of this book. Our intention is to present an overview of the areas we consider to be especially pertinent to training the severely handicapped and to provide direction for assessment and remediation.

Establishing a Desire to Communicate

Communication occurs when people interact in some way (verbally or nonverbally) so that a message passes from one person to another and a response is given in return. In most circumstances, one person intends to send a message and the other person intends to receive it.

Severely handicapped clients may be discouraged from communicating because of the great effort (e.g., physically) it takes and because their needs are anticipated by others. McLean and Synder-McLean (1978) note that children who have older siblings may develop expressive language skills later than expected due to the older siblings' "... tendency to interpret and respond to nonverbal communicative efforts (which) alleviates the younger child's need or reason for using language" (p. 48). This tendency to interpret and anticipate clients' needs by parents and training personnel may likewise reduce the severely handicapped client's desire to communicate.

Guess, Sailor, and Baer (1977) stress the need for demonstrating that the client can gain control over his or her environment through expressive language. Their program, entitled *Functional Speech and Language Training for the Severely Handicapped*,[1] was developed along five dimensions: *reference, control, self-extended control, integration*, and *reception*. The *reference* dimension establishes the fact that words or signs represent an object or event. The dimension of *control* teaches a variety of requesting behaviors (e.g., "I want (object)" or "I want you to (action-with-object)" to illustrate to the client the "power of language." Once the client realizes his or her ability to initiate communication (verbally, gesturally, or symbolically), then *self-extended control* becomes the next goal. At this point the client learns to ask for more information by asking, "What is this?" *Integration* requires the client to chain together previously learned skills to converse about an object or event. It should be noted that *reception*, or understanding, is taught after production in this program in order to stress the immediate need for speaking or communicating rather than simple instruction following.

Children who have withdrawn from communicating with others in their environment (e.g., autistic or emotionally disturbed) require special techniques to establish communication interactions. Searcy, Opat, and Welch (1979) describe the Mercy Approach to Theraplay,[2] which ". . . focuses on developing the child's desire to communicate within an accepting, intrusive, nurturing and boundary defining setting" (p. 3). Their approach is based on Jernberg's (1979) "Theraplay" techniques designed for emotionally disturbed children. The "Theraplay" procedures use structured play to establish communication interactions between a primary therapist and the child. Gradually these newly established interactions are transferred to parent and child. The parents receive counseling and become involved in training through observation and gradual participation in the "Theraplay" setting. The psychological needs of the handicapped child are carefully considered to help create a comfortable environment for successful communication. The ultimate mode of communication may be vocal or non-vocal, but the basic desire and rewards of communication are illustrated to the child.

Thus, establishing the desire to communicate may be considered a prerequisite to language training. The trainer must create an environment and relationship with the client which demonstrates a caring, accepting atmosphere for the client to develop control over the environment through using communication skills. Many programs which emphasize responding in the absence of contextual support and communicative intent may not elicit this desire. For example, asking "What is this?" when it is clear that the trainer knows what "this" is may not stimulate the desire to communicate.

---

1. See Appendices A and B and Chapter 6 for more information about this program.
2. The Mercy Approach to Theraplay is being developed at Mercy Hospital and Medical Center in Chicago, Illinois.

Allowing the client to select an item (e.g., from a bag or box) out of the trainer's view and then asking him "what do you have?" may be a more functional task.

In summary, the general atmosphere of the training and home environments may enhance the client's desire to communicate. Developing training tasks that are functional and demonstrate to the client that there is a reason for communicating may also encourage initiation of communication.

Eliminating Interfering Behaviors

Some severely handicapped individuals exhibit undesirable behavior which interferes to varying degrees with their ability to participate in expected daily activities and formal training programs. Two major types of interfering behaviors will be discussed in this section:

1. *Self-stimulating behavior*: such as body-rocking, hand-gazing, obsessions for particular objects (e.g., lights, water) and repetitive movements of a body part (e.g., hand-waving, clapping, foot-tapping) (Azrin, Kaplan, and Foxx 1973; Dolan and Burton 1976; Kent 1974; Woolman 1980).

2. *Self-injurious behaviors*: such as head-banging, hand-biting, and body-pinching (Gaylord-Ross 1977).

These types of behavior may threaten the health of the client or may preoccupy the client so that learning new skills is seriously impeded (Gaylord-Ross 1977). Therefore, it is necessary for the trainer to identify self-stimulating and self-injurious behavior and attempt to eliminate or control it. Once some control or reduction in frequency of this behavior is established, new skill training can be initiated or continued with less interruption.

The primary means of assessing interfering behavior is careful clinical observation by a trainer who observes the client and documents any self-stimulating or self-injurious behavior. It is helpful to note during what types of situations this behavior occurs and the frequency of its occurrence. These observations should be made over a period of several days at various times of the day and in different activities. This baseline information is then used to design procedures for reducing the interfering behavior.

The trainer may employ a variety of procedures to eliminate or reduce interfering behavior. Teaching alternate behavior is a procedure suggested by Dolan and Burton (1976) and by Sapon et al. (1976) as a means of controlling self-stimulating behaviors. Substituting an acceptable movement such as rocking in a rocking chair for general body-rocking is one approach toward reducing body-rocking in other situations. The client gradually learns when rocking is acceptable. Also, for example, if a client engages in hand-gazing, a ring or colorful water soluble tatoo can be put on his hand to attract attention and to stimulate comments about what the client is looking at. If a client is fascinated by lights or playing with water, a flashlight or short period of water play could be introduced as reinforcement for successfully completing a task. Thus, the teaching of alternate behavior approach is one of positive reinforcement and environmental manipulation to provide the client with more acceptable patterns of behaving.

Azrin et al. (1973) and Kent (1974) advocate contingent punishment to eliminate interfering behavior. Their techniques utilize a reversal procedure which requires the client to engage in postures which are incompatible with the client's self-stimulating behavior. Instructions and physical assistance are presented to move the client through the incompatible postures; for example, to eliminate lateral head-weaving, the client is required to move alternately from the position of head up to head straight to head down for 20 minutes (Kent 1974). This activity is presumably aversive to the client and serves to punish a previously emitted interfering response. The time interval is reduced as the interfering behavior occurs less frequently, until only a verbal warning need be issued to remind the client to stop the interfering behavior.

Koegel and Covert (1972) found that with autistic children who exhibited self-stimulating behavior with their hands, a quick slap on the hands or the trainer moving the client's hand(s) down with the command, "No, hands down," worked best to eliminate the hand movements. This procedure, if effective, may be more practical in a classroom situation where personnel is limited than using the 20 minute reversal procedure. Woolman (1980) also found the reversal procedures advocated by Kent (1974) too time consuming and suggested that they did not focus enough on the desired behavior.

Gaylord-Ross (1977) conducted a study to test the effectiveness of four treatment procedures to eliminate self-injurious behavior demonstrated by severely handicapped clients (i.e., autistic, psychotic, and profoundly retarded) in three special schools. The four procedures used in the study were:

1. *overcorrection*, in which the client is physically restrained from making the injurious movement;
2. *reinforcement withdrawal*, in which the trainer's attention is removed from the client;
3. *differential reinforcement*, in which the client is rewarded for appropriate behavior that is incompatible with the injurious behavior;
4. *omission training*, in which the client is reinforced for not engaging in the injurious behavior for certain periods of time.

The results of this study indicated that the *overcorrection* procedure was most successful, as the use of contingent restraint was both punishing and helpful in establishing a counter-controlling function for the client. A verbal command (e.g., "No, hands down") gradually became the only reminder needed to stop the client's undesirable behavior.

This section has presented several treatment procedures designed to eliminate or reduce self-stimulating or self-injurious behavior by severely handicapped clients. The reversal procedure (Azrin et al. 1973; Kent 1974) and the overcorrection procedure (Foxx and Azrin 1973a; Gaylord-Ross 1977) require the trainer to spend extra time with the client, but have been demonstrated to yield positive results. Whatever the choice of procedure, eliminating interfering behavior will increase the client's attentiveness to other activities and enhance learning. In most cases such training will be taught concurrently with other training goals. Because an interfering behavior interrupts a training task, the trainer must deal with it immediately and before resuming the original goal of the session.

Improving Attention

Attempting to test or train a non-compliant, distractible, hyperactive, withdrawn and/or uninterested child is a challenge to the evaluator or trainer. In developing attending skills, the trainer must not allow a power struggle to develop between the trainer and client. This can happen if the training procedures involve tasks of little interest to the client and require unreasonable lengths of time (e.g., client must maintain eye contact with trainer for 30 seconds). Therefore, the trainer should consider the client's general level of physical and psychological development when determining specific training criteria for the client. This section on improving attention will focus on physical attention and visual attention. There is no intention to imply that these are totally separate behaviors. In actual training they may be taught concurrently. Within this section physical attending includes establishing sitting, attending to trainer, and on-task attending. Visual attending includes visual fixation, visual tracking, and visual scanning skills.

Physical Attention

Quiet sitting on the trainer's lap or sitting on a cushion on the floor may be the first step in establishing independent chair sitting for more structured training sessions with some clients. It is crucial that the client have something to do while remaining relatively quiet and in the appropriate sitting position. Bricker and Dennison (1978) suggest a three phase attending program. This involves: Phase 1—sitting in a chair while playing with toys; Phase 2—looking at the trainer as a prerequisite for later motor imitation training; and Phase 3—working on-task to determine and increase the length of time a client can stay working on a task. The trainer must become skilled in anticipating when the client will tire of an activity and change the activity or cease the lesson *before* the client stops attending.

Five preliminary precommunication skills (attention, sitting, on-task behavior, object permanence, and gesture communication) are assessed through caretaker interview and observation of the child during testing, using the *Environmental Prelanguage Battery* (Horstmeier and MacDonald 1978a). Specific training suggestions for these five skills are offered in their *Ready, Set, Go: Talk to Me* program (Horstmeier and MacDonald 1978b).[3]

Woolman (1980) divided the attending section of her Presymbolic Training Program into two sections: (1) Physical attending—(a) sitting in a chair, (b) eliminating interfering behavior, and (c) sitting at a table; (2) Visual

---

3. See Chapter 6 and Appendix A for more information.

attending—(a) establishing eye contact, (b) attending to three objects (p. 348). Each of these tasks has a mastery criterion of attending at the specified level for 30-second trials without participating in another activity. In addition, the client is required to maintain a fixed position with back straight against the back of a chair, feet flat on floor, and knees together. Obviously this procedure might not be physically appropriate or realistic for some severely handicapped clients.

Simmons and Williams (1976) present in their attending program tasks divided into small steps with increased time criteria (e.g., attends for one to five seconds with continuous cueing) to encourage client success. The authors include programs for responding to auditory, nonverbal cues; responding to name; establishing eye contact; attending for five seconds with continuous cueing; and attending with a time lapse between cue and response.

For the severely handicapped client who is confined to a wheelchair or bed, physical attending may be enhanced by proper body positioning (Bigge 1977). Once body position is adjusted for optimal comfort, visual attention tasks may be employed.

Visual Attention

Most training programs for the severely handicapped assume that the client has adequate or corrected vision as a prerequisite for entering the program. Moreover, visual attending skills such as visual fixation, visual tracking, and visual scanning may be overlooked during initial areas of training when trainers are anxious to extablish communication. However, for the severely physically impaired client, the development of visual attending skills may be the key to establishing a communication system, via eye gaze and scanning procedures. This becomes particularly important if a non-vocal system is selected, such as a communication board or electronic communication aid. This section will offer definitions of the terms visual fixation, visual tracking, and visual scanning and present some suggested training activities to develop these skills.

Visual fixation

Robinson and Robinson (1978) define visual fixation as " . . . regard of a stimulus which is held in a fixed position" (p. 115). Their criterion for establishing visual fixation is that the client must look at an object within one to ten seconds after its presentation and maintain eye contact with it for ten to fifteen seconds. They note that if the trainer is unsure whether the child is visually fixating, he or she may check for reflection of the stimulus in the client's pupil(s).

Several aspects which may be considered during assessment and training of visual attending skills include the following:

1. *Stimulus*—developmentally, children respond first to light sources, and later to patterned stimuli such as faces (Fantz and Nevis, 1967); thus, "Look at me" may not be an appropriate initial goal;
2. *Distance*—it will be necessary for the client to learn to attend to

objects, people, and events that are out of reach as well as those within reach;

3. *Latency*—it may be helpful to determine how long it takes the client to respond to a visual stimulus, then to reduce this latency so that he or she will be able to attend to events of short duration (Robinson and Robinson, 1978);

4. *Positioning*—conjugate gaze, in which both eyes are focused on the same point, is most likely if there is sufficient support for the head to be stable and centered at midline (Robinson and Robinson, 1978; Sternat et al. 1977);

5. *Cue(s)*—It may initially be necessary to supplement the visual stimulus with some type of cue, such as a verbalization ("Look, Jenny), a vocalization ("ooooh"), a noise (using a rattle as the stimulus), or a gesture (moving the stimulus or pointing to it).

One or more of these factors may be systematically altered as needed to extend the child's visual attending skills.

Visual tracking

Visual tracking involves following a moving object. An operational training definition of tracking is following an object that is moved slowly through a horizontal, vertical, or circular path (Scheuerman et al. 1976; Robinson and Robinson, 1978). Visual tracking is vital to the development of other skills such as object permanence and social and play interactions (Scheuerman et al.).

When introducing a tracking task the trainer should stand or sit so that the client does not become distracted by looking at the trainer when an item is presented for tracking. The client may move just his or her eyes or, more commonly, move the head and eyes simultaneously to follow the object. Using a mirror for the client to follow his own image may be a helpful technique. A variety of activities can be employed throughout the day to check tracking skills. Examples of naturalized activities include the following:

1. Rolling balls from one location to another;
2. Dropping objects into water or into a container;
3. Watching liquids being poured at meal time.

Using barriers to partially or fully hide objects is a higher level task involving visual tracking skill whereby the client must follow an object until it stops, then maintain a gaze at the point where the object stopped or disappeared (Scheuerman et al. 1976).

Some clients may have physical problems such as poor head or oculomotor control which may make visual tracking difficult. For a client who is physically unable to accomplish smooth motor movements during tracking, an alternate response could be a shift in gaze from one object to another (Robinson and Robinson 1978)

Programs for teaching tracking skills to severely handicapped people are presented in Robinson and Robinson (1978) and Scheuerman et al. Some considerations during assessment and training of tracking skills are listed below:

1. *Stimulus*—the size, color, pattern, and complexity (e.g., presence of moving parts) may affect learning;
2. *Location*—this involves the distance (within reach or out of reach) and the level (above, below, or at eye level);
3. *Range*—this could be from a few degrees, to 90° and return, to 180°; the starting point and whether or not the stimulus crosses the client's midline are also important;
4. *Cue(s)*—as with visual fixation, vocal, verbal, auditory, or gestural cues can be added;
5. *Speed*—this could range from slow to fast;
6. *Path*—potential paths include horizontal, vertical, diagonal, continuous, circular, and random;
7. *Barriers*—use of transparent, translucent, or opaque barriers would make this a more difficult task, introducing object permanence training.

These factors could be systematically manipulated during training to provide for optimal generalization.

Visual scanning

Visual scanning involves a visual search of parts of an object or the individual components of an array of objects (Scheuerman et al. 1976). Skill in scanning is vital to allowing the handicapped person choices within his or her immediate environment. A variety of non-vocal communication aids are available which permit the client to select a message by a scanning response (e.g., head, eye, hand, or foot movement) from items presented by a person or communication aid (Harris-Vanderheiden and Handerheiden 1977). The *Zygo Communication Board Program* (Hall, O'Grady, and Talkington 1978) provides a systematic training program for establishing scanning skill on that commercially available device. Scanning requires tracking ability, as the client must look across or down a series of items presented and then react in some way to stop on the desired item (e.g., press a switch to stop a light on the appropriate item).

The *Visual Symbol Communication Instruction* Program (Elder 1978) provides a very structured approach to teaching initial visual scanning and discrimination skills. A Visual Communication Display is used. This acrylite board has four pockets which may hold symbol cards. Initially, the client is required to scan the four pockets to determine which contains a blank card, while the remaining three pockets are empty. The position of the card is then rotated between two pockets. Next, a symbol card and blank card are rotated between two pockets, and the client is required to find the symbol card. Finally, a symbol card is rotated with three blank cards, so that the client must scan all four positions to make the correct choice. This basic procedure is repeated with other symbol cards, after which two-symbol discrimination is initiated.

Initial scanning training can be implemented during individual sessions (e.g., during training for a specific scanning device) or as part of other activities (e.g., during table preparation for a meal, the client indicates which chair or utensils are missing). Scheuerman et al. (1976) suggest a number of other scanning activities that can be practiced within the natural environment, such as,

1. having the client indicate empty spaces of an egg carton;
2. purposely leaving crumbs on the table following a meal and having the client indicate where to clean.

Physical and visual attention are preliminary skills that can be taught concurrently with each other and with other tasks. For example, when training identification of objects, the trainer may chart length of attending for on-task behavior or may record visual tracking responses involving the object once the object is identified appropriately.

Though many of the programs designed for teaching attending skills are artificially-structured, they may often be modified by using naturally-structured activities such as those suggested by Scheuerman et al. (1976). Using naturally-structured activities, natural settings, and a variety of trainers should ensure that newly learned attending skills are generalized and that they serve to facilitate communication.

Increasing Cognitive Skills

Piaget's theory of intellectual development (Piaget 1954; 1963) which delineates a series of invariant stages for normal cognitive development in children has been borrowed by many disciplines (e.g., special education, speech-language pathology) in developing programming for handicapped individuals. Piaget's theory has been used as the basis for devising both assessment tools (Chappell and Johnson 1976; Miller et al. 1980; Shane and Bashir 1980; Uzgiris and Hunt 1975) and training programs (Bricker and Dennison 1978; Chapman and Miller 1980; Chappell and Johnson 1976; Robinson and Robinson 1978; Tilton, Liska, and Bourland 1977).

Piaget's theory can be briefly summarized in terms of four primary stages:

1. *Sensorimotor stage*—ages 0–2 years,[4] in which cognitive behavior (or thought) is determined by sensory and motor interactions with the environment;
2. *Preoperational stage*—ages 2–7 years, in which cognitive behavior is characterized by rote and preliminary cognitive strategies in which logic is not well developed;
3. *Concrete operations*—ages 7–11 years, in which cognitive behavior is systematic and the child is capable of concrete problem solving;
4. *Formal operations*—ages 11–upward, in which cognitive behavior is abstract and mental operations of logic become established.

The primary focus on cognitive development for severely handicapped individuals is at the sensorimotor and early preoperational (2–4 year) stages.

---

4. The age ranges used in this section with reference to Piaget's stages or substages are approximate and are for normally developing children.

The sensorimotor stage can be divided into six substages. The first three substages encompass the ages of 0–8 months and concern unplanned or unintentional activities. Two examples of unintentional activities would be simple reflex activities like kicking or repeating motions that accidentally cause an interesting event (randomly hitting a mobile). The second three substages involve the development of planned or intentional activities. An example of an intentional activity is deferred imitation, such as when a child sweeps with a broom when he or she has not recently seen someone sweeping.

Chapman and Miller (1980) discuss the "intentional sensorimotor child," encompassing sensorimotor stages (substages) 4, 5, and 6. Following is a brief list of behaviors seen in each of these three stages. Further examples and discussion of these stages can be found in Chapman and Miller (1980), Ginsburg and Opper (1969), and Piaget and Inhelder (1969):

1. *Stage* 4 (8–12 months)—children at this stage can anticipate actions and imitate actions already in their repertoires; they also actively search for objects which vanish, indicating development of object permanence; although clients at this stage do not talk, they produce differentiated vocalizations and syllabic babbling;
2. *Stage* 5 (12–18 months)—at this stage children learn new means to achieve familiar goals and become capable of systematic imitation of new models; object permanence is more firmly established; clients begin to comprehend single words in context and produce performatives, in which a gesture accompanies a vocalization or word;
3. *Stage* 6 (18–24 months)—children at this stage are beginning to demonstrate representational thought, as seen in understanding words when the referent is not present and producing two word combinations.

This brief summary of stages 4, 5, and 6 should help clarify general behavior characteristics to be expected at each stage. We will continue to refer to these three sensorimotor stages and the preoperational stage throughout the remainder of this book, without further definition.

Functional Object Use

Many authors view the development of functional use of objects as a prerequisite skill for understanding the language employed to describe the use of the objects (Chappell and Johnson 1976; Bricker and Dennison 1978; Miller et al. 1980). The exploratory action of young infants to put most objects into their mouths is gradually replaced by the discriminative use of objects whereby the child learns that an object can be manipulated in a variety of ways (Bricker and Dennison 1978). Chappell and Johnson view such "sensorimotor exploration" (p. 18) as Level 1 of three developmental levels of children's responses to objects. Level 2 involves "imitative self-utilization of items,"; for example, when the child places a spoon to his or her mouth without food on it. Level 3 is labeled "primitive play application," whereby the child engages in symbolic play (e.g., pretending to give a doll a drink). A client who demonstrates primarily Level 1 exploration of objects may then be encouraged in training to imitate the trainer's use of the object. Although training in these areas of cognitive development may be considered prerequisite to language training, concurrent stimulation in verbal labeling of objects and their manipulations is encouraged. For example, during a Level 2 activity when the client is playing with a phone, the trainer may say, "see the phone", "pick up the phone", "say hello." As an example of a Level 3 activity in using a phone, the trainer may say, "give dolly the phone" or "have dolly call Daddy."

Chappell discusses the use of props in training by reviewing a study by Overton and Jackson (1973) regarding pretend behavior in two and three year-olds. They found that two-year-olds needed the object in order to demonstrate the object's use, while three-year-olds were able to pretend to use an absent object. (With most severely handicapped clients, actual objects should be used in training and are preferable to minature toy substitutes).

A number of sources describe programs or steps designed to train functional use of objects (Bricker and Dennison 1978; Horstmeier and MacDonald 1978b; Lyon et al. 1977). Functional object use may be taught concurrently with communication training. As the child explores the use of objects, the trainer simultaneously describes what the child is doing.

Object Permanence

Object permanence, or the awareness that an object still exists when it is not in sight, is an important cognitive skill accomplished during Piaget's sensorimotor stages. A number of authors have devised training programs to increase skills in this area (Kahn 1978; Horstmeier and MacDonald 1978b; Nietupski et al. 1977; Robinson and Robinson, 1978).

Robinson and Robinson (1978) describe a series of three object permanence tasks that increase in complexity:

1. *Prerequisite object permanence skills*—requiring the client to visually follow an object to a place where it is partially hidden and eventually retrieve it, if the client is physically able to do so;
2. *Simple object permanence problems*—requiring the client to observe an object being completely hidden from view and to search for and retrieve it;
3. *Complex object permanence problems*—requiring the client to search and recover an object when its location is unknown.

During all these activities, the client is learning to manipulate the environment physically. The need for a non-vocal client to develop object permanence skill is very important for his use of a symbolic communication aid when at times some items might be covered by the client's arm or, on a multiple sheet device, may be on another page. The client needs to realize that the items are still available.

Several other authors present strategies for accelerating object permanence (e.g., Nietupski et al. 1977; Tilton et al. 1977). Again, the communication specialist should consider whether it is efficient to focus on this target as a prerequisite or to present it as part of a concurrent communication program.

Other Early Cognitive Skills

Discriminating characteristics of objects through matching and sorting tasks may also be considered a preliminary skill to later language learning. Being able to construct a whole from pieces, as in puzzle manipulation, demonstrates the emergence of problem-solving skills. McCormack and Chalmers (1978) have developed teaching sequences entitled *Early Cognitive Instruction for the Moderately and Severely Handicapped*. Their program includes an assessment device and detailed training strategies to teach the following early cognitive skills: matching, sorting, constructing, recognizing (receptive language), identifying (expressive language), memory, and sequencing.

Establishing Motor Imitation

Some prelanguage and language programs provide sequences for teaching motor imitation skills as preliminary skills. Typically, gross motor movements are taught initially and include such activities as clapping, waving "bye-bye," and touching body parts (Baer 1978; Bricker and Dennison 1978; Harris 1975; Horstmeier and MacDonald 1978b; Kent 1974; Striefel 1977). Gradually, fine motor movements of the mouth may be imitated (Harris 1975; Sloane, Johnston, and Harris 1968) before presenting vocalizations for imitation.

The choice of types of motor movements that should be taught or which are easiest to teach has received consideration by several authors (Bricker and Dennison 1978; Harris 1975; Kent 1974). Kent (1974) recommends teaching motor responses that are specifically needed as responses for other portions of her program (e.g., pointing to body parts and objects on table). In her program the use of the verbal or the signed command "Do this" is presented before the motor movement is demonstrated. The child is physically assisted through the expected movement.

Kent (1974) also offers suggestions about altering the movements to be imitated if a child is unsuccessful with the initially presented movements. She suggests that tasks involving manipulation of an object are easiest to accomplish (e.g., pushing a toy car). Movements involving both hands or both feet are assumed to be easier to perform than one-limb movements. It is also presumed to be easier to perform movements that are completely visible to the child (e.g., wiping hands versus touching ear).

Bricker and Dennison (1978) suggest that the motor tasks selected for initial imitation should already be in the child's repertoire. These authors use the term "imitation chains" (p. 169) to describe the technique in which the trainer repeats a movement the child has performed spontaneously. Once the child imitates the trainer's imitation of a movement the child has initiated, the child may then imitate familiar movements initiated by the trainer. Gradually, unfamiliar movements initiated by the trainer are presented for imitation.

Some authors (St. Louis, Rejzer, and Cone 1980) suggest that if motor imitation is being trained, it is more useful to train functional movements like drinking from a cup, wiping hands with a towel, or some initial communicative gestures or signs (e.g., wave "bye-bye," the sign for "more") than motor tasks such as tapping a table or clapping hands. Bricker and Dennison (1978) recommend encouraging motor imitation in practical situations such as pushing elevator buttons, opening doors, and moving a light switch.

Once motor imitation is established, it may lead to developing vocal or verbal imitation, although there is little research to document this hypothesis. Kent (1974) suggests that motor imitation be used as a last attempt to accomplish vocal imitation if other techniques have failed to elicit vocalizations. This procedure would have the client imitate a chain of events, beginning with motor movements and ending with a vocalization (e.g., tap table, stand up, say "hi"). Gradually the motor movements should be faded and only the vocalization required. There is some controversy as to the role of motor imitation in the eventual establishment of verbal imitation (see Harris 1975 for a review). However, with some clients this chaining procedure may be useful.

When a non-vocal communication mode is being considered as a primary communication system, the client's ability to imitate motor movements may facilitate acquiring proficiency in using the system. If a gestural communication system is being taught, new vocabulary can be taught through the imitation of signs or gestures introduced by the trainer. Symbolic communications systems usually rely on a motor movement (e.g., pointing, activating a switch) to indicate the message to be transmitted. During initial training having the client imitate the movements to select appropriate items on a communication device may aid in his or her establishing a generalized means of indicating on the device. Specific programming for using gestural and symbolic communication will be discussed in later chapters along with further discussion of the issue of imitation in training the use of non-vocal modes.

The trainer should be aware of the client's physical abilities and limitations before initiating motor imitation training. Consultation with the client's physician, as well as with occupational and/or physical therapist, should be sought to assist in program planning.

Developing Oral-Motor Control

The communication specialist working with clients having neurological disorders, such as cerebral palsy and speech impairments related to aphasia (e.g., dysarthria and apraxia), will need to consider the client's control of his or her oral mechanism for producing intelligible speech. The potential to improve oral-motor control is a vital consideration in deciding on the use of vocal communication as the primary communication mode for a client. Some researchers have investigated the relationship between feeding problems and speech performance in cerebral palsied children (Love, Hagerman, and Taimi 1980; Sheppard 1964). They found a suggestive positive relationship between abnormal oral reflexes (e.g., rooting reflex, sucking reflex), or feeding problems, and speech proficiency. However, there is some question as to the relationship of oral movements for feeding and movements for speech production. Bosma (1975) indicates that in normally developing children there does not appear to be a direct relationship between feeding and early speech gestures. However, developing a feeding program continues to be a part of prespeech training for children with cerebral palsy (Liebman 1977; Mueller 1975a). Although it cannot be substantiated that feeding training will develop specific oral movements for speech production, such training may foster more rapid and efficient eating (Love et al. 1980). This section will briefly present some prespeech and feeding training suggestions which may help develop a client's oral-motor control for eating and possibly strengthen control for later speech production. The areas to be presented are: positioning, breathing, inhibiting oral reflexes, oral sensory stimulation, inhibiting drooling, drinking from a cup, and spoon feeding. The suggestions offered in this section are exemplary of techniques used with cerebral palsied children and are not to be considered as complete programming.

Positioning for Feeding and Speech Production

The position of the cerebral palsied client for feeding and speech production is crucial to allow for adequate swallowing of food and breath support for vocalizations. Depending upon the severity of the client's neuromuscular condition, he or she should be positioned in particular ways. An assessment of gross and fine motor skills should be completed before training begins, using a device such as the *Developmental Profiles* by Herst et al. (1976). Then a comprehensive program for positioning the client for varied activities (e.g., eating, sleeping) should be designed (Utley, Holvoet, and Barnes 1977; High 1977). Generally, the trainer should try not to control the client's head by placing a hand behind the head at the neck, because that may cause the client to tense and resist positioning by pushing the head back (Mueller 1975a).

Proper positioning for speech is critical in developing adequate breath support for vocalization (Golbin 1977). For a young child, sitting in a straddle position on the parent's or trainer's lap may be most comfortable. A pillow or wedgeboard could be placed between the child's back and a table to provide needed support. For an older child, a specially equipped chair with head, arm, and leg supports may be useful in initially placing the client in a suitable position for proper eating and vocalizing. Physical and occupational therapists may work toward developing positioning independent of adaptive devices.

Training for developing breath control for speech involves not only developing good posture but also training the client to inhale and exhale properly to sustain vocalizations (McDonald and Crane 1964; Mueller 1975b).

Inhibiting Oral Reflexes

The persistence of primitive oral reflexes such as the sucking, biting, and lip reflexes can interfere with adequate feeding and in articulating speech. Appendix D presents several sources for assessing oral reflex patterns. Control of the lower jaw needs to be established for eating (before a spoon or cup is introduced). The trainer can help establish jaw control by placing his or her middle finger under the client's chin, the index finger under the lower lip, and the thumb on the client's cheek. The pressure of the middle finger " . . . enables tongue functioning to be indirectly controlled thus helping swallowing to be more normal" (Mueller 1975a, p. 119). The client may resist the trainer's attempts to manipulate his or her jaw. It may be necessary to desensitize the child gradually so that the trainer can touch his or her face and mouth area without provoking severe tension or spasms.

To inhibit the lip reflex (involuntary movements of the lips in a pouting or closed lip position), McDonald and Crane (1964) suggest stimulating the reflex by tapping the corner of the client's lips and then holding the lips with fingers to prevent involuntary movements.

Oral Sensory Stimulation

During normal motor development, a child places many objects in and around his mouth as one means of exploring the environment. Severely physically impaired children may be unable to bring things to their mouths and, therefore, may have been deprived of oral sensations. Liebman (1977) suggests that parents make oral stimulation part of their play time with their child. Bringing different textures to the cheeks and lips (e.g., rubbing a fuzzy stuffed toy on the client's cheek or allowing a rubber toy to touch the lips) will provide the child with tactile information and possibly help desensitize him or her to oral manipulation. Utley et al. (1977) present additional suggestions for desensitization.

Inhibiting Drooling

Many clients with cerebral palsy or other neuromuscular disorders may exhibit abnormal swallowing patterns (i.e., tongue thrust) and drooling. If a client has poor posture and has difficulty holding up his or her head, drooling may occur. A client whose mouth is habitually open with tongue carried forward in the mouth may also drool. It is important to note that it is not advisable initially to verbally correct the client who drools. Obviously once the saliva is out of the mouth, it is beyond the client's control. It is preferable to attempt to prevent drooling. Teaching correct mouth positioning and developing a more normal swallowing pattern may reduce drooling (Crickmay 1966). Reduction of drooling, even if vocal communication is not a realistic goal, helps the client in his general appearance and may enhance his or her social interactions.

Drinking From a Cup

Drinking from a cup requires patience and practice for many severely physically handicapped individuals. Taking liquid from a cup involves lip closure as well as control of the head and jaw. Starting with thickened liquids (e.g., flavored yogurt) in a plastic cup with a portion of the cup cut out for the nose will make the task of drinking easier for the client (Liebman 1977; Mueller 1975a; Utley et al; 1977). Straw sucking is a difficult task and should not be introduced until cup drinking is well established, and then only to increase lip mobility (Mueller 1975a).

Spoon Feeding

When introducing spoon feeding, the trainer or parent must insure that the spoon is placed on the midline of the tongue with enough pressure to inhibit protrusion of the tongue. It is important to try to stimulate the upper lip to scrape the food off the spoon rather than allow the client to scrape the food off with the teeth or gums (Liebman 1977; Mueller 1975a). The spoon used in early training should have a bowl that is fairly flat with a rounded tip. The handle of the spoon can be modified to allow for easier entry into the mouth when the client begins to self-feed (e.g., handle bent at a right angle).

Summary

All of the preliminary behavior discussed in this chapter is related to the eventual establishment of a means of communicating regardless of communication mode. Most current authors recommend teaching this behavior concurrently with a language program, as mentioned in the introduction. In any case, we wish to stress that it is important not to wait for the client to be "ready" for training. We believe that part of the educator's, therapist's (physical, occupational and/or speech-language), and parents' role is to take the client at whatever level he or she can function and create experiences that lead him or her toward reaching his or her optimal potential.

Chapter 5: Supportive Services

Introduction

The development and utilization of support services are crucial to meeting the needs of the severely handicapped client. Primary support systems include parents and other caregivers, professionals, paraprofessionals, and specialized service agencies or organizations.

The Team Approach

Although several authors (Allen et al. 1978; Beck 1977; Cohen, Montgomery, and Yoder 1979; Hart 1977; Silverman, McNaughton, and Kates 1978) have stressed the importance of involving professionals from various disciplines, they do not agree on a specific model for the team approach. Hart (1977) describes the following models:

1. The *multi-disciplinary approach*, based on the medical model, in which experts in diverse areas share information about each client;
2. The *inter-disciplinary approach*, in which team members share information and attempt to unify their findings;

3. The *transdisciplinary approach*, in which the team assigns a primary therapist to the client.

Hart cautions that the relative degree of importance attached to the information collected by the various team members may be determined by the type of setting (medical, psychotherapeutic, educational), by the person who collates the information, and by the manner in which the data are shared (staffing, report to teacher). She also warns that both the multi and inter-disciplinary approaches "often lack an important step in their models: immediate and ongoing feedback with responsible follow-up of the recommendations" (p. 392). Therefore, she recommends using the transdisciplinary approach.

Although professionals may disagree with Hart's classification, they should recognize that there are different team approaches. Their choice will depend on a variety of factors. The clients served will have some influence, at least with respect to the team members included. Roos (1977) asserts that every team, regardless of the model chosen, should include the client's parent(s) or spouse.

The stage of the assessment/intervention process may also affect the team members, and possibly the approach. For example, teams involved in cleft palate rehabilitation often follow a developmental approach, in which professionals from various disciplines enter and leave the team when appropriate to the client's current needs (Koepp-Baker 1971; Krogman 1979). An example of this with regard to the severely handicapped population would be inclusion of a vocational rehabilitation specialist when the client is ready for job training. These professionals would likely be consulted at earlier points in the process but would not be added to the team until the situation warranted. Similarly, the pediatrician might be a central member of a team for an infant or young child but would leave the team as his or her services were no longer needed. In this way the number of team members at any one time could be kept to a minimum, yielding a more realistic and manageable grouping. It may also be useful to utilize a multi or inter-disciplinary approach for the initial evaluation, then shift to a transdisciplinary approach for the intervention phase, to avoid as much as possible the lack of follow-up noted by several authors (Allen et al. 1978; Beck 1977; Hart 1977).

The background and orientation of the various team members may also contribute to determining an approach. As with the entire decision process, this should be brought to a level of awareness so that an inappropriate approach is not selected simply because that approach has become the one routinely used.

Finally, the resources available should be considered in choosing a team model. Beck (1977) notes that inter-disciplinary team evaluations " . . . have always included recommendations for intervention, but the resources for implementing them have been unavailable in most communities" (p. 397). In such situations the transdisciplinary model might be the most appropriate since it can be implemented by only one team member. However, both Hart (1977) and Beck (1977) stress that the person with primary responsibility (typically the teacher) must have an adequate background in each of the disciplines included on the team in order to ask appropriate questions, interpret data, and carry out specific intervention tactics suggested by the ancillary personnel.

In conclusion, there are several ways to approach the use of a team in serving the severely handicapped. Any of these approaches may be appropriate in certain situations. It is important that the team maintain a flexible attitude in order to best serve the clients' needs in a variety of different situations. Regardless of the the team approach utilized, group dynamics will be an important consideration. Several resources are available to help the team develop cohesiveness (Holm and McCartin 1978; Rubin, Plovnick, and Fry 1975; Bassin and Kreeb 1978).

Parents and Other Primary Caregivers[1]

There is general agreement about the need to actively involve parents in the intervention process for their severely handicapped children. Recently, several authors have designed special communication programs to satisfy this need (Harris 1976; Horstmeier and MacDonald 1978b; Schumaker and Sherman 1978). This increased involvement of parents requires that we reassess our roles in relation to parents, the parents' roles in relation to their children, and the programs which serve those children.

Responsibilities of Professionals in Relation to Parents

Although professionals have many responsibilities to the parents of their severely handicapped clients, the primary ones include sharing information with the parents, giving them emotional support and directing their training.

Sharing information traditionally includes explaining the nature of the child's problem(s), interpreting the test results, and describing the diagnostic and therapeutic procedures. However, parents should also be told how recent litigation (Mills v. Board of Education 1972; Pennsylvania 1972) and legislation (PL 94-142) affects their rights and responsibilities.[2] They should be encouraged to contact other local, regional, and national agencies and organizations which offer further information and support.[3] As noted, this responsibility implies a two-way exchange of information in which a partnership develops between parent and professional. Roos (1977), of the National Association for Retarded Citizens, cautions that parents " . . . sometimes feel that any suggestion made by a parent regarding his own child is categorically dismissed" (p. 73). Parents can share their views by rating the importance of various services. Cansler, Martin, and Valand (1975) designed a form to rate such areas as training in classroom activities and teaching methods, coun-

---

1. "Other primary caregivers" refers here to persons such as foster parents, houseparents for residential centers, or others who have primary responsibility for the care and nurturing of clients.
2. Turnbull (1978) offers a brief review of these areas.
3. See Appendix C of this book for a list of organizations, with descriptions of services provided by each.

seling for family problems, and transportation services. A similar form could be prepared to allow parents to rate the importance of communication-related services such as training parents to carry out specific programs, training parents to assist in generalization of school programs, training siblings to communicate more effectively, and providing opportunities for discussion with other parents of communication-impaired children.

A second responsibility for the professional working with parents of severely handicapped children is *support*. This may take a broader and more concrete form than that required for parents of less handicapped children. For example, moving through the emotional adjustment process might be more prolonged and more intense for parents of the severely handicapped. Many local, regional, and national organizations offer parent-support groups. Professionals should be aware of these services as they can direct parents to them. If a parent group is not available in the community, one could be established through various agencies such as public or private clinics and schools or through a local chapter of an organization such as the Association for Retarded Citizens. Some organizations and authorities have published guidelines for setting up parent programs (Arnold 1978; Auenback 1968; Bassin and Kreeb 1978; Cansler et al. 1975; Project WISP/Outreach 1979).

Support from parent groups does not replace personal support from the professional. Parents can reveal their special concerns through use of a rating sheet. Turnbull (1978) suggests that their principal concerns may be emotional adjustment, socialization for the child, relationships with siblings, and financial management, such as estate planning and guardianship. Although he suggests several ways to deal with each of these areas, he also recommends referring the parents to another professional, such as a lawyer, if necessary.

As with information sharing, support should be mutual, in which parents also demonstrate support for professionals. The professional can encourage this support by including parents in the decision process and by providing sufficient data to back up program suggestions. For example, a major suggestion, such as election of a non-vocal augmentative communication system, could be supported by presenting Silverman's (1980) data on the impact of non-vocal communication and by explaining Shane's and Bashir's (1980) decision matrix used in selecting a non-vocal system (see Chapter 2).

Training of parents is another major role for the communication specialist. Use of parents as primary or secondary intervention agents is widely recommended (Baker 1976; Horstmeier and MacDonald 1978a,b; Roos 1977; Schumaker and Sherman 1978; Turnball 1978). Turnball suggests a number of reasons why parents should be encouraged to serve as trainers of their handicapped children:

1. Parents are powerful reinforcing agents;
2. Parents know their children better than others and generally spend more time with their children than do professionals;
3. The effectiveness of intervention can be increased if parents follow up at home on the skills being taught at school;

4. Teaching children at home lowers costs;
5. Parents receive gratification from contributing to the development of their child.

Baker (1976) suggests that there is an especially strong rationale for parental involvement because language development typically takes place during infancy and early childhood and because language skills are so basic to the development of other skills. Whether they serve as primary or secondary trainers for their children some training and supervision will likely be needed for all parents, if only to teach them to sustain communication skills which the children have learned in the classroom. Some communication systems (e.g., most sign systems) may require considerable training merely to enable parents to interpret their child's communication attempts.

Group training sessions may reduce the work load for the professional as well as provide another means of support to the parents. Horstmeier and MacDonald (1978b) present models for group and individual parent language programming. Each model includes general suggestions regarding content and procedures for each parent training session. Baker (1976) suggests several models for training parents, providing general descriptions and reviews of specific projects. Baker also presents a review of the results of a number of parent programs. He concludes that, " . . . although parent training has been generally demonstrated to be effective, the empirical basis for specific procedural decisions remains fragmented at best" (p. 716). Therefore, he stresses that any parent training program should include sound procedures for assessing its effectiveness. Baker asserts that " . . . few families make a consistent and serious effort to carry out programs and still fail. Hence, encouraging participation becomes the paramount issue" (p. 717). He describes and reviews several program incentives which may increase family participation:

1. *Social pressure and social support,* such as writing and signing specific performance contracts with the trainer;
2. *Money,* such as a "contract deposit" which is refunded contingent on completion of agreed-upon performance;
3. *Reinforcement by family members,* such as agreeing on special activities (e.g., a picnic) following specific gains in child performance;
4. *Contingent professional resources,* such as cards for use in a toy-lending library, training time being contingent on supplying data on child performance.

(pp. 721–22)

Professionals should also listen to suggestions from parents concerning successful ways which they have found to deal with their handicapped children.

The traditional roles of sharing information with, supporting, and training parents must be expanded to meet the greater needs of parents and to conform to the partnership concept imposed by changes in law and current thought. More specific suggestions for working with parents and other caregivers will be presented in the chapters dealing with related behaviors and specific communications systems.

Responsibilities of Parents

Like professionals, parents of severely handicapped children may fulfill several roles. Turnball (1978) asserts the need for parents to *be parents*, dealing with problems such as emotional adjustment and socialization. The role of parents as *teachers of their children* is widely recognized. Parents also have an important role as *advocates*, or agents of social change (Roos 1977; Turnbull 1978), working alone or through organizations toward changes in law (such as PL 94-142), policy (for example, school policy on segregation of handicapped students), and public attitudes in general. Each of these parental roles will require the professional to assume an appropriate role in response. The roles of parents and professionals are varied and interwoven, changing as the situation warrants. If professionals are to establish effective parent-professional interactions, they must be cognizant of all these roles.

Supportive personnel

Several authors suggest that we may anticipate an increase in the use of supportive personnel, including paraprofessionals and volunteers, in the field of special education (e.g., Committee of Supportive Personnel, American Speech-Language-Hearing Association [ASHA] 1979; Sigelman and Bensberg 1976; Smith and Smith 1978; Tucker and Horner 1977). Several reasons for this increase are as follows:

1. The impact of PL 94-142, which requires free services for all children who need them and forbids the use of waiting lists;
2. Increased public awareness regarding the need for more extensive services to a wider population;
3. Problems related to fiscal and program accountability (Sigelman and Bensberg 1976);
4. A movement toward performance-based criteria of certification, hiring, and advancement, rather than relying solely on degrees (ibid);
5. The trend toward community-based services, yielding less centralization of services (ibid.).

The discussion here centers on the paraprofessional with direct training duties, specifically in the area of communication. The ASHA guidelines recommend that this person be called a "communication assistant" and propose specific guidelines for the definition, role, qualifications, training, and supervision of such an assistant. An article by Tucker and Horner (1977) offers a model for training paraprofessionals, including academic and practicum courses as well as training methods. Both sets of guidelines suggest extensive competency-based training, although the Tucker and Horner guidelines are more specific than those proposed by the ASHA Committee on Supportive Personnel. It should be noted that the Tucker and Horner guidelines are specific to the severely handicapped population, but not to the area of communication, while the ASHA guidelines are directed toward communication problems but not specifically toward the severely handicapped. Thus the trainer planning to implement a program with para-professionals might want to combine features from both sets of guidelines.

The supervision of paraprofessionals will likely be determined to a great extent by the discipline of the supervising professional. For example, speech-language pathologists will fall under the guidelines of their national organi-zation, the American Speech-Language-Hearing Association (ASHA). Re-gardless of the discipline, supervision will be an important issue since the ultimate responsibility for clients will rest with supervising professional.

Sigelman and Bensberg (1975) discuss the problem of motivating para-professionals. They report a number of successful strategies and suggest a variety of meaningful rewards such as the following:

1. Providing knowledge of results;
2. Devising competition between various groups of paraprofessionals, using criteria such as client progress or number of training sessions;
3. Providing written praise (from administrators, parents, professionals) for successful results;
4. Giving rewards contingent on client improvements, including money, time off from work, special events, and so forth.

Several of these methods will greatly depend on cooperation from administrators and may not be realistic in some situations. However, it seems worthwhile to make the effort to design strategies appropriate for the situation since the relevant literature clearly demonstrates the success of such strategies in terms of client improvement (Sigelman and Bensberg 1976).

A number of recent communication programs were designed for—or can be adapted for—implementation by paraprofessionals (Carrier and Peak 1975; Elder 1978; Guess, Sailor, and Baer 1976; Horstmeier and MacDonald 1978b). Appendix B of this book covers a variety of vocal and non-vocal programs, indicating which are appropriate for use by paraprofessionals. Paraprofessionals have been widely used with a range of populations,[4] and this trend is likely to continue. Administrators and those who currently provide direct services to the severely handicapped must be prepared to train and effectively work with paraprofessionals to meet ethical and legal stan-dards of service to the severely handicapped.

Environmental Support and Involvement

Several authors have noted that a major factor in the success of a communi-cation program is the involvement of those in the client's environment (Kopchick and Lloyd 1976; Sigelman and Bensberg 1976). This may be of even greater importance with regard to non-vocal modes of communication since the communication partner(s) must invest more time and effort into

---

4. See Gershon and Biller (1977), Reid and Reid (1974), or Sigelman and Bensberg (1976) for a review of this topic.

decoding the message. Many communication systems must be learned by the partner, including most sign systems and, to a lesser extent, symbol systems such as Rebus or Blissymbols. This may require more effort than those in the environment are willing to make. In addition, unless the communication system has voice output capability, the partner must pay full attention to the user. Silverman (1980) discusses problems related to lack of support from the people in the client's environment. This problem may be examined with regard to initiating a communication system, especially in a non-vocal mode, or generalizing a system which the client is learning. Each area will be discussed separately.

Gaining Support for Initiating a System

The overall approach to gaining acceptance and support for introducing a system would seem to be advance planning. That is, the trainer must anticipate potential objections or resistance and defuse them before they yield significant opposition. The potential user, parents, and others in the environment should be involved as much as possible in the decision process so that the suggestion of a new system will not come as a complete surprise. Thus the first strategy for gaining support is *early involvement* by all who will be affected by such a major decision.

It is difficult to make an informed decision without the proper background. Therefore, the second strategy is *providing information*. This may include general information (e.g., about non-vocal systems in general) and specific information (e.g., about the system(s) deemed most appropriate for this client). The information should not be highly technical but should help provide a basis for decision-making.

A number of concerns might be expressed by the people with whom the client will communicate. In fact, it might be necessary to *ask for a discussion of concerns* if this does not happen spontaneously. Silverman (1980) recognizes several common attitudes (e.g., "The clinician has given up on improving [or developing] the person's speech," p. 208), and suggests ways to deal with these attitudes. Primary methods include providing information about the concern (such as the reviews of studies showing the impact of non-vocal systems, e.g. Silverman 1980, pp. 32–35, 40–44) and giving reassurance (e.g., that the trainer will continue to work on speech).

We recommend that trainers use additional methods for providing reassurance, such as acquainting those concerned with *demonstrations of successes* with clients using comparable systems, through readings, films, or personal visits. The exact information provided will depend to some extent on the system to be implemented.[5] For example, numerous films and pamphlets are available through Blissymbolics Communication Institute regarding Blissymbols and through the Office of Cued Speech, Gallaudet College, regarding that system. Newsletters produced by various organizations often

---

5. See Appendix C of this book for sources of information regarding various populations and systems.

contain articles which are appropriate for this purpose(e.g., Blissymbolics Communication Institute's *Newsletter* and *Bulletin*, the *Cued Speech Newsletter*, and *Communication Outlook*). If use of a commercial device is considered, information can also generally be obtained in advance. For example, HC Electronics has the following information available at no cost concerning their Phonic Mirror HandiVoice (an electronic speech synthesizer): brochures, a film entitled "Breaking Through the Wall," and a newsletter, *Echo On*. A personal visit with a user of the potential system could be an excellent means of gaining support.

Finally, the current and future uses of the proposed system(s) should be discussed, *focusing on implementation with the specific client*. For example, if the primary system selected is Signing Exact English, it could be helpful to explain that this system should provide a good foundation for future acquisition of reading skills as it parallels spoken and written English.

It may be necessary initially to gain support by having a trial period of implementation. The time span for this trial therapy would depend on considerations such as the amount of support provided by the environment and the client's rate of learning. It is hoped that these strategies will be sufficient to develop support for initiating a communication system, especially when a relatively novel system is suggested.

Gaining Support for Implementing a System

The preceding section pertained mainly to non-vocal systems of communication. It generally is easier to gain support for initiating a vocal language program than a non-vocal program simply because vocal language is more universally accepted. However, implementation of a vocal language program may pose problems as well simply because it will require time from everyone involved with the client. Initially, at least, it may take less effort and time to anticipate a client's needs than to wait for the client to express those needs. Other potential demands on staff and parent time by the client who is developing communication skills are an increased demand for attention, the need for direct training, and the need for individual attention during communication with many clients using non-vocal systems (e.g., sign systems, pointing systems). All of these problems are compounded if staff and/or parents are resistant or indifferent to communication training programs. Areas in which support must be gained are listed below:

1. Communicating effectively with the client, including interpreting the client's messages;
2. Training the client (directly or indirectly);
3. Setting up and monitoring generalization programs.

Since these areas are somewhat specific to the system used, they will be discussed in more detail where appropriate throughout the book. Several general strategies will be suggested here.

The first general strategy is to *provide group training*. Persons attending training sessions may include parents, siblings, teachers, paraprofessionals, volunteers, and peers. This type of training has been used successfully by a number of researchers (e.g., Abkarian et al. 1978; Ebert 1979; Harris-Vanderheiden 1976; Horstmeier and McDonald 1978b). The content of training sessions would vary considerably depending on the system used and the level of the audience.

A strategy especially suited to carry over with staff would be to *assign ultimate responsibility to one individual,* who would serve as a Communication Generalization Coordinator. This practice follows the example of Foxx and Azrin (1973b) in their toilet training program. It is especially suited to needs in a residential setting but could also be accomplished in school settings. Duties of this coordinator would be carefully specified, including such areas as keeping records and monitoring training and generalization programs.

It may be difficult to gain the support of a staff member to serve as coordinator unless that person, in turn, is provided with support. A strategy to accomplish this end is to *enlist the support of the administrator* (e.g., special education director, school principal), again as suggested by Foxx and Azrin. Some of the tactics suggested earlier relative to gaining initial support should be helpful here. The communication specialist could ask the administrator for concrete recognition such as a written declaration of support for the goals of the program, release time for staff to attend training sessions, relief from some duties and/or additional pay for the person designated as coordinator, acknowledgment of program success in the form of memos or some of the rewards suggested in the section on motivating paraprofessionals. We are aware that these suggestions may be somewhat idealistic. However, we believe that they are worth trying. We have found that, when given specific requests for support such as those described here, many administrators have been surprisingly helpful.

One final strategy for increasing the involvement of those in the environment is to arrange for *sharing sessions or idea exchange letters* (Harris-Vanderheiden 1976). These would be exchanged among parents, staff members, and others who have found effective ways to meet the needs of communication training and generalization of skills with severely handicapped clients or with a specific population communication system, or client.

Funding

It is difficult to review the topic of funding for communication serivces to the severely handicapped. First, the resources rapidly change as new federal, state, and local funds become available and old sources of funding become unavailable. Changes in legislation or federal regulations, for example, allow different items and service to be eligible at different times. Medicare, for instance, currently funds therapy services for non-vocal clients but does not allow funds for most prosthetic communication devices. In addition, many regulations may be interpreted differently by different regions or agencies, and some services are optional under the enabling legislation. An example would be prosthetic devices (including hearing aids) in state plans for Medicaid. Another important consideration is whether sources are needed for funding entire projects or single communication aids, although some of the sources will be the same for both.

Montgomery (1979) lists a number of potential funding sources. A modification of this list follows:

1. *Grants* (to set up centers or programs)—sources include governmental agencies such as the Department of Education, Bureau of Education for the Handicapped, and contract agreements with private colleges;
2. *Public agencies*—these include Crippled Children's Services, Department of Rehabilitation (for disabled adults with employment potential), Medicare, Medicaid, and PL 94-142 monies, in which use is determined by local decisions;
3. *Private agencies*—sources include private insurance companies and foundations;
4. *Local service organizations*—this includes advocacy groups such as the Association for Retarded Citizens, churches, Parent Teacher Associations and Parent Teacher Organizations, service organizations (e.g., Sertoma Club, Quota Club, Telephone Pioneers of America), college fraternities or sororities which provide services to people with communication handicaps, high school or college clubs;
5. *Contributions*—these may come from private individuals and businesses (e.g., IBM provides matching funds for some equipment);
6. *Rental or leasing agreements*—many commercial firms allow clients to rent or lease products to determine if they are appropriate for the client;
7. *Used equipment*—although not a funding source, this option may substantially reduce costs; sources of used equipment are manufacturers and newsletters such as the one published by the Pacific Northwest Non Vocal Communication Group.

Manufacturers are often quite knowledgeable regarding funding and can offer further suggestions about sources.

Some controversy exists concerning the use of local funding sources such as service organizationas and private contributors. The main concern is that continued reliance upon these sources may tend to cause agencies such as the local school systems, Medicare, and private insurance companies to ignore the responsibilities regarding funding. In addition, gaining funding haphazardly may give the impression that the projects funded are trivial (Judy Montgomery, personal communication). Professionals in the field of communication disabilities seem to have two possibly conflicting responsibilities:

1. We must ensure that our clients receive the best possible equipment as soon as possible;
2. We must pursue greater support of services for our clients, taking care not to set precedents that will misleadingly suggest to the public sector and private insurance companies that their assistance is not needed.

There are a number of guides to funding sources. Several newsletters, such as *Communication Outlook*, issue frequent reports on funding. Several guides to funding sources are listed in the summer, 1978, and fall, 1978, issues of *Communication Outlook* (see Appendix C). Another information source is The Foundation Center, also described in Appendix C. Most states have a foundation center, usually located at a major university. These centers provide access to computer listings of funding sources appropriate for the need.

For information on federal funding sources the *Catalog of Federal Domestic Assistance* is recommended (see Appendix A). It covers funding sources such as Crippled Children's Services, Medicare, and Medicaid. Information on Medicare and Medicaid can also be obtained from local branches of federal and state agencies such as the Social Security Administration and the Department of Welfare. For example, a 62 page booklet, *Your Medicare Handbook*, is available from most Social Security Administration offices. The American Speech-Language-Hearing Association also provides informational packets on Medicare and Medicaid as they relate to speech-language pathology and audiology services. In addition, an ASHA Task Force has prepared *A Report of Third Party Reimbursement of Speech-language Pathology and Audiology Services* (1980). This covers public and private insurance programs and information on dealing with insurance claims. ASHA has also initiated a quarterly publication, *Governmental Affairs Review*. It will cover areas such as developments in federal legislation (including funding components such as Medicare and PL 94-142), federal regulations (such as those concerning Medicare home health cost limits), and sources of further information.

The application process may often be enhanced by personally contacting a representative of the potential funding organization. For example, if a claim which appears to be eligible is turned down, the communication specialist might contact a representative and request a review.

The previous discussion on funding is intended to serve as an introduction. Readers are referred to the references listed in this section and to Appendix C for more comprehensive information.

Part Two: Vocal Systems

Chapter 6: Vocal Communication Strategies

Introduction

This chapter provides an overview of 24 vocal language programs available to special educators and communication specialists. The general issues (e.g., models, methodology, role of imitation, and so forth) involved in examining a communication system, which are presented in Chapter 3, will be discussed in this chapter as they relate to vocal language programs and to the various stages or sequences which programs follow in developing vocal communication skills. The role of parents or other primary caregivers in a client's home environment will be discussed in terms of overall program planning and of establishing generalized language skills.

The decision process, as presented in Chapter 2, does not end with selecting a mode of communication or a particular training program. The process must be ongoing, and the decision must be frequently assessed so that significant changes in the client's language abilities and living environment can be used to direct future programming. Moreover, the mandated requirement of developing an Individualized Educational Plan (I.E.P.) for each client in the public schools stresses the individuality of each client, and, in most cases, a single vocal program will not meet a client's particular needs. The trainer must consider blending portions of several programs to meet the client's needs optimally.

Vocal Language Programs: An Overview

Once the decision is made to train the client to use vocal communication as the primary system, the trainer must then design specific goals and tasks to teach the client appropriate vocal language skills. The trainer must use all the observational data, test results, and reported information gathered from the primary caregiver(s) during the assessment process to develop an Individualized Educational Plan for that client.

Many vocal language programs are available commercially. Twenty-four such programs are listed in table 6-1. For easy reference they will be referred to by the number assigned in table 6-1 throughout the rest of this chapter. Note that each program is annotated in Appendix A and that selected ones are further described in Appendix B.

Table 6-1 does not represent an exhaustive listing of vocal language programs. These 24 programs are included becuase of their general availability for use within public school and institutional programs. Most of the programs are relatively inexpensive, requiring simply a manual for implementation. In these programs, the trainer typically supplies all of the stimulus materials although a few programs do provide such materials (e.g., table 6-1: 4, 5, 14) in the form of pictures, puzzles, puppets, and so forth.

Ten of the language programs were developed as part of comprehensive skill training procedures for severely handicapped clients (Table 6-1: 1, 3, 6, 8, 17, 18, 19, 21, 22, 23). For example, Volume II of Teaching the Moderately and Severely Handicapped (table 6-1:1) contains communication training plus socialization, safety, and leisure time skills. It is important to note that Volumes I and III (Bender and Valletutti 1976a; Bender, Valletutti, and Bender 1976) are also available for use in other areas such as behavior, self-care, motor skills, and functional academics for the mildly and moderately handicapped. Since communication training is not contained in Volumes I and III, they are not included in table 6-1.

The remaining fourteen programs (table 6-1: 2, 4, 5, 7, 9, 10, 11, 12, 13, 14, 15, 16, 20, 24) were developed solely as language training procedures for clients with mildly to severely disordered language abilities. Although several of these language programs were developed for mildly handicapped clients

Table 6-1

Vocal Language Programs

Program	Author	Appendices A	Appendices B
1. Teaching the Moderately and Severely Handicapped: Volume II	Bender & Valletutti (1976b)	x	x
2. A Language Intervention Program for Developmentally Young Children	Bricker et al. (1976)	x	
3. Portage Guide to Early Education	Bluma et al. (1976)	x	x
4. Peabody Language Development Kits	Dunn & Smith (1965, 1969)	x	
5. Distar Language I	Engelmann & Osborn (1976)	x	
6. The Teaching Research Curriculum for Moderately and Severely Handicapped	Fredericks et al. (1976)	x	x
7. A Language Program for the Nonlanguage Child	Gray & Ryan (1973)	x	
8. S.T.E.P.: Sequential Testing and Educational Programming	Greenberger & Thum (1975)		x
9. Functional Speech and Language Training for the Severely Handicapped	Guess et al. (1976)	x	x
10. Teaching Speech to a Nonverbal Child	Harris (1976)	x	x
11. A Milieu Approach to Teaching Language	Hart & Rogers-Warren (1978)	x	
12. Emerging Language 2	Hatten et al. (1976)	x	
13. Ready, Set, Go: Talk To Me	Horstmeier & MacDonald (1978)	x	x
14. GOAL: Language Development	Karnes (1972)	x	
15. Language Acquisition Program for the Retarded and Multiply Impaired	Kent (1974)	x	x
16. A Language Development Program: Imitative Gestures to Basic Syntactic Structures	Murdock & Hartmann (1975)	x	x
17. A Prescriptive and Behavioral Checklist for the Severely and Profoundly Retarded	Popovich (1977)	x	
18. WVS: Receptive Language Curriculum for the Moderately, Severely, and Profoundly Handicapped	St. Louis et al. (1980)		x
19. WVS: Expressive Language Curriculum for the Moderately, Severely, and Profoundly Handicapped	St. Louis et al. (1980)		x
20. A Behavioral-Psycholinguistic Approach to Language Training	Stremel & Waryas (1974)	x	
21. Behavioral Characteristics Progression (BCP)	Struck (1977)	x	x
22. Guide to Early Developmental Training	Tilton et al. (1977)		x
23. Volume 1: Communication—Minimum Objective System for Pupils With Severe Handicaps	Williams & Fox (1977)		x
24. Sourcebook for Language Learning Activities	Worthley (1978)	x	

(table 6-1: 4, 5, 7, 14, 24), they are included in this overview because the materials and/or procedures are often used in language stimulation and generalization training for the severely handicapped.

Prognostic Factors

The key to training any type of behavior is making sure that the client experiences success in his or her attempts to perform the required behavior. The trainer must carefully consider the client's present abilities and attempt to predict how successful he or she will be in establishing new behavior patterns. In establishing vocal language, at least ten prognostic factors should be considered. Table 6-2 presents an outline of these factors listed according to an assumed order of importance. These factors, although not yet validated, may serve as initial considerations.

One of the most important factors in teaching vocal language is the *client's physical ability to produce speech sounds*. Shane and Bashir (1978) assert ". . .that persistent oral reflexes suggest an extremely poor prognosis for oral speech development". They suggest that the client's eating patterns, drooling (if present), vocal repertoire, and neuromuscular status of the oral mechanism should be evaluated carefully. Love, Hagerman, and Taimi (1980) call for careful assessment of the neuromuscular status of the oral mechanism in cerebral palsied clients. They found that poor articulation and overall reduced speech proficiency occurred in subjects having frequent feeding problems caused by neuromuscular impairment, although the frequency of feeding problem was less severe than expected. A severely physically impaired cerebral palsied client may not have sufficient control of the oral musculature

Table 6-2
Prognostic factors for success with vocal language

1. Physical ability to produce speech sounds	(Guess, Sailor, Baer 1977; Love, Hagerman, and Taimi 1980; Shane and Bashir 1980)
2. Level of cognitive development	(Miller and Yoder 1974)
3. Motivation and communication intent	(Miller and Yoder 1974; McLean and Snyder-McLean 1978; Bloom and Lahey 1978; Siegel and Spradlin 1978)
4. Age of less than five years at initiation of training	(Harris 1975; Hayden and McGinness 1977)
5. Ability to imitate words verbally	(Guess et al. 1977; Lovaas 1973)
6. Ability to attend to trainer	(Kent 1974)
7. Echolalia as observed in autism	(Harris 1975)
8. Previous speaking as in selective mutism	(Harris 1975)
9. Adequate hearing	(Guess, et al. 1977)
10. Adequate vision	(Guess, et al. 1977)

to produce intelligible speech. A client with verbal or oral apraxia may be able to vocalize and produce selected sound patterns but may be extremely frustrated by his or her inability to produce words correctly.[1]

Factor two, *level of cognitive development*, implies that, given adequate physical ability to vocalize, the higher the client's level of cognitive development the more likely will be the development of vocal language. Miller and Yoder (1974) indicate that engaging in imaginative and representational play are foundations for cognitive development. A client who manipulates objects properly and interacts with his or her environment will likely understand the function of language and demonstrate a need to communicate with other people.

The third prognostic factor, *motivation*, relates closely to communication intent. Current research interest in pragmatics related to language acquisition focuses on communicative interactions and the functional use of gestures or words to convey messages. Many authors (McLean and Snyder-McLean 1978; Bloom and Lahey 1978; Siegel and Spradlin 1978) view communication intent as vital to language training. A client who has been unsuccesful in communicating needs and desires may cease trying. In some situations the caregivers in the client's environment may anticipate the client's needs or may quickly interpret gross movements or sounds without discriminating the actual intention of the client's attempt at communication. Misinterpretation of these attempts can be devastating to a non-vocal client or one who is using limited vocalizations. Bigge (1977) discusses a way to avoid or lessen "deadlock" situations where the message giver and message receiver find their attempts at communication lost. Empathy conveyed in a statement like, "I don't understand what you mean. It sure makes me feel sad. Let's try again," may help the client continue to try.

The fourth factor to be considered is the *age at which training is initiated*. Harris (1975) concludes from the studies she reviewed "that children who fail to develop speech by five years of age have a poorer prognosis than do those who have language by that time". Hayden and McGinness (1977) advocate early intervention with children at high risk for developmental disabilities. They assert that "failure to provide a stimulating early environment leads not only to a continuation of the developmental *status quo*, but to actual atrophy of sensory abilities and to developmental regression" (p. 153). They stress that there are critical periods for development of certain skills; therefore, early intervention may help tap these critical times.

Most educators agree that early intervention is best, but educators are frequently confronted with the challenge of training teen-age clients with little or no functional speech. Williams and Fox (Table 6-1: 23) indicate that the trainer must consider how many years it may take to establish speech as the major communication mode. An augmentative means of communicating might then be the preferred choice of treatment (see Chapters 8 and 9).

---

1. For a systematic screening procedure to assess the oral mechanism see St. Louis, K.O. and Ruscello, D.M., *Oral Speech Mechanism Screening Examination*. Baltimore, Maryland: University Park Press (in press).

The next prognostic factor presented in Table 6-2 is the *ability to imitate words verbally*. Guess, Sailor, and Baer (1977) state that verbal imitation is the most important factor for entrance into their functional language program (Table 6-1: 9). During the field-test portion of their program development, they found that about 30 to 40% of the severely handicapped children participating in the training program fail to develop verbal imitation. A few nonimitative children did succeed in the language training sequences, but the authors noted that those children appeared to have ". . .more of a motivational problem than a lack of imitative ability" (p. 365). Lovaas (1973) also notes that imitation is a key factor in predicting success in training speech. A more detailed discussion of the role of imitation in language development is presented in Chapter 3 and in the imitation section of this chapter.

Factor six indicates that the client needs to be able to *attend to the trainer and stimulus*. Kent (table 6-1: 15) devotes a portion of her program to preverbal skills. She assumes that skills such as attending and eliminating interfering behavior should be established before entrance into her language program. In fact, many language programs attempt to establish attending (table 6-1: 1, 2, 3, 6, 8, 10, 13, 17, 18, 19, 21, 23) before initiating direct language training. Other programs assume that attending is well established before entrance into the program (as in table 6-1: 5, 7, 9, 11, 12, 14, 24). In addition, several pre-language programs are available for training skills such as attending (Simmons and Williams 1976; Woolman 1980). These programs are discussed in Chapter 4.

Factors seven and eight, *echolalia* and *previous speaking experience*, are presented in Harris' (1975) review of the literature as predictors for establishing speech with training. She indicates that researchers have found it easier to train children who at some point have had speech than those who have not. Examples are autistic children who are echoic and persons who are selectively mute. If a client previously possessed speaking ability, he or she is more likely to have a foundation for communication interaction and a strong desire to regain the ability to speak. Although the client's vocalizations may be extremely limited, some previous knowledge of language form and content can typically be utilized to help train speech again.

Factors nine and ten, *adequate hearing* and *adequate vision*, are listed as prerequisite skills for entrance into the Guess, Sailor, and Baer program (table 6-1:9). It is important to note that most of the vocal language programs in table 6-1 require normal hearing and normal or corrected vision, although these criteria are usually assumed and are not stated as specific prerequisites. Some of the programs (table 6-1:1, 15, 19, 21, 22, 23) provide suggestions for adapting the programs for manual communication to accommodate the severely hearing impaired as well as non-vocal normal hearing clients. All of the vocal programs discussed in this chapter use visual stimuli in the form of objects, pictures, or other symbols as the focus for training. A client with blindness as his or her only handicapping condition could be expected to develop speech normally, although he or she might demonstrate problems in conceptual development. A client who is deaf and blind or blind and severely physically impaired would require very specialized adapted training (see Chapters 8 and 9).

To summarize, the ten prognostic factors presented in table 6-2 should be considered carefully when designing a communication system for a specific client. Difficulty or impairment in one or more factors does not mean automatic rejection of vocal language training, but it does indicate that training procedures will need to be modified appropriately to meet the needs of the particular client. If it is determined that the client has a very poor prognosis for developing functional speech, then the introduction of a non-vocal approach to communication should be considered at least initially.

Assessment

Part of the decision process described in Chapter 2 revolves around careful assessment of the client's current level of language functioning as well as evaluation of physical, mental, and emotional development. Each of the prognostic factors discussed in the previous section should be considered during assessment of vocal communication potential. The factors may be assessed both formally and informally. For example, physical ability to produce speech sounds could be assessed in the following ways: directly, through an observation of speech sound production under spontaneous, imitative, and elicited conditions; and indirectly, through assessment of feeding, oral-motor movements, infantile oral reflexes, and so forth. Each of these sub-areas could also be assessed directly or indirectly. For example, the specific procedures described by Love et al. (1980) could be used in addition to informal observation and parental reports, to assess feeding skills.

The use of formal standardized or criterion-referenced tests is usually recommended if reliable responses can be obtained. However, most tests are designed for a compliant, physically normal, auditorily and visually alert client. Most severely handicapped individuals have multiple handicapping conditions which may make it difficult to use many assessment tools exactly as they were intended. A skilled evaluator will use formal tests only as one reference point in the total assessment process. Appendix D offers an overview of some available assessment devices. In the following section of this chapter a general evaluation of vocal language assessment strategies will be presented. Part of this section will focus on prescriptive assessment procedures which accompany some of the specific language programs listed in table 6-1.

General Assessment Strategies

Reichle and Yoder (1979) suggest using three general assessment strategies to evaluate the language abilities of a language disordered client. One strategy involves transcribing a child's emitted communication behavior (vocal as well as gestural) in a "free operating environment." This can be time-consuming if the client speaks or attempts to communicate only infrequently within a given time period. Strategy two is an observational assessment procedure by which the evaluator observes the client in a variety of situations and notes communication interactions. This procedure also can be very time-consuming and may yield limited information. The third strategy is interviewing the client's main caregivers (e.g., classroom personnel, ward staff, and parents). Riechle and Yoder (1979) have found in their review of literature pertaining to assessment strategies that interviewing can be as reliable as the first two strategies and, when used with transcribed samples and observational data, can supplement or support those findings. Using all three strategies will obviously yield the most complete information for designing a comprehensive intervention program for a client.

As mentioned, most formal assessment devices require compliance to commands as part of the desired response. Huttenlocher (1974) has indicated that until a developmental level of at least twelve months is reached, compliance may not be established and formal testing may be fruitless. Thus, for example, a teen-age client functioning at an estimated six to eight-month level will probably not be able to handle most formal test items. Smith (1972) found that pointing to pictures, a common test response mode, was not in the repertoire of normally developing children until the 18-month level. Chapman (1974) suggests that the use of a question-asking strategy, which also is a common testing procedure, is not effective until at least the 24-month level.

Miller, Reichle, and Rettie (1977) found in their study of 15 to 20-month-old normally developing children that, when asked to locate an object, these children made one of three responses: they either (1) ignored the stimulus, (2) looked at the object, or (3) pointed or vocalized. Thus, when evaluating low-functioning clients, the evaluator should record not only the occurrence of expected response, but an observational note as to what other type of response occurred (e.g., child turned head away from the stimulus).

It is difficult to imagine a child who is totally unresponsive to his or her environment or who is totally uncommunicative. Therefore, the evaluator must be sensitive to a child's subtle responses to the environment. Soltman and Reike (1977) present suggestions for a systematic observation and recording procedure with a non-responsive child. Their procedure allows a communication specialist to carefully document environmental antecedent events, client responses, client initiations, and staff responses to the client's initiations. They emphasize the need for a team approach (including parents) in the evaluation process. For example, understanding what annoys or frustrates the staff, parents, and client provides valuable information for program planning.

Prescriptive Assessment Devices

For the purposes of the following discussion, prescriptive assessment devices are defined as testing procedures included in a specific language teaching program which will help the trainer determine if the program is appropriate for the client and, if so, at what point in the program training should begin. There are four ways in which the 24 vocal language programs listed in table 6-1 can be catagorized regarding the use of prescriptive assessment devices:

1. Programs based on or coordinated with other separately published assessment devices;
2. Programs that contain a detailed assessment device labeled as an inventory, checklist, or strand;
3. Programs designed in very specific training steps usually labeled as objectives, where each step or objective serves as its own pretest and posttest to determine movement through the program;
4. Programs that do not provide or recommend specific assessment procedures.

Table 6-3 is a compilation of the 24 vocal language programs divided into these assessment categories. Note that several programs are included in more than one category.

Prescriptive assessment procedures, whether they are general inventories or involve specific objectives, may also be used as reassessment devices to chart progress and reevaluate training priorities. Many of the programs are useful in generating Individualized Educational Programs, using the general skill areas targeted for treatment as long term goals and selecting specific objectives within that area as short term goals (table 6-3: 18, 19, 21).

In summary, preselection of a standard assessment battery is not appropriate for the severely handicapped population. The communication specialist must utilize a variety of assessment tools and techniques as part of an ongoing decision process. These assessment procedures may be a part of— or separate from—the vocal language program(s) to be used.

Stages of Vocal Programs

Several authors (e.g., Garcia and DeHaven 1974; Harris 1975; Risley, Hart, and Doke 1972) have noted that many language acquisition programs for the severely handicapped utilize a series of stages, though not all programs include all stages. Harris (1975), in her review of language training for non-verbal children, identified four commonly used stages:

1. Attention;
2. Non-verbal imitation—which may include imitation of body movements and vocal sounds but not meaningful words;
3. Verbal imitation;
4. Functional language.

Attending and Motor Imitation

Training the client to attend and establishing motor imitation are often considered prerequisite skills to entering a language program. These stages are discussed in more detail in Chapter 4. Some of the vocal language programs reviewed in this chapter present training sequences for establish-

Table 6-3

Vocal Language Programs—Assessment Categories*

Programs based on other assessment devices	Programs that contain a detailed assessment device	Programs designed with each object serving as a pretest and post-test	Programs that do not provide specific assessment procedures
13. Ready, Set, Go: Talk to Me (Environmental Prelanguage Battery and Environmental Language Inventory)**	3. Portage Guide to Early Intervention	1. Teaching the Moderately and Severely Handicapped: Vol. II	4. Peabody Language Kits
14. GOAL: Language Development (Illinois Test of Psycholinguistic Abilities)*	5. Distar Language I	2. A Language Intervention Program for Developmentally Young Children	12. A Milieu Approach to Language Training
18.* WVS: Receptive Language Curriculum (The West Virginia Assessment and Tracking System)*	8. S.T.E.P.	6. The Teaching Research Curriculum	
19.* WVS: Expressive Language Curriculum (The West Virginia Assessment and Tracking System)*	13. Ready, Set, Go: Talk To Me	7. A Language Program for the Nonlanguage Child	
	15. Language Acquisition Program	9. Functional Speech and Language Training	
	16. A Language Development Program	10. Teaching Speech to a Nonverbal Child	
	17. A Prescriptive Behavioral Checklist	12. Emerging Language 2	
	21. Behavioral Characteristics Progression (BCP)	18. WVS: Receptive Language Curriculum	
	22. Guide to Early Developmental Training	19. WVS: Expressive Language Cirrculum	
	23. Vol. I: Communication Minimum Objectives System	20. A Behavioral-Psycholinguistic Approach to Language Traning	
		21. Behavioral Characteristics Progression	
		22. Guide to Early Developmental Training	
		24. Sourcebook of Language Learning Activities	

*All numbers correspond to the program listing in table 6-1.
**These assessment devices are included in Appendix D.

ing attending and motor imitation (table 6-1:1, 2, 3, 6, 8, 10, 13, 15, 16, 17, 19, 21, 22, 23). Stage 3, verbal imitation, and Stage 4, functional language, are the main focus of this chapter.

Vocal and Verbal Imitation

Motor imitation, vocal imitation, and verbal imitation[2] are sometimes trained as successive skills. Rieke, Lynch, and Soltman (1977), in their presentation of language strategies, indicate that the goal of imitation training is for the client to imitate the action, sound, or word spontaneously without prompting or reinforcement. They caution that over-reinforcing imitative acts once the client is producing them spontaneously may be detrimental because it may discourage the client from imitating vocalizations.

Some authors suggest that motor and vocal imitation can be taught concurrently (Reichle and Yoder 1979; table 6-1:6, 13, 15, 19) rather than as consecutive skills. The use of a chaining procedure by which the client is required to imitate a series of motor tasks ending with a vocalization allows the client to use previously learned movements with a new skill of vocalizing (Kent 1974).

A number of authors (e.g., Bloom and Lahey 1978; Reichle and Yoder 1979; Schumaker and Sherman 1978) suggest strategies for training vocal imitation. The latter recommend beginning by increasing vocalizations in infants through verbal praise (such as "good girl!") and tactile stimulation (such as rubbing the infant's cheek). They define vocalizations as ". . . any sound a chld makes with the vocal apparatus, excluding crying and reflexive coughs, sneezes, and hiccups" (p. 291).

Reichle and Yoder (1979) discuss the training of "mutual imitation." The trainer imitates a sound or word made by the client, and the client is credited and reinforced if he or she repeats the utterance again after the trainer says it. The goal here is to bring sounds or words already in the client's repertoire under stimulus control. Bricker and Dennison (1978) also use this technique, which they refer to as "imitation chains" (p. 169). Once the client understands turn-taking activity, unfamiliar stimuli can be introduced for imitation. Schumaker and Sherman (1978) suggest a number of steps to be followed in training vocal and verbal imitation. Their procedures are intended for use by parents with their infants but could be adapted for use by other trainers or with older clients.

Bricker, Dennison, and Bricker (1975) and Bricker and Dennison (1978) developed a training procedure whereby the trainer capitalizes on spontaneous utterances made by the client during natural interactions at play or during other activities. One of their suggested procedures is to increase the amount of action play (such as swinging, tickling) that is physically stimulating to the client and may evoke vocalizations which can be imitated by the trainer and for which the client can be reinforced.

---

2. "Vocal imitation" refers to imitation of sounds or nonmeaningful sound sequences, while "verbal imitation" refers to imitation of words.

Of the 24 programs listed in table 6-1, nine assume that the client has some functional verbal language and that imitation skills are already established before the program is begun (table 6-1:4, 5, 7, 9, 11, 12, 14, 20, 24). Fourteen of the programs cited provide some sequences designed to train imitative skills (table 6-1:1, 2, 3, 6, 8, 10, 13, 15, 16, 17, 19, 21, 22, 23).

In summary, many vocal language programs suggest that attending and motor imitation be established before or during the training of vocal or verbal skills. Imitative training is a frequently used vehicle for developing verbal skills within the programs reviewed. Functional language, the final stage of most vocal language programs, will be discussed throughout the remainder of this chapter relative to specific issues in language training.

Issues in Selecting a Vocal Program

The general issues involved in selecting a program discussed in Chapter 3, models, methodology, comprehension and production content, context, and generalization, will now be presented as they specifically relate to vocal communication training.

Models

Language programming seems to pivot on the assumption that expressive (vocal or non-vocal) language allows a person control over his or her environment. Two theoretical models based on developmental logic and remedial logic were discussed in Chapter 3. Most language programs (table 6-1:2, 3, 6, 12, 15, 17, 22) are designed primarily from developmental data on normally developing children. Caution must be exercised in relying entirely on developmental norms because there is evidence of a large variation in normal development (Siegel and Spradlin 1978; Waryas and Stremel-Campbell 1978; Bloom and Lahey 1978).

Guess, Sailor, and Baer (1978) describe the choice of a remedial model for their functional language program (table 6-1: 9) as an attempt to meet the immediate needs of the handicapped individual. They attempt to train the client to control his or her environment by expressive language as soon as possible, suggesting that such control will be reinforcing in itself and thus will stimulate more language. However, it is not clear how the trainer is to proceed once the client progresses beyond the early stages of communicating. It appears that the choice of units taught in this program (persons, possession, and so forth) is influenced by normal developmental patterns and by data from severely handicapped learners who have completed the program. The communication program developed by Williams and Fox (table 6-1: 23) illustrates a program which uses both the developmental and remedial models. The authors use a developmental milestone chart to help assess and place clients into their program but emphasize that the actual teaching objectives must be revised on the basis of information about the performance of handicapped clients as they progress through the program. Siegel and Spradlin (1978) assert that the two models (remedial and developmental) are not precise enough to allow a clear choice between them. Therefore, they suggest that both approaches should be blended so as to design an adequate individualized program for each client.

Methodology

The methods by which a language program is introduced to a client may vary, depending upon the type of reinforcement employed and the setting in which the program is conducted. The two major methods used in the 24 programs in table 6-1 are based on the following:

1. *Artificially structured techniques* (primarily using operant technology in individual training sessions);
2. *Naturally structured techniques* (primarily utilizing the natural language environment to stimulate language in group training sessions or during activities of daily living).

Artificially structured techniques employed by many programs (e.g., table 6-1: 1, 2, 5, 9, 10, 15, 16, 17, 18, 19, 20, 21, 23) are typically conducted in individual training sessions employing carefully controlled data collecting procedures. *The West Virginia System Curricula*, (table 6-1: 18, 19), for example, employ a Universal Data Sheet for recording trial responses in order to assess acquisition of skills during sessions and maintenance of these skills between sessions. The *Functional Speech and Language Training for the Severely Handicapped* (table 6-1:9) also employs an extensive data record form to chart each session.

An example of an artificially structured approach designed primarily for group administration is the *Distar Language I Program* (table 6-1:5). Although individual responses for each child in the group are not recorded, the trainer is given very specific instructions on how to manipulate the program materials, present lessons, correct errors, and to reinforce group participation and individual responses. On the basis of the student's group and periodic individual responses, the trainer must decide whether to recycle a student or group through a previous lesson or continue on to a new lesson.

Naturally structured techniques are typically based on less rigid or structured training and data collecting procedures. The general setting for this type of approach is in a group language session or the natural environment. The natural environment would include classroom and home daily living situations (e.g., eating, toileting, interacting with siblings and peers, and so forth) rather than specific 10 to 20 minute individual training sessions. Group sessions allow the client to receive language models from peers as well as from trainers. In addition, staff time may be more efficiently used. The trainer must be skilled in group techniques to encourage all group members to participate to the best of their ability.

The severity of the client's handicapping condition often seems to dictate the language training environment. Group lessons are typically not chosen for clients with severely handicapping conditions. However, as discussed in

Chapter 3, several recent studies (Flavell et al. 1978; Storm and Willis 1978) found group training to be an effective format for training some skills, even with the severely and profoundly retarded.

It is very important for severely handicapped clients to be included in a "talking environment." Dolan and Burton (1976) have indicated that it is vital that parents and trainers continue to talk to non-vocal clients even if progress in speech seems extremely limited and the client appears not to be interested in language. Unfortunately, in classes for the severely and profoundly retarded or physically handicapped, language is sometimes only programmed into specific language sessions. The trainers receive so little communication feedback from the students that they may not attempt communication with some clients unless it is included in the training schedule. This lack of language interaction may exist also with family members of non-communicating children or adults. To avoid this type of situation, a program such as the *Milieu Approach to Language Learning* (table 6-1: 11) may be useful. It is based on the premise that language must be taught in a "talking environment." Hart and Rogers-Warren (1978) compare the individual training session approach with their milieu model and conclude that their model

1. is less expensive;
2. is more conducive to generalizing behavior because the child does not leave the normal flow of verbal-social activities;
3. teaches the function of language, not just the form.

As discussed earlier, Brown, Nietupski, and Hamre-Nietupski (1976) also present a case for less individual training and more language concentration in groups or in the natural environment. They indicate that individual training may be appropriate for some part of the day but not as the only structured language training. In a class for the severely and profoundly retarded, an aide could be assigned to organize group interactions while the teacher is conducting an individual session. Too often, while individual training is going on the other class members are left on their own, which may result in perpetuating self-stimulating behavior or continuing social isolation.

Again, it may be unnecessary to make an either/or choice between artificially and naturally structured approaches. The communication specialist can plan the day to allow time for both types of approaches. In addition, the naturally structured approach may also be carefully planned; the trainer can set up an activity in which goals are pre-set and data is collected on one client at a time within a group setting.

Comprehension and Production

The issue of whether to train comprehension before requiring production from severely handicapped clients is presented in Chapter 3. Careful scrutiny of the vocal language programs reviewed in this chapter reveals that during the assessment process most programs divide test items into receptive language tasks and expressive language tasks. This may lead to separate training of these skills. Until recently there has been little disagreement among researchers on the issue that normally developing children and communication disordered children appear to understand language before they can express themselves. It has been discovered that the first words spoken are not necessarily the first words understood (Bloom and Lahey 1978).

Most language programs are likewise divided into sections in which receptive language training tasks are presented separately from expressive language tasks. This ordering appears to follow the premise that comprehension precedes production.

Language programs that divide training objectives into receptive language training and expressive language training typically do not require that a client progress through the training sequence in all the receptive objectives before beginning expressive training. However, Siegel and Spradlin (1978) strongly support a need for concurrent training of receptive and expressive language material. In Kent's program (table 6-1: 15) the client moves from the verbal-receptive section to the verbal-expressive section as vocabulary expands and as a review of material previously learned is undertaken.

Guess, Sailor, and Baer's program (table 6-1: 9) begins with the naming of objects in Step 1. Step 2 requires recognition of the objects learned in Step 1. Their premise is that verbal expression best allows a client to manipulate and control his or her environment and therefore is in itself immediately reinforcing. Each new area of content is approached in this manner.

The *Distar Language I Program* (table 6-1:5) also begins, in the first lesson, to require object labeling with comprehension tasks interspersed in the form of a comprehension review, such as asking the client, "Is this a (object name)?"

The *Emerging Language Program* (table 6-1: 12) contains 136 expressive language objectives. The instructor is encouraged to rephrase the objectives to require demonstration that the client understands the vocabulary presented if the client fails the expressive task. For example, Objective 1 in the program states: "The child will name the following ten objects . . . ". If the child had difficulty, the objective could be rewritten as a receptive task such as this: "the child will point to the following ten objects."

Thus different training programs handle the comprehension—production issue differently. We agree with Siegel and Spradlin (1978) that concurrent training will yield the most immediately functional program. However, as with other issues, the capabilities and limitations of the individual clients must be considered.

Content

Most of the programs reviewed stress the need to select carefully the content or specific vocabulary to teach severely handicapped clients. The actual responsibility for selecting the most functional language for any individual client generally lies with the trainer, who must coordinate input from caregivers and consider all the settings in which the client must communicate. When a non-vocal language system is selected, particuarly a communication board, the number of words that can be utilized is restricted significantly by the physical make-up of the system (see Chapter 9). This is not the case with a vocal language program, where there is an almost infinite choice of words that could be taught.

Researchers in language acquisition of normal and disordered speakers have attempted to suggest rules for selecting an initial lexicon (vocabulary) for training functional language (Holland 1975; Lahey and Bloom 1977; Bloom and Lahey 1978). Relevant findings in this area are presented in Chapter 3. The realization that knowledge about specific objects and actions is dependent upon age, interest, and actual experiences of the client makes the selection of words an ongoing process. As the client's experiences increase, so will the need for expansion of his or her vocabulary to allow for communication interaction in new situations. The strategies presented in Chapter 3 for selecting initial content should be considered relative to choosing words as the entries (e.g., client preference, frequency of occurrence). In addition, strategies specific to vocal language or vocal language programs will be discussed in this section.

Functional language, the language needed by the client to meet his or her immediate needs, is the primary concern when planning a program for a handicapped client. For example, Lahey and Bloom (1977) reject the use of color words in training language disordered clients because they have little communication value. Special education classrooms have often overemphasized color training becase color words are easily illustrated. Nevertheless, color attributes are not as simple as they may appear. The question can be raised, "Is the client discriminating the color name from the physical characteristics of the colored object, or might the client be interpreting the color label to be that particular object (when shown a red ball and given "red" and the stimulus word)?"

Horstmeier and MacDonald (table 6-1:13) suggest that insisting on social phrases like "please" or "thank you" too early with the language impaired client may limit his or her use of appropriate labels. It may be easier for the child to say "please" and point to what is wanted rather than use the correct word.

As mentioned, input from caregivers is vital in selecting initial content for training. After words are selected, they must be used consistently when communicating with the client in all settings (e.g., at home and at school). For example, toileting skills can become confusing if the label for the voiding receptacle is varied (e.g., "toilet," "potty," "pot," "commode").

Several factors should be considered in determining the ease of production and discrimination of training words. Bloom and Lahey (1978) note that there are no definitive guidelines on which word configurations are easiest to produce and discriminate. Nevertheless, they suggest the following:

1. Consider those sounds a child is already producing;
2. Consider using short words because they are easier to produce than polysyllabic words (the first words of normally developing children

tend to be of one syllable such as "no," or a repetition of one syllable, as in "dada");

3. Consider selecting words that are acoustically distinct from each other in order to reduce confusion (e.g., do not include "stop" and "shop" in the same training session).

Content selection involves many decisions based on input by caregivers, training staff, and the client's particular needs and desires. With the severely handicapped, learning a limited number of words may be necessary, but it is vital that those words be functional and allow for combining the words for a variety of messages.

Context

The actual setting and circumstances that accompany a communication attempt represent the context of that language event. McLean and Snyder-McLean (1978) suggest that two bases of context must be considered when planning intervention strategies: (1) instrumental physical context and (2) instrumental communication context. Instrumental physical context means that the trainer must arrange a setting that provides increased opportunity for the child to manipulate materials in many ways, such as shaking, disassembling as well as assembling objects, pouring, and so forth. Instrumental communication context requires that there be someone with whom the child can communicate regarding situations that occur within that environment. This often involves careful arrangement of a classroom to present opportunities for optimal communication. McLean and Snyder-McLean (1978) suggest creating natural environment learning corners (e.g., toy kitchen or bedroom) and role playing natural actions within these settings.

Hart and Roger-Warren's milieu therapy approach (table 6-1: 11) capitalizes also on the natural environment for stimulating and modeling functional language. In their view, the generalization of new language content may be facilitated by demonstrating and emphasizing the immediate use of words and actions. Creating situations in which the child needs to ask for assistance helps demonstrate the function of language. For example, the trainer in a play kitchen setting might have a series of clear plastic containers with desirable edible items within view of the client. The containers could be sealed so that the client must seek assistance to open the containers. This type of interaction within a natural setting is a way to begin a training strategy, discussed by Reike, Lynch, and Soltman (1977), of establishing "initiating behaviors." The goal of the activity would be to create a situation in which the child spontaneously attempts communication. The attempt might be initially reaching for or touching the container to indicate a desire to seek what is inside. Then, in the attempt to seek help to open it, the client is reinforced for any gesture or vocalization (e.g., changes in vowel intonations or word attempts) directed toward a person who might assist in opening the container. McLean and Snyder-McLean (1978) suggest that for lower functioning children, developing context around basic daily living skills would be most beneficial (e.g., having the child specifically indicate clothing to be worn rather than having the parent automatically dress the child).

The trainer within this type of setting is available to respond by commenting, answering, and reinforcing the communication attempt. Rieke, Lynch, and Soltman (1977) caution that the trainer must resist talking too much. The role of the trainer is summed up in the "3Rs" of their strategy, whereby the trainer responds, reiterates, and reinforces the behavior the client initiates (p. 33).

As discussed earlier, language training should not be confined only to quiet individual training sessions but integrated into the entire daily program so that few instances are lost to react to a client's emerging attempts at communication. The natural environment context allows for the most obvious demonstration that language is useful, which in itself is reinforcing. Moreover, it is important to note that the communication interaction that takes place in a group setting or in a natural environment setting will generally be a one-to-one (client to other client, client to trainer, or client to parent), as are most communication interactions with normal speakers in a group.

The role of a communication specialist in a class for the severely handicapped may follow several models. The communication specialist may serve primarily as a consultant to the classroom staff in assisting in program planning and evaluation of progress. When a milieu approach is utilized, language training is an integral part of all daily activities. Thus the classroom staff must insure that instruction is continual. Individual therapy sessions may be conducted by the communication specialist on a regular basis or as trial sessions to experiment with new techniques with a particular client or to demonstrate varied techniques to the other staff so that they may incorporate these techniques into their daily activities.

The team approach to training the severely handicapped, as presented in Chapter 5 (support services), focuses on the people involved in program planning and implementation. The context of training involves a variety of settings in which the client must function and the variety of people with whom the client must interact. The staff should be open to flexible roles and flexible scheduling to allow for the blending of individualized training and stimulating language growth in a more natural interactive environment.

Generalization

As stated previously, creating as natural an environment as possible in which communication attempts can be nurtured is most likely to enhance the generalization of new behavior. Siegel and Spradlin (1978) state that "Training across settings involves teaching and reinforcing the child for emitting certain behaviors in situation after situation until the child can demonstrate the skill in a situation never previously encountered, without additional training" (p. 390). It is vital that the initial trainer not be involved in all the new situations, as the child must learn to perform independently of the trainer and the original training environment.

Stokes and Baer (1977) use the term "training loosely" to stress the features of planning generalization procedures requiring the trainer to be flexible and creative in changing the stimuli from trial to trial, session to session, and in differing settings to determine if generalization has occurred.

To the question, "Can generalization actually be trained?" there is no clear answer. A review of the 24 vocal programs presented in table 6-1, permits the observation that most authors believe that attempts must be made to encourage the use of new skills across settings and among people. It is difficult to program these interactions so that systematic data can be collected to actually prove that a certain situation evoked use of a newly acquired skill. Guess, Sailor, and Baer's program (table 6-1:9) very carefully outlines 60 training steps. At the end of each step a statement regarding generalization is presented. These statements suggest that items taught during the individual sessions be given to parents, parent-surrogates, teachers, and others (siblings or institutional peers) and that they be directed to check periodically to determine whether or not the client can use the items in their particular setting. This brief directive does not offer much help in giving parents or others suggestions of what to do, when, where, and how to do it.

Horstmeier and MacDonald (table 6-1:13) offer parents more specific help in alerting them to watch for specific skills taught in school being performed at home. They present a suggested form for noting specific behaviors at home and suggest that a reminder sheet be placed in a convenient and noticeable spot (e.g., the refrigerator door) to remind all household members of what to expect from the client.

Within the classroom, group activities can be designed to reinforce concepts initially taught in individual sessions. Selected lessons from general language stimulation programs such as the *Peabody Language Kits* and *GOAL Program* (table 6-1:4, 14) can be used by the trainer to promote generalization. The mechanics of recording data to chart generalization progress may pose some problems due to the unstructured and often spontaneous nature of reviewing skills in different settings. The use of a paraprofessional as group leader might allow the teacher to act periodically as observer and record specific comments about each child's interaction in the particular activity. The mastery assessment form designed by Williams and Fox (table 6-1:23) and reprinted in Chapter 3 of this book may help the trainer to keep data on several aspects of generalization.

The ultimate goal of any training procedure is to teach a concept or a skill that the client will be able to use in a variety of situations with a variety of people. Evidence of this generalized use of new information is most positive when the client spontaneously uses the concept or skill without assistance and completely on his or her own initiative. This is a difficult task with the severely handicapped and requires careful planning and encouragement from everyone involved with the client.

Parent Involvement

Parents play an important role in encouraging their children and reporting to school staff the generalization of content taught at school. Quite often trainers express frustration in comments such as this: "If only the parents would follow through with what we do at school, then the child would progress faster." This places a heavy burden on the parents and relieves the trainer of responsibility for the client's growth. It is an idealistic assumption that complete coordination between home and school will assure rapid or sustained growth in communication skills with severely or profoundly retarded clients or the multiply impaired.

McCormack and Audette (1977) view training severely handicapped learners as a twenty-four hour job. They stress that programming must involve "whole person planning" (p. 210) which considers the client's physical, emotional, social, and intellectual needs. Integrated and cooperative planning must be implemented by establishing a relationship between school and home environments (family or institutional). Striving for cooperative involvement of home caregivers is important, but the trainer must recognize that commitments (e.g., jobs, other children, illness) will play a part in the quality and quantity of time available for carrying out specific programs or charting specific behaviors at home.

Parents should be involved in the programming from the beginning to help in selecting vocabulary and in describing family routines and family interests. This family-oriented information can be used by the trainer in selecting the content and contexts that will be meaningful to the child when he or she is at home.

Shumaker and Sherman (1978) view parents as intervention agents who interact with their children quite naturally. They offer many suggestions to enrich present interactions rather than to interrupt daily activities with specific, scheduled language-training sessions. They regard "incidental teaching episodes" as more effective in establishing spontaneous use of language than structured training sessions. The key to home teaching is making the activities enjoyable not only for the child but for the parent too. Too much pressure on the child that *now* is the time to talk can have an adverse effect. It is better to create a desire to speak than to demand speech.

Parents, especially fathers, may indicate that they do not know what to say to their infant or severely handicapped child. Schumaker and Sherman (1978) suggest that they can describe what they are doing when that are bathing, dressing, changing, feeding, consoling, and playing with their children. Other situations, such as driving in the car, shopping, and commenting on or discussing television programs viewed together, could be added to the list of times parents can encourage language sharing.

Parents of children with limited speech are deprived of the natural reinforcement of vocal feedback from their children. Talking around the child may become the pattern at home rather than making an effort to include the child in ordinary conversation.

Of all the programs reviewed in this chapter, the *Ready, Set, Go: Talk To Me*

Program (table 6-1:13) offers the most clear and useful tool for targeting language intervention at home. It is written for parents by professionals, including the parent of a handicapped child. The program attempts to assist the parents in capitalizing on daily events to reinforce vocal communication. Harris' program (table 6-1:10) is also intended for use by parents. The target population for her program is autistic children.

Since most of the other programs listed in table 6-1 use technical terminology and detailed record keeping designs, many parents might not be prepared to implement them. For specific suggestions on parent intervention strategies, the reader is referred to Schumaker and Sherman (1978). They offer several strategies and suggest numerous examples for parents in the following areas: increasing vocalization in infants, teaching the infant to imitate, prompting spontaneous word usage, expansions, extensions, and prompting spontaneous utterances of several words.

In summary, the skilled communication specialist will utilize many features of selected programs to help devise suggestions for parents to use at home. Basically, parents need to know that they are already doing much to influence and encourage their child. Supporting their efforts in providing a variety of experiences and explanations about these experiences becomes an important supplemental role of the trainer. Just as planning language training for a client must be individualized, so should planning the involvement of parents or caregivers. Each home represents a unique environment for language enrichment. Each family usually has several people who interact with the client. Initially the trainer may solicit the help of one family member to implement an activity or report about communication interactions at home. Then, gradually, other family members should be instructed and encouraged to participate to assure generalization across settings and people.

Part Three: Non-vocal Systems

Chapter 7: Non-vocal Systems: An Overview

Introduction

"If you want to know what it is like not being able to speak, there is a way. Go to a party and don't talk. Play mute. Use your hands if you wish but don't use paper and pencil. Paper and pencil are not always handy for a mute person. Here is what you will find:
> People talking.
> Talking behind, beside, around, over, under,
>   through, and even for you.
> But never with you.
> You are ignored until finally you feel like a
>   piece of the furniture.

If you are working with nonspeech people I challenge you to experience this. Then you will have an idea of what it is like for nonspeech people."

Creech 1979.

This suggestion comes from a person who has been non-vocal throughout his life. He feels strongly that those working with non-vocal people should attempt this in order to develop a better understanding of the needs and feelings of non-vocal people. Clearly, such a temporary simulation cannot provide a full picture of the needs and frustrations of non-vocal people, but it may help to develop understanding and identify areas of concern. At the least, this experience should help the individual develop more appropriate ways of interacting with non-vocal people.

The recent surge of interest in non-vocal communication options is staggering. The last five years has seen a tremendous growth in the number of articles, pamphlets, newsletters, and textbooks relating to use of non-vocal approaches. The number and variety of communication prostheses has also increased dramatically, with formation of new companies and laboratories and expansion of already existing ones. This interest is apparent also in the popular media. Human interest stories concerning use of non-vocal approaches have appeared in such varied sources as a national magazine, the *Reader's Digest* (May, 1980), a major newspaper, the *Miami Herald* (February, 1980), and a popular television show, *That's Incredible* (May, 1980). Unfortunately, in each of those cases the reader/viewer was tantalized with fascinating descriptions of amazing technology without being provided specific facts or references to sources for more information. Thus, although members of the general public may begin to be informed that vocal language is not the only communication option, it is unlikely that they will know where to seek help or for whom augmentative systems should be considered. A number of major organizations dealing with the handicapped provide information about non-vocal communication. These organizations, and the services provided by each, are covered in Appendix C of this book. This Chapter and Chapters 8 and 9 will attempt to synthesize and explore existing information on non-vocal systems and approaches.

Functions of Non-vocal Systems

A variety of different functions have been suggested for non-vocal communication systems. The following have been found to be appropriate uses of non-vocal systems:

1. A *primary communication system*, thus substituting to some extent for a vocal mode; this may be viewed as temporary for a client who is learning to use vocal communication; the goal here is one of transmitting information through non-vocal means;
2. A *supplement* to vocal communication for the client who has difficulty with formulation or intelligibility but who has some useable speech; the term *augmentative* is often used to describe this function;
3. A *facilitator* of communication, with emphasis on speech intelligibility, output and organization of language, and/or general communication skills.

The first function listed may indicate that the non-vocal system is being used as a substitute for vocal language, a position which some researchers (Harris and Vanderheiden 1980) find untenable. However, if we are truly concerned about being communication-oriented, as Silverman (1980) recommends, and if our primary concern is interaction, as Harris and Vanderheiden suggest, transmitting information is an acceptable function, at least initially. In addition, a non-vocal system may serve a primary function as an interim communication system for a client who is receiving speech therapy, such as a laryngectomee.

The *supplemental function* is inherent to some communication systems, such as Cued Speech and Beukelman's and Yorkston's (1977) alphabet-number board. These systems, by their very nature, are augmentative and must be combined with speech. Other sysems, such as Blissymbolics or Signed English, can be made supplemental, either by using the system plus vocal language simultaneously, as in signed speech (e.g., Schaeffer 1980), or by employing them to provide context or to clarify utterances (e.g., Abkarian, Dworkin, and Brown 1978).

Use of non-vocal systems as primary communication systems or as supplemental to vocal language was represented visually on the non-vocal/vocal continuum presented in Chapter 2. As that continuum indicated, the difference between a primary and a supplemental system may be to a great extent a matter of degree. The possible change in emphasis across time was also illustrated on that continuum.

There is, understandably, a great deal of interest in the use of non-vocal systems *to facilitate a variety of behavior*. Non-vocal systems have been found to increase speech intelligibility (e.g., Beukelman and Yorkston 1977), improve the ability to communicate (see Silverman 1980, table 2-1, for a review of a number of studies), and increase attempts at speech communication (see Silverman, 1980 table 2-2, for a review of a number of studies). In addition, Shane (in press) suggests that some non-vocal systems, particularly symbolic systems, may help the client to organize language output through their explicit visual content, such as the Fitzgerald Key (Fitzgerald, 1949). Concerning all these studies, Silverman (1980) asserts that ". . .intervention with nonspeech communication modes can be rationalized for the purpose of speech facilitation as well as improving message transmission" (p. 45).

In summary, non-vocal communication systems may serve a variety of functions for the individual. As with other issues discussed in this book (e.g., developmental versus remedial model), perhaps a compromise may be reached in which non-vocal communication systems serve any or all of the functions discussed at different times in the client's life.

Implications of Using Non-vocal Systems

We must be aware that electing to use a non-vocal system will have definite implications for our clients. For example, people in the client's environment may consider that we have "given up" on speech and may do likewise by not encouraging the client to vocalize. Ways to avoid or deal with this situation were suggested in Chapter 5. Persons in the environment will likely interact with the client differently and will have to be taught appropriate means of interacting. These implications will be discussed briefly in the following two chapters.

Another major implication of using a non-vocal system is that, as Harris and Vanderheiden (1980) point out, "Nonvocal techniques are not a direct substitute for speech, and communication and interaction patterns as well as the overall communication development process may follow different courses for vocal and nonvocal children." They assert also that ". . .communication interaction patterns are very specific to the *speed* of communication, much more so in fact than they are to the *mode* of communication" (p. 245). The difference in speed, the time it takes to transmit a message, means that normal communication routines and strategies will not be directly translated to non-vocal systems. This is somewhat dependent on the non-vocal system chosen. For example, some of the manual communication systems can parallel spoken language, at least in utterances produced if not in time span. The parallels to spoken English in terms of propositions, sentence structure, and transmission time, will be discussed separately for each non-vocal system presented in Chapters 8 and 9.

All of the implications mentioned relate to using a non-vocal system, as opposed to vocal language. Obviously, for the client who has no successful, standardized communication system, introduction of a non-vocal system may have many highly desirable implications. The potential impact on intelligibility, speech attempts, and so forth were noted earlier and are considered in more detail in Silverman (1980). Silverman also reports a number of other positive impacts of non-vocal communication modes, such as increased attention span and reduced frustration (1980, table 2.3).

Clearly, awareness and consideration of both positive and negative potential implications should help in implementing non-vocal systems and in avoiding or confronting resulting problems.

Gestural and Symbolic Modes

The next two chapters describe and discuss the use of gestural and symbolic communication modes, respectively. *Gestural communication* includes systems which necessitate movement of the body, typcially the arms and hands, but do not require access to equipment or devices separate from the body. Examples are sign languages, sign systems, and pantomime. *Symbolic communication* comprises systems which require access to a symbol system separate from the body, such as Blissymbols, rebuses, or words. In making the selection of the mode (vocal or non-vocal, gestural or symbolic), the reader is referred back to Stages I and II of the decision process model presented in Chapter 2. For those clients who could use either a gestural or a symbolic communication mode, the primary considerations presented in table 7-1, such as cost, mobility, and adaptability, should be especially helpful in making the decision. It should be stressed again that the trainer may choose to teach the use of more than one system. Harris and Vanderheiden (1980) point out that the non-vocal person ". . .does not usually have access to any one technique that can be as primary and powerful as speech is for the vocal child" (p. 246). For example, non-vocal systems differ in their portability, speed, possible audience, and physical stress on the user. Thus a client might use a communication board with a printed or vocal output in the classroom and a combination of vocalizations and Amer-Ind when communicating with

Table 7-1

Primary considerations in selecting a gestural or symbolic communication system*.

Feature	Gestural Systems	Symbolic Systems
Cost	There may be a need to pay for special training of teachers; this could involve travel costs and tuition fees. Sign instruction books and/or glossaries may have to be purchased.	Implementation of some symbol systems may require special training (e.g., Non-SLIP, Blissymbolics). Commercial devices (e.g., prepared communication boards, lap trays) may be expensive. Added options (e.g., output options, electronic switches) may have to be purchased.
Mobility	Gestural systems are quite mobile; however, use of sign may interfere with use of hands for other activities (e.g., eating, driving).	Symbol boards may be less mobile, due to factors such as weight, size, power source, and the client's physical problems (it may be difficult to transport a board while walking with crutches). Smaller and/or more portable versions of boards may be devised for use in various settings.
Adaptability	Gestural systems may need to be adapted due to the client's physical limitations. Examples of adaptations are use of one-handed vs. two-handed signs; use of gross vs. fine motor signs. Adaptations may also be made in response to the child's cognitive/experiential limitations. Examples of these adaptations are limitation of sign content (e.g., fewer, more concrete signs) & use of gross vs. fine motor signs.	Numerous physical adaptations are available: a variety of switches may be used to provide a means to indicate; options may also be selected to provide vocal, printed, or video output; adaptations of type of device can be made to suit the client's needs in various settings such as classroom or field trip. Cognitive/experiential adaptations include modification of symbol type (e.g., Blissymbols vs. pictures), content, and organization (e.g., single vs. multiple display).
Message	The gestural system (e.g., Signed English) must be taught to all persons who are to communicate with the client. This could be especially difficult if the client lives in an "open environment" (e.g., lives at home, goes to public school, has many non-handicapped friends). No options are available within the various sign systems to allow delayed reception (e.g., for homework) or a permanent record. Thus the client must learn another system, such as traditional orthography.	Some symbol systems (e.g., Blissymbols) require regular orthography below each symbol to help eliminate the need for special training of message receivers. Some confusion may persist due to words or ideas formed through combinations of symbols. Vocal or printed output is available to help clarify message reception. This also provides a message that can be read at leisure and can yield a permanent record. Persons in the environment must be trained to request and expect certain types of responses, depending upon the type of communication device used.
Social Interaction	Use of signs requires the client to attend to the "speaker" in order to see the signs. This may enhance eye contact & general interaction.	The message receiver must concentrate on the communication board unless a special output (e.g., vocal) is utilized. This reduces eye contact and makes it difficult to communicate in a group setting.
Flexibility	Vocabulary can be increased spontaneously (i.e., the client can make up new signs as needed). Grammatical structure may be taught, though exact parallel to English may not be realistic due to physical limitations (e.g., speed of signing) or cognitive limitations.	Vocabulary is limited due to lack of space on many boards; supplementary notebooks may help increase vocabulary, or the client may have alphabets or phonemes with which to produce new words. Grammatical structure may be indicated to some degree (e.g., inflectional markers on board). Again, exact parallel to English may be unrealistic due to physical or cognitive limitations

*Adapted in part from Harris-Vanderheiden and Vanderheiden (1977), Harris and Vanderheiden (1979); Kohl et al. (1977), and Williams and Fox (1977).

friends. These decisions will be based on the same factors which resulted in selecting the primary communication system. Finally, the trainer must decide whether to teach systems concurrently or to train one system to a specified level of performance before beginning with the next (Fristoe, Lloyd, and Wilbur 1977).

The decision process model presented in Chapter 2 will be used as a basis for examining gestural and symbolic communication systems in Chapters 8 and 9. In most cases a decision on system selection cannot be made until the communication specialist has considered features of each of these systems.

Chapter 8: Gestural Communication Strategies

Introduction

An ever-growing list of publications documents the success of gestural communication systems with the severely handicapped. Some types of gestural system have been used with nearly every type of severely handicapped population, including both children and adults. Considerable success has been reported with a wide variety of clients, ranging from preschool mentally retarded children (Simpson and McDade 1979) to adolescent autistic clients (Schaeffer 1980) to adult aphasics (Skelly and Schinsky 1979). Within and across handicapped populations, different effects of introducing gestural communication can be seen, particularly in communication and emotional adjustment.

In some cases clients gain only a core vocabulary for expressing basic needs (Hobson and Duncan 1979), while in other cases they achieve communication skills which parallel spoken English (Skelly and Schinsky 1979) or appear to facilitate spoken English (Grinnell, Detamore, and Lipke 1976). Gestural training has been found only minimally useful for some clients (Kimble 1975). Consequently, this mode, while not a panacea for all clients, appears to have considerable usefulness with many clients.

This chapter will cover several primary concerns in gestural communication: types of gestural systems, content of gestural systems, and methods of training. These areas are illustrated in figure 8-1.

Assessment for Use of a Gestural System

Primary questions to be answered when assessing a client for use of a gestural communication system include:

1. What *type* of gestural system is most appropriate for the client?
2. What is the *content* of the gestures to be taught?
3. What *methods of training* are best suited to this system and this client?

Each of these three concerns will be considered in the appropriate sections of this chapter. For example, for each gestural system covered in detail the requirements for use (e.g., physical, cognitive, academic) will be presented. Appendix D provides an overview of major areas of assessment.

Several authors have suggested predictive indicators of success in gestural training programs. Hobson and Duncan (1979) observe that a pretest of the client's receptive abilities may predict ability to learn sign language. They found that initial scores on the *Peabody Picture Vocabulary Test* (Dunn 1959) correlated significantly with: (1) vocabulary learned after six weeks, and (2) retention after two months. The subjects in that study were nine profoundly retarded, institutionalized persons.

Topper-Zweiban (1977) found that the Manual Expression Subtest of the *Illinois Test of Psycholinguistic Abilities* (Kirk, McCarthy, and Kirk 1968) appeared to be the most reliable indicator of success for the non-vocal profoundly retarded subjects in her study. She suggested that the client's Manual Expression Age could be used in the following ways:

1. *To determine priority*—clients with higher Manual Expression Ages would receive higher priority for training;
2. *To group for instructional purposes*—clients with similar Manual Expression Ages could be grouped for instruction;
3. *To estimate the length of therapy*—lower scores would suggest the need for more intensive therapy.

She noted certain difficulties regarding use of this test, especially with severely handicapped populations. First, some of the items are uncommon, particularly in institutions (e.g., eggbeater). Also, adjustments may have to be made in the testing procedure. She suggests that instructions could be presented verbally for visually impaired clients or through pantomime for hearing impaired clients.

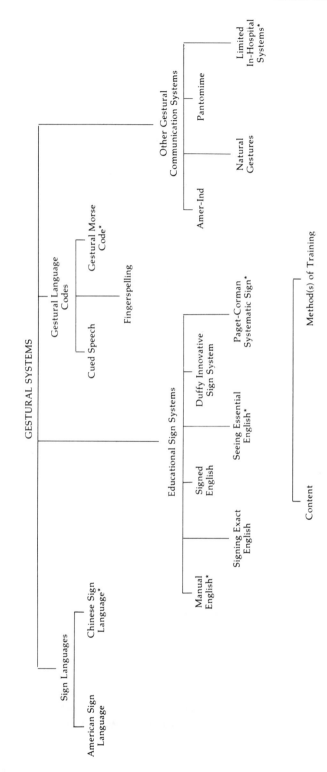

Figure 8-1
The Decision Process Model: Gestural systems.

*Indicates communication systems which are not covered in depth in this book.

Skelly and Schinsky (1979) discuss the issue of predicting success relative to training in the use of Amer-Ind. They report that, for their tests, no reliable correlation has been found regarding client success or failure. The tests used in the studies they report include The *Porch Index of Communicative Abilities* (Porch 1971), the *Sklar Aphasia Scale* (Sklar 1973), and the *Aphasia Language Performance Scale* (Keenan 1975). They recommend that "Action should be used in the tests, both as input and output" (p. 79). Therefore, Skelly has devised the *Amer-Ind Scale*, the *Action Test of Amer-Ind Signal Comprehension*, and the *Skelly Action Test of Auditory Reception of Language*. The *Skelly Action Test of Auditory Reception of Language* may provide useful information regarding the client's response to reality-based action situations involving the necessity to follow directions. The commands given require gestural responses; therefore, the examiner could use the results to assess the client's auditory reception of language and gestural abilities simultaneously, though it would be difficult to separate the two abilities.

Thus, although some indicators may help predict success for some populations, these indicators should not be relied on solely. Nevertheless, they may provide useful input for programming.

Types of Gestural Systems

A number of gestural communication systems have evolved or have been designed to serve the needs of the severely communication handicapped, especially the deaf. These systems may be divided into categories based on the origin, type, and intent of the systems:

1. *Sign languages,* such as American Sign Language, British Sign Language, and Chinese Sign Language; these have developed out of a need to communicate and are not universal; that is, each has its own structure and rules;
2. *Educational sign systems,* such as Signed English, Signing Exact English, and Duffy's System; these have been developed fairly recently to represent spoken English; many of these systems are based to some extent on American Sign Language and/or the American Manual Alphabet;
3. *Gestural language codes,* such as Cued Speech, fingerspelling, and gestural Morse Code; these serve to represent the letters or sounds of a language such as English;
4. *Other gestural communication systems,* such as Amer-Ind, natural gestures, pantomime, and limited in-hospital systems; these consist of a wide range of formal and informal systems.

Matching these systems to the needs and capabilities of clients is a difficult task which requires that the trainer have a thorough understanding of the available systems. The following discussion will focus on a number of gestural systems which have been or could be used with the severely handicapped. For each major system the following information will be presented:

1. *What*—a description of the system, including features such as history, content, and structure;
2. *Why*—a consideration of the functions of the system;
3. *Who*—a consideration of potential candidates and appropriate audience, plus a brief review of the literature on applications to various populations;
4. *How*—a discussion of training methodology concerning learning by both trainers and clients;
5. *When*—a suggestion of the time period for optimum introduction;
6. *Where*—a brief list of sources of further information regarding the system and its implementation.

Several authors have compared and contrasted the linguistic and functional characteristics of various gestural systems (Bornstein 1973, 1979; Mayberry 1976; Wilbur 1976, 1979). This section reviews their observations and discusses how the systems are used.

Sign Languages: American Sign Language

A number of sign languages have developed in various countries to serve as vehicles of communication for the deaf. Woodward (1976) has identified several sign families. For example, the French sign language family includes sign languages currently used in three countries (France, Denmark, and the United States). However, sign languages from the same family are not mutually intelligible. Thus sign languages cannot be considered to be universal but must be studied as distinct languages. This chapter will cover only one sign language, American Sign Language, since it is the principal system used in the United States and Canada.

What. American Sign Language (ASL), or Ameslan, is the language used among most deaf adults in the United States. In fact, it is the fourth most common language in the country (Mayberry 1978). Traditionally, ASL is reported to have been brought to the United States by Thomas Gallaudet, an educator who went to Europe to learn about methods for educating the deaf, and Laurent Clerc, a deaf French man. Gallaudet and Clerc established a school for the deaf in America, using a sign language based on Old French Sign (Lane 1977; Wilbur 1976). However, Woodward (1976; 1978) presents sociological and linguistic evidence suggesting that many of the signs in ASL were derived from signed languages already used by American deaf people before Old French Sign was introduced. It is important to recognize that ASL is a language, not merely a code to represent English or any other language. Thus there is often not a one-to-one correspondence between ASL signs and English, French, or German words. In addition, even if one assigns the best English gloss to each ASL sign, word-by-word translations from one language to the other would not be equivalent since the structure of the two languages differs as well. For example, the ASL signed sequences THEY FINISH

EAT NIGHT[1] or FINISH EAT NIGHT THEY could be translated in English as "They have already eaten their dinner" (Mayberry 1976). Each of these is an acceptable utterance relative to its own language, but they are clearly not parallel in structure.

Signs in ASL can generally be described by three components or elements, with a fourth needed to distinguish some sign pairs:

1. *Tab*, the *location* where a sign begins and ends with relation to the signer's body, also termed the *place of articulation* (example: chest);
2. *Dez*, the distinctive *handshape(s)* or *configuration(s)* used to make the sign (example: flat hand);
3. *Sig*, the *movement* involved in making the sign (example: circular);
4. *Orientation*, or plane(s) of the palm of the hand (example: palm up).

Adapted from Siple (1978, pp. 6–7)
and Stokoe (1980, p. 128)

Klima and Bellugi (1979) observe that the *Dictionary of American Sign Language* (Stokoe, Casterline, and Croneberg 1978) describes 19 hand configurations, 12 places of articulation, and 24 types of movement (which can combine in clusters). Markowicz (1977) notes that the exact number of each of these may vary, as do the number of vowels in spoken English, depending on the dialect. As with other languages, ASL has formational rules that specify the possible combinations for signs.

Each of the four elements can illustrate minimal contrasts. For example, the signs CANDY, APPLE, and JEALOUS are all formed with the same place of articulation, movement, and orientation; only the hand configuration distinguishes among the three signs (Klima and Bellugi 1979, p. 42). Similar examples could be provided for other parameters of sign formation.

Baker and Padden (1978a) and Frishberg (1979) review a number of modifications in signs (specifically, ASL signs) intended to aid production or reception. For example, Frishberg notes that many signs that once required body and head movement, facial gesture, or environmental contact in their *citation forms*[2] are currently limited to movements of the hands only (e.g., COMPARE). This allows for easier production by the signer. Baker and Padden report that a larger number of signs are located in the high visibility area of the signer's head and neck than at other locations. Again, in some cases, older signs made on the waist or chest have changed through time, and are now made further up on the body, aiding in reception. In summary, Baker and Padden assert that "ASL signs are 'natural'—they are shaped to be seen and efficiently produced by the human body" (p. 11).

Just as shades of meaning can be provided to spoken language through voice-related qualities such as pitch, stress, and intonation, a variety of simultaneous behaviors can add nuances of meaning to sign language. Baker and Padden (1978b) review a number of studies which, as they state ". . .have

---

1. This book follows the convention of capitalizing words that represent signs, signals, or gestures; using lower case with quotes to represent spoken words; and using lower case without quotes to represent English words.
2. *Citation forms* are the forms of signs isolated from context and produced alone.

clearly revealed the fallacy of assuming the hands to be the only carriers of linguistic information in signed discourse" (pp. 27–28). For example, some lexical items are formed or supplemented by facial expressions, such as SAD (with a sad facial expression) and BITE (often accompanied by a biting motion of the mouth). Nonmanual signals can also code grammatical functions, as will be discussed later in this chapter.

Klima and Bellugi (1979) report that ". . .though signs are produced at half the rate of words, the rate of producing propositions does not differ in the two modes" (p. 194). This is true for ASL but not necessarily for other sign systems. ASL economizes by omitting the kinds of grammatical morphemes that English uses. However, the information coded in those morphemes is not lost in ASL, as can be demonstrated through translation from English to ASL and then from ASL back to English. A variety of methods are used for compacting linguistic information in ASL so that the language is made more efficient while still retaining its effectiveness in coding messages. As Wilbur (1976) points out, ". . .what needs to be indicated sequentially in auditory languages, by using markers and word order, often can be indicated simultaneously in ASL" (p. 194). Numerous examples of this efficiency can be provided. Klima and Bellugi (1979) report several general procedures for compacting linguistic information.

The first procedure is the *structured use of space*. For example, in a narrative, a sign central to the meaning may be made in the first sentence (e.g., the sign DOG) and followed by a classifier sign (e.g., ANIMAL). Subsequently, that locus in space may be reserved, and later signs (e.g., FEED and PAT) may be directed toward the locus reserved for the dog. This saves time because the signer is not required to sign DOG each time the animal is referred to. A *time line* may also be used ". . .such that the space more or less parallel to the side of the body indicates present tense, the space forward of the body indicates future, and the space behind the body indicates past" (Wilbur 1979, p. 437). Thus tense can be indicated simultaneous with production of a sign. The preceding examples are only two of the ways in which the structured use of space can increase efficiency in ASL.

Another procedure for increasing efficiency is the *superimposed modulations of the movement of signs* (Klima and Bellugi 1979). For example, native signers could observe various productions of the sign SCARED and could determine, through qualitative changes in the movement, whether the signer intended translation of "was scared" or "became scared." Similarly, slight modulations of movement may be seen in noun-verb pairs, in which the manner of movement is restrained and movement is repeated for the noun (e.g., FLY/AIRPLANE, SWEEP/ BROOM) [Suppalla and Newport 1978].

A third procedure for simultaneous coding is the *simultaneous use of facial expression for grammatical purposes*. For example, an otherwise positive statement may be negated through use of a negative facial expression.

Several authors (Baker and Padden 1978b; Liddell 1978) discuss the variety of *nonmanual signals* used in ASL. For example, Baker and Padden analyzed several nonmanual behavioral changes (face, brows, head, blink, gaze, hands, body). They noted that many synchronous behaviors occur during signing of conditional sentences. They concluded that it is configurations of these nonmanual behaviors, rather than any single behavior, that carry meaning.

This issue of nonmanual signals is important in selecting a sign system for use with a severely handicapped client. If the client is expected to use ASL as a communication system (rather than as a short-term language facilitation system only), it will be important for the client to be able to capitalize on using these nonmanual behaviors as well as the manual signs. Indeed, Baker and Padden (1978a) suggest that nonmanual behaviors be considered as basic building blocks of ASL, along with manual components such as handshapes.

Why. As with other gestural systems, ASL can serve as a facilitator of language and has been found successful (Simpson and McDade 1979). Since it is a rich and complex language, ASL can also serve as a long-term communication system and in fact does fill this role for the adult deaf community in the United States. Thus there is an already-existing audience of ASL users and a large number of potential teachers. Its capabilities for simultaneous coding of several pieces of linguistic information makes ASL desirable from the aspect of efficiency. This is a positive feature since more time is required for forming a sign than for uttering a word. Wilbur (1979) suggests that this feature might prove to be very helpful to clients at the single-sign stage in either reception or expression.

Who. As noted, American Sign Language developed as a communication system for the deaf and is widely used by that population in the United States and Canada. Success has been reported in use of ASL with a variety of other populations, including the mildly to profoundly retarded (Hobson and Duncan 1979; Simpson and McDade 1979; Stremel-Campbell, Cantrell, and Halle 1977); the autistic (Bonvillian and Nelson 1976; Carr et al. 1978; Fulwiler and Fouts 1976; Konstantareas, Oxman, and Webster 1978); and other non-vocal individuals who are multihandicapped or who have undiagnosed etiologies (Koselka et al. 1975; Konstantareas et al. 1978). However, in many cases the clients in these studies have demonstrated success with lexical entries of ASL in isolation, or with two and three-sign strings only, rather than with ASL as a total system (Hobson and Duncan 1979; Simpson and McDade 1979). In addition, Stremel-Campbell reports using ASL signs, but in English word order. We are not suggesting that severely handicapped clients other than the deaf *cannot* make full use of ASL as a language, but merely that to date it has been used in a limited fashion in most cases.

Candidates for ASL should possess the following skills or should be expected to acquire them:

1. *Good motor control of both hands,* in order to produce the 19 basic hand configurations;
2. *Good range of motion with both arms,* in order to produce signs at a variety of places of articulation and with a number of movement patterns;
3. *Good control over facial musculature,* in order to achieve nuances of meaning through facial expressions;

4. *Good visual acuity and visual discrimination,* if the client is to receive as well as produce sign;

5. *Sensorimotor Stage 5 or 6 intelligence.* (Chapman and Miller 1980)

The question of *who* should also be concerned with who will be able to interpret the client's utterances if ASL is to be used as the primary means of communication. Baker and Padden (1978a) report that ASL is used by approximately one-half million deaf Americans and Canadians of all ages, thus providing a large population of potential communication partners. However, the non-vocal hearing client may not have access to a deaf community. Thus it may be necessary to train communication partners for the client.

Signs have traditionally been described as *transparent.* Transparency refers to how well a sign's meaning can be understood from its form alone. Klima and Bellugi (1979) have studied the transparency of commonly used ASL signs such as APPLE, BOY, EARTH, and WEEK presented to subjects who knew no signs. They found that 81 of the 90 signs were not guessed by any of the ten hearing subjects. A second group of ten hearing subjects scored no better than chance in selecting signs on a multiple-choice test. Thus it is apparent that most of the ASL signs on this list were not readily transparent. However, they demonstrated that many signs may be considered *translucent*: "that is, nonsigners essentially agree on the basis for the relation between the sign and its meaning" (p. 10). In addition, iconicity in signs can often be stressed or invented to serve as aids in remembering signs. Thus, although it will be necessary for those in the client's environment to directly learn most signs, once meanings have been taught they will, in most cases, be relatively easy to remember. However, native speakers of English will have to learn the syntax of ASL in addition to the vocabulary. This may be more difficult if they do not have frequent access to persons fluent in ASL. Thus finding or training an audience for the client who becomes fluent in ASL may be a significant problem.

How. As with most sign systems used with the severely handicapped other than the deaf, ASL is "taught" rather than learned as a natural language. More than most other sign systems, ASL would seem to be appropriate for learning as a natural language, through an environmental approach, since it is a true language. Wilbur (1976) reviews studies which demonstrate that ASL may be acquired spontaneously by hearing and deaf children who are exposed to it. Unfortunately, most parents would have some difficulty in this respect because learning ASL as an adult constitutes learning a second language (Stokoe 1980). That is, it is unlikely that most families of hearing, but severely handicapped, children would choose to use ASL as their primary communication system. In addition, the hearing non-vocal client may not have any peers who use ASL.

If specific therapy sessions are to be used, training is similar in many respects to training for other sign systems, to be discussed in this chapter. However, the differences in structure of ASL suggest that trainers should employ specialized techniques for training use of ASL versus, for example, Signing Exact English. Naturally, client factors such as hearing status, cognitive status, age, and the intended function of ASL will also help determine training strategies. If ASL is intended to serve as a full communication system for the client, the structure specific to ASL must be considered. In addition, nonmanual signals such as facial expressions, body orientation, and eye gaze which are related to the lexical entries and structures of ASL may require specific training. For example, it may be helpful to carefully model the combination of behavior that signals production of a yes-no question (head and shoulders leaned forward, chin forward far enough to keep the face vertical, and eyebrows raised) [Liddell 1978]) in contrast to behavior that signals a WH-question (brows raised and drawn together) [Baker and Padden 1978a]. Baker and Padden (1978b) present a list of some functions of eye movements and facial movements in ASL discourse which may help bring this behavior to a level of consciousness for the trainer and the client.

The preceding discussion on training nuances of ASL assumes that the trainer is a fluent user of ASL. This may be far from true for those of us who have learned signs from a book and/or a course and have little or no opportunity to practice in discourse with native ASL users. Stokoe (1980) asserts that " . . . if a teacher of the deaf has a genuine desire to learn Sign, the problem is not to find one who knows it but to persuade those who know it that using Sign is permissible and will not be punished overtly or covertly" (p. 149). This may be true for people with ready access to a deaf community. However, for communication specialists living in rural areas it may be more of a problem. A number of manuals are available to help a potential trainer learn ASL (Babbini 1974a,b; Fant 1977; O'Rourke 1973; Riekehof 1978; see annotations in Appendix A of this book). The communication specialist who is not bilingual in English and ASL may want to consider a number of alternatives:

1. *Increase fluency in ASL* through further course-work and, preferably, practice with a native ASL signer prior to or concurrent with beginning training of clients;
2. *Locate a fluent ASL user to serve as the trainer,* at least temporarily;[3]
3. *Limit ASL training* to teaching of vocabulary and basic syntax either as a facilitative or early language system or as a system for a client whose language is not expected to reach a high level of complexity;
4. *Select a system* whose structure more closely parallels English (e.g., Signing Exact English, Cued Speech), so that it is not necessary to learn a new structure as well as new vocabulary forms.

Several training programs have been designed or adapted for teaching ASL or ASL signs to various populations. For example, Snell (1974) provides an ASL modification of Kent's (1974) language program for the retarded or multiply impaired. Other training programs have been designed specifically to teach ASL signs to the severely handicapped (Wilson, Goodman, and Wood 1975). These types of programs typically have a very limited scope. The

---

3. Contact the Registry of Interpreters for the Deaf, listed in Appendix C.

communication specialist teaching ASL to clients having higher-level language skills might find a second-language approach helpful. This would be especially true for clients who became non-vocal after acquiring language (e.g., adult aphasics or laryngectomees).

When. Since ASL is a true language, its use may be initiated in a natural language approach with infants. If ASL is to be taught as a second language, it could be introduced after the client is proficient in one language.

Where. A great amount of information is available on ASL as a system (Kilma and Bellugi 1978; Stokoe et al. 1978; Wilbur 1979). A number of manuals are also available for learning ASL signs and/or ASL structure, as indicated in the previous section (see Appendix A for more information). Several curricula are available for use in teaching ASL to severely handicapped clients (e.g., Snell 1974; Wilson et al. 1975, reviewed in Appendix B). A more advanced ASL curriculum is being prepared by the Department for Deaf-Blind Children, Perkins School for the Blind (Regional Centers for Services to Deaf-Blind Children, see Appendix C). Many of these resources, plus additional information and materials (e.g., games, flash cards, and translation exercises) may be obtained from the following sources: Gallaudet College, the National Association of the Deaf, and Regional Centers for Services to Deaf-Blind Children. Addresses and further information are presented in Appendix C.

Discussion and Summary. There are a number of myths and misconceptions concerning American Sign Language, such as the myth that it is ungrammatical (Markowicz 1977). This brief presentation may help to eliminate some of these misconceptions. Many of the myths can be laid to rest simply by recognizing that ASL is a language, not just a coded representation of another language, such as English. Viewing it as a separate language, we can see that—

1. *ASL is not a universal language,* it is merely the sign language used by most deaf persons of the United States and Canada; the deaf of other countries (e.g., Japan, Denmark) use sign languages which differ from each other, just as spoken languages differ;
2. *ASL is no more concept-based than other languages,* such as English; in fact, both words and signs are based on concepts;
3. *ASL is not ungrammatical,* though utterances translated from ASL to English may appear ungrammatical, just as utterances translated from French or Italian frequently appear ungrammatical; ASL is based on a large number of grammatical rules which govern its use.

Markowicz (1977)

As a language of the deaf, ASL has a rich history of use, dating back more than 160 years. Its use with other non-vocal severely handicapped populations is of much more recent origin. In a limited fashion ASL has been demonstrated successful with clients having a wide range of handicaps. There is a future for more extensive use of ASL with some severely handicapped populations, due in part to its efficiency and the large audience of ASL users.

Educationally-based sign systems, often termed *pedagogical systems*, are those designed to meet certain educational needs. As discussed in the previous section, American Sign Language has its own structure and vocabulary, which often do not parallel English. Therefore, several systems have been designed to represent spoken English for educational purposes. Examples of these systems are Seeing Essential English, Signing Exact English, Manual English, Signed English, Linguistics of Visual English, and Paget-Gorman Systematic Sign. Other systems have been created to serve other needs. For example, Duffy's System was developed for the severely physically handicapped. Several educational sign systems (e.g., Manual English, Seeing Essential English, Signing Exact English, Signed English) have some features in common since they are based to some extent on American Sign Language and the American Manual Alphabet. The educationally-based sign systems utilize many ASL signs, with new signs added as required, based on the logic of the system. Word order and use of inflections generally help to distinguish between ASL and the newer educational systems.

Although there are similarities among some of the sign systems, there are also many differences. The extent of these differences varies according to the systems compared. Fristoe and Lloyd (1978) and Goodman, Wilson, and Bornstein (1978) sent questionnaires to special educators, the majority of whom worked in programs serving the severely mentally retarded. These questionnaires dealt with the use of non-vocal (primarily sign) systems in special education programs. One important finding was that many persons reported that they used ASL, while in fact they were using ASL signs in English word order. Fristoe and Lloyd (1978) suggest "either that they do not recognize that there are differences in sign systems or else that they are not aware of the importance of the differences" (p. 101). They also note that respondents often gave misinformed reasons for choosing one system over another, for example stating that Signing Exact English is simpler than other systems (in fact, Signed English is less complex). Therefore, the communication specialist should be aware of the distinctions among systems when selecting the sign system most appropriate for a specific client. Sign systems included in this section are those which have been or could be used with non-vocal severely handicapped clients. The systems covered according to the outline presented earlier are Signed English, Signing Exact English, and Duffy's System.[4] Several systems which are less widely used in the United States or are less appropriate to the needs of the severely handicapped are covered briefly. This category includes Paget-Gorman Systematic Sign, Seeing Essential English, Manual English, and the Linguistics of Visual English.

---

4. Duffy's (1977) unnamed system will be referred to as Duffy's System for ease of reference.

Paget-Gorman Systematic Sign

This system was the first English-based educational sign system. It was developed by Sir Richard Paget (1951) in England, who intended that its use be discarded when the child no longer needed it for communication (Wilbur 1979). This system does not use ASL signs but is based on pantomimic signs which include combinations of 21 standard hand positions and 39 basic signs. The basic signs serve to group signs with a common concept, such as FOOD and ANIMAL, while the hand configurations indicate specific entries within each group. For example, "dentist" is formed by PERSON + TOOTH, while "lion" consists of ANIMAL + ROAR. In addition to those meaningful signs, several functional signs represent affixes such as possessive, adverb (-LY), and present progressive (-ING). Wilbur (1979) notes that this system attempts to avoid the various problems (e.g., internal inconsistency) that most other systems have in forming complex and compound signs. This is handled by establishing a set of morphological rules which generally do not parallel English rules. An example is the productive formation of signs through combinations of basic signs and standard hand configurations. Thus, rather than adding an affix (-IST) to the root word ("dent" or TOOTH) to represent the word "dentist," Paget-Gorman Systematic Sign uses PERSON + TOOTH. Wilbur (1979) reports that Craig (1976) suggests that, while this logical pattern of using basic signs may not aid children in sign language acquisition, it may be very helpful to hearing adults learning the system.

In summary, Paget-Gorman Systematic Sign differs considerably from most of the other sign systems described within this chapter since it is not based on American Sign Language and does not use English morphological structures. Further information on this system may be found in Craig (1976) or Wilbur (1979).

Seeing Essential English

Seeing Essential English (SEE 1) was the first educational sign system in the United States. It was developed by David Anthony (1966; 1971) as a simplified system for use with the mentally retarded deaf. Two sign systems, Linguistics of Visual English and Signing Exact English, were derived from Seeing Essential English. This book will not cover Seeing Essential English, as it is not widely available and does not seem to have gained widespread use with the severely handicapped. See Anthony (1971) or Bornstein (1973) for a further descriptions of this system.

Manual English

Manual English was developed by the Total Communication Program at the Washington State School for the Deaf (1972). The purpose of this project was to provide a manual system that would approximate English enough that the two could be used in simultaneous communication. Wilbur (1979) notes that Manual English uses more fingerspelling than does Signing Exact English and allows users options such as whether to use VERB + TENSE or VERB + E + D to form a past tense. A number of ASL signs as well as many initialized[5] signs are used. Manual English uses one sign for each meaning, similar to Paget-Gorman Systematic Sign and unlike Signing Exact English. Further information on this system may be found in Wilbur (1979).

Linguistics of Visual English

This sign system is intended for use with preschool and kindergarten children. It is a morpheme-based system. Signs are intended to represent morphemes rather than word roots, prefixes, and suffixes. Morphemes are distinguished on the basis of similarity in two of three characteristics: sound, spelling, and meaning. The signs of ASL are paired with English bound and unbound morphemes. For example, Mayberry (1976) notes that the word "carpet" would be made through the ASL signs CAR + PET (translated "auto" + "physically stroke"). Linguistics of Visual English follows English word order and uses English function words and inflections such as pronouns, articles, tense markers, and auxiliaries. Further information on this system may be found in Mayberry (1976) or Wilbur (1979).

Signed English

What. Signed English[6] is a manual system which, according to Wilbur (1976), is an outgrowth of the ASL-English pidginization process.[7] It results from the work of several groups of investigators, which accounts in part for the variation and confusion surrounding the system in the literature. Mayberry suggests that the terms "signed English," "manual English," "visual English," and "siglish" do not refer to a specific manual communication system. Basically, signed English consists of ASL signs in English word order, with or without the use of fingerspelling or selected grammatical inflections. The amount of fingerspelling and the number of inflections used will greatly depend on the formality of the discourse situation. Thus increased use of fingerspelling and inflections may yield utterances that more closely parallel spoken English in formal situations. Wilbur (1979) also notes that signed English may refer to " . . . the signing that is used by hearing people who have learned signs but have not received instruction in ASL syntax and thus put the signs together in English order and fingerspell whatever signs they do not know" (p. 205).

The purpose of Signed English as conceived by Bornstein and his colleagues (1973; 1974) is " . . . to facilitate the English language development of the preschool child by providing him with a reasonable semantic approximation to the usual language environment of the hearing child" (p. 330).

The target language was determined by collecting weekly logs of the oral language used by and with hearing preschool children of middle-class parents having a wide range of language competence and formal education. Then the

---

5. *Initialized signs* begin with the first letter of the desired word. For example, the basic sign for "group" can be initialized to form more specific words such as "family," "class," or "team" (Riekehof 1978).

6. "Signed English" is used as a generic term to refer to the category of which Bornstein's "Signed English" is an example.

7. This refers to the process of incorporating the vocabularies of two or more languages, in this case English and ASL.

vocabulary used, needed, and judged appropriate was determined, using input from parents and preschool teachers. Existing ASL signs were chosen to represent approximately 1700 of these words. The remaining 800 sign words were either invented or taken from other systems. Additional vocabulary will be added in a forthcoming revision of *Signed English Dictionary* (Bornstein, personal communication). Unlike some of the other educational systems (e.g., Linguistics of Visual English, Seeing Essential English), Signed English does not change the form of ASL words to match English words. As Bornstein explains, sign words in Signed English parallel whole English words in meaning only.

Fourteen sign markers are used in Signed English. Three of these are class markers, in which one sign represents a class of structural change; for example, a single sign marker indicates production of any past irregular verb. Thus production of GO plus this sign marker would indicate the past tense verb "went." The remaining nine markers represent specific inflections such as past tense regular -ED, as in "walked," or third person singular -S, as in "walks." Although it is recommended that all markers be used in communication, Bornstein notes that some signers will be unable or unwilling to use the full system. Therefore, two possible reductions in the number of markers have been suggested. The first set would omit only three markers (irregular past, irregular plural, -ING verb form), while the second set would retain only the five most needed markers (past regular -ED, agent, regular plural -S, and comparatives -ER and -EST). In general, only one sign marker can be added to each sign word so as to maintain the simple structure considered necessary for use with and by preschool children. Bornstein recommends that finger-spelling be used for words and word forms not covered by the vocabulary and sign markers. Another way in which this system was modified to meet the needs of preschool children was to include separate signs for contractions such as "don't" since preschool children encounter and learn them as single words.

Why. Signed English has been successfully used as a communication system as well as for speech and language facilitation with the severely handicapped (e.g., Abkarian, Dworkin, and Brown 1978; Kimble 1975; Kopchick and Lloyd 1976; Schaeffer 1980). Factors which may make this system especially desirable for some clients are its focus on a limited vocabulary appropriate to young children, paralleling of English word order, and use of a limited set of sign markers.

Who. Signed English candidates should meet the same requirements as candidates for ASL, with the exception that good control of facial musculature is less crucial. This is because nonmanual behavior does not code as much linguistic information in Signed English since it used English structure. Signed English has been used or advocated for use with a variety of populations, including the severely mentally retarded (Kimble 1975; Kopchick and Lloyd 1976), the autistic (Schaeffer 1980), and the adventitiously nonverbal (Abkarian, Dworkin, and Brown 1978). It could be an appropriate system for others for whom a sign system was being considered, providing that the nature and size of the vocabulary and the number of sign markers were sufficient.

With regard to communication partners, signs in this system would likely not be transparent since many are based on ASL signs. Thus, it would be necessary for parents, teachers, and others to directly learn the system. However, several factors should theoretically make it easier to learn than ASL for competent speakers of English. First, since it is designed to parallel English, it will basically be necessary to learn only a vocabulary of signs based on English words rather than a new set of grammatical rules. Second, the vocabulary is restricted to 2500 entries and the sign markers to 14, in contrast, for example, to the more than 5200 signs in ASL (Bornstein 1974). These two features would, of course, also make Signed English relatively easy to learn for clients having competency in English, such as spastic dysphonics. As Bornstein points out, "It is for adults, primarily, that the logic of the manual supplement [Signed English] was purposely kept simple and straightforward" (p. 339). Therefore, it is feasible to consider learning Signed English from one of the many available books (see the *where* section).

When. It is generally suggested that exposure begin as early as possible, for example as soon as a child is diagnosed as deaf. However, recall that Chapman and Miller (1980) assert that sensorimotor Stage 5 or 6 is necessary for a client to benefit from sign training. This again brings up the issue of training preliminary behaviors, discussed in Chapter 4. Signed English could likely be used as input to clients with cognitive skills below Stage 5; however, output would not be expected initially for those clients.

How. As always, training procedures will depend primarily on the needs of the client and the realities of the environment. Training procedures specific to use of Signed English, especially for preschool or mentally retarded clients, involve use of some of the many teaching aids available from the Gallaudet College Bookstore. Varied formats are provided, such as posters, storybooks, nursery rhymes, and songbooks. According to Bornstein, each teaching aid uses pictures to present the client with " . . . a consistent and accurate relationship between the printed word, signed word, and appearance of the lips" (p. 340). In addition, each teaching aid is self-contained so that it may be used without the need of other materials. Thus parents can learn Signed English and become primary teachers of the system for their children.

Where. Information about Signed English may be obtained by writing to the Gallaudet College Press for a free guide to the system. Teaching aids such as storybooks may be purchased from the Gallaudet College Bookstore (see Appendix C). The reader may also wish to review Bornstein, Saulnier, and Hamilton (1980), which presents a first evaluation of the system.

Discussion and summary. The Signed English system is an attempt to represent English manually. However, it is a more limited and less complex system than several of the other educational systems reviewed in this chapter, such as Signing Exact English. Bornstein, (personal communication) questions whether a more complex system is truly workable. The potential of Signed

English for use with the severely handicapped appears quite broad, due in great measure to its simplicity.

Signing Exact English

What. Signing Exact English, often referred to as SEE 2, is based on David Anthony's development of Seeing Essential English (SEE 1) [Anthony 1966; 1971]. Initially there was considerable similarity between the two systems; for example, Bornstein (1973) estimated an overlap between the two as 75 percent for general vocabulary only to 80 percent with inclusion of affixes, pronouns, and BE-verbs. However, the most recent manual for Signing Exact English (Gustason, Pfetzing, and Zawolkow 1980) includes approximately 1000 signs not included in earlier editions. Thus the two SEE systems seem to be evolving separately.

A brief history of the development of SEE 2 is very instructive. Bornstein (1973) reports that the developers were former members of the Seeing Essential English group who felt that that system could be improved. The three women primarily responsible for developing materials for SEE 2 have had considerable involvement with the deaf. One author was deafened at age six and has taught extensively in various programs for the deaf, including the one at Gallaudet College. The second author was the mother of a deaf child and served as Head Interpreter in a public school. The third author, the daughter of deaf parents, grew up using American Sign Language and now serves as an interpreter in a public school and as consultant to many programs using sign systems.

Signing Exact English currently consists of nearly 4000 signs, including a large number of the most commonly used English affixes. Words in SEE 2 are considered basic, compound, or complex. Basic words are root words with no additions, such as GIRL, TALK, or SIT. Compound words are formed by joining two or more basic words, such as CHALKBOARD or UNDERCOOK. Complex words are formed by adding an inflection or affix to basic words such as GIRLS, TALKED, SITTING.

Signs for *basic words* are determined through use of a *two-out-of-three principle.* This states that the same sign is used for two English words if two of the three word features, (pronunciation, spelling, and meaning) are the same. Thus there is only one sign for "right" (as in right shoe) and "right" (as in correct), but the English words "write" and "rite" would each have separate signs.

For *complex words* an affix is added in signs if one is added in English, regardless of meaning. Wilbur (1979) points out that this results in the same -EN inflection added in forming REDDEN and CHICKEN, even though the meaning of the -EN is radically different.

The primary rule involving *compound words* is that they are signed as two signs only if the meaning of the compound word is related to the meanings of the separate words, such as COWBOY and UNDERCOOK. If the meanings are not related, as in FORGET and UNDERSTAND, the sign is treated as a basic word, and the ASL sign is used or a new sign is invented.

Wilbur (1979) points out a number of inconsistent applications of these basic rules. She notes that there are instances in which, for no apparent reason, the rules are not followed. For example, rather than following the two-out-of-three principle, some words are broken down into morpheme divisions (e.g., "height" = HIGH + T), or syllable divisions (e.g., "jewelry" = JEWEL + R + Y). These deviations from the rule do not appear to be systematic, and it is difficult to see how they were determined since this is a sign system rather than a naturally evolving language such as ASL or English.

Why. The SEE 2 system was developed as a manual communication system to represent English for educational purposes. The use of a large number of affixes and a large vocabulary of English words is intended to help the user develop a good base for understanding and producing idiomatic standard English, whether signed, spoken, or written. SEE 2 should also be easier to use than ASL in a simultaneous manner (speech + signs) since it can be made to closely approximate spoken English.

Who. The SEE 2 system was designed for use with deaf children or as a second language. Candidates for this system should meet the same basic requirements as for Signed English, with one exception. The relatively greater emphasis on use of pronouns and affixes will require that the client be expected to develop to a fairly high level of English competence. Thus, its use would seem to be less appropriate for the severely mentally retarded.

Since it parallels English to a great extent, SEE 2 might be a desirable system for use with those who have acquired competence in English but cannot produce it for some reason (e.g., vocal fold paralysis). This feature of SEE 2, its close approximation to English, should make SEE 2 simpler for hearing adults to learn than ASL, assuming that full use of the structure is desired. Due again to its close relationship to English, this system should be appropriate for clients who are expected to develop reading skills, although this premise has not yet been proven.

When. As with the other sign systems presented in this chapter, Signing Exact English is intended for use, at least regarding input, as soon as feasible. Chapman and Miller (1980) suggest that this should be when the client reaches sensorimotor Stage 5 or 6.

How. Again, teaching methods will depend to a great extent on client features such as current level of linguistic competence and the intended function of the system (e.g., as a second language system for the adventitiously non-vocal). Several materials and training methods have been developed specifically for this system, such as dictionaries, vocabulary development kits, and a teaching manual with suggestions for use, games, and record-keeping charts. Suggestions are also provided for creatively using American Sign Language principles while signing as exactly as possible what is being spoken in English.

Since the word order and sentence structure parallel English to a great extent, it should be possible to learn SEE 2 through manuals and introductory sign courses, followed by extensive practice.

Where. The materials and training suggestions are available through the National Association of the Deaf (See Appendix C).

Duffy's System

What. This sign system is the result of a master's thesis by a special education teacher in a class for trainable mentally retarded/physically handicapped children (Duffy 1977). The system was developed following observation and trial therapy with severely handicapped clients. Each sign was then tested on four subjects, ages 7 to 15, who were medically diagnosed as quadriplegic, athetoid cerebral palsied. The speech of these subjects was limited to vowel sounds and a few consonants (/b/, /p/, /m/, /n/).

The sign system comprises 471 signs which are formed by gross gestures such as raising one hand or placing one hand on the knee or the wheelchair armrest. Some signs are accompanied by vocalizations. For example ONE = "un" + raise one hand, while TWO = "ooo" + raise two hands. A few of the entries are only vocalizations. An example is the letter "U," which is indicated by the sound /u/. For some signs alternate methods of production are suggested; for example, K can be indicated by touching the chin with the hand or touching the chin on the wheelchair armrest. Wherever possible signs are iconic, such as crossing the legs for X or pantomiming pulling up pants for PANTS.

The system is logically organized. Many of the categories are preceded by a general sign. For example, the general sign for time precedes most time-category signs (e.g., 1:00 = TIME + 1). A general sign can also be used to indicate "I am spelling" or "numbers will follow". Within lexical groupings a logical base can also be seen. Days of the week are formed by the sign for "day" plus the number of the day (Sunday = DAY + 1, Monday = DAY + 2). Similarly, months are indicated by the sign for time plus the first letter of the month and another letter (December = TIME + D + "eee"; May = TIME + M + "aaah"). Questions are indicated by making the sign QUESTION followed by the appropriate sign (WHO, WHAT, WHERE). Facial movements and whole body movements are often used in expressing feelings. For example, one set of feelings requires the client to bounce up and down in the chair while executing arm movements and/or facial expressions (EXCITED, UPSET, SUR-PRISE, LUCKY). In addition to the categories of letters, numbers, time, and emotions, a wide variety of other categories are covered. Examples are persons, places, adjectives, prepositions, verbs, and pronouns. With the exception of producing questions by using QUESTION + question word (e.g., WHY), no structural rules specific to this system are presented.

Why. This system has been used successfully with four cerebral palsied clients. Of all the sign systems presented in this chapter, this one requires the least motor control. It would likely be used only as an output system, since clients who could decode this system, with its emphasis on numbers and letters, could likely decode speech or a non-vocal system presented at a faster rate (e.g., fingerspelling or American Sign Language). Duffy (personal communication) suggests that this system might be used as an interim system while vocal communication skills are being developed. It may prove to facilitate speech since many of the signs involve vocalization. She reports that two of the four subjects in her study are now using speech as their primary communication mode. Duffy's System could also be used as a supplement to another communication system (e.g., a symbolic communication board using Blissymbols) since it is portable and requires learning a relatively small number of signs.

Who. This system was designed for the physically handicapped, particularly the cerebral palsied. Execution of signs requires the following:

1. *Volitional control over gross motor movements of all limbs,* since some signs are two-handed (TIME) and some involve active use of the legs (X);
2. *High level of cognitive-academic development,* if the spelling aspect is to be used; however, many signs based on numbers or letters could be memorized without regard to their component parts;
3. *Moderate control over facial musculature,* since some signs involve use of the lips (F) or facial expressions (ANGRY);
4. *Volitional control over some vocalizations,* primarily vowels, since some signs require supplemental use of vocalization (CUP, MAY).

Although this approach is apparently most suited to the physically handicapped, especially the cerebral palsied, it may be of some use to hemiplegic clients with symbolic deficiencies (e.g., aphasics) since many signs are iconic and all require only gross motor movement.

This would not be a difficult system for those in the client's environment to learn. The small number of signs, the iconicity of many signs, and the logical basis of the system should aid in rapid acquisition by non-impaired adults.

When. A number of the simple, iconic signs (PANTS, CUP) could be taught to a young child or client with cognitive development at about the sensorimotor Stage 5 or 6. Some of the more academic signs (e.g., letters, numbers, time) could be taught if and when the client demonstrated readiness.

How. Duffy recommends that the trainer initially teach from a wheelchair because several of the signs involve touching a part of the wheelchair (WHEELCHAIR, K). In addition, for clients who are in wheelchairs, this will provide an appropriate model of positioning. Other teaching procedures follow general sign training methods, with adaptations made according to the client's physical limitations.

Where. Duffy has prepared the following materials related to this sign system: a text describing the need and the project and presenting all 471 signs, with illustrations where necessary; a 10-minute slide presentation including 72 slides, an 18-page script, and a cassette tape; and a short videotape demonstrating use of the system with three physically handicapped clients. The text and the slide set are available through the University of Nevada, Las Vegas, library.[8] The videotape is available from Laurel Duffy.[9]

Discussion and summary. Duffy's System currently consists of 471 gross motor signs, with some signs supplemented by vocalizations. Although this system has not yet achieved widespread use, it does appear to be a viable choice for

---

8. Request the following call numbers: LC/4580/D8 (text) and LC/4580/D81 (script and slide set).
9. 3175 Marsford Place, Las Vegas, Nevada, 89102.

some physically handicapped clients. Rate of output would likely be slow due to the necessity in many cases, of producing several gestures to encode one concept. However, this feature also makes the system more applicable to the physically handicapped since a relatively small number of gross motor movements are combined to form 471 signs. Thus, for clients who are motorically unable to use a more extensive gestural system such as Signed English, this could be a very useful system.

Gestural Language Codes

Gestural language codes are systems which allow the user to code a specific language, such as English or Finnish. Amer-Ind, to be described later in this chapter, would not fit into this category since it does not code a language. In the systems included here gestures represent segments of a spoken language (e.g., phonemes, syllables) or a written language (letters of the alphabet). For each of these gestural language codes the structure is that of the language it represents. The codes presented in this section are intended to represent English or other languages based on the Roman alphabet.[10] Modifications can be made for applying the codes to other languages, such as Russian.

Fingerspelling

What. Fingerspelling is a code which uses 26 distinct handshapes to represent the 26 letters of the Roman alphabet, as illustrated in figure 8-2. Thus the major parameter to be considered is configuration, although motion is important for the letters J and Z. A left-handed manual alphabet has been developed (Chen 1968; 1971), in which the gestures depict English letters as much as possible. Wilbur (1979) notes that fingerspelling is slow in comparison to signing or speech.

Moores (1980) reports that the use of fingerspelling as a tool in deaf education has been documented as far back as 1620. Simultaneous use of speech and fingerspelling is referred to as the *Rochester Method* in the United States and *neo-oralism* in the Soviet Union.

Regarding the execution of fingerspelling, Wilbur notes that skilled fingerspellers form words as units rather than as simple sequences of letters. This may create a perceptual problem for the message receiver because the center letters of a word may be assimilated to the surrounding letters and the formation of the letters may be blurred. Thus she asserts that one must make successive guesses regarding what is being perceived, much as one does in speechreading. A thorough knowledge of the grammar of the language is required in order to narrow the possible choices of the words being presented.

Why. Moores (1980) reports that " . . . investigators comparing fingerspelling with oral-only programs and with oral-manual programs consistently favor the use of fingerspelling with speech but without signs" (p. 42). He reviews several studies concerning this issue, all conducted with deaf or hearing-

---

10. The Roman alphabet is the basis for languages such as English, French, and Italian.

Figure 8-2
The American Manual Alphabet.

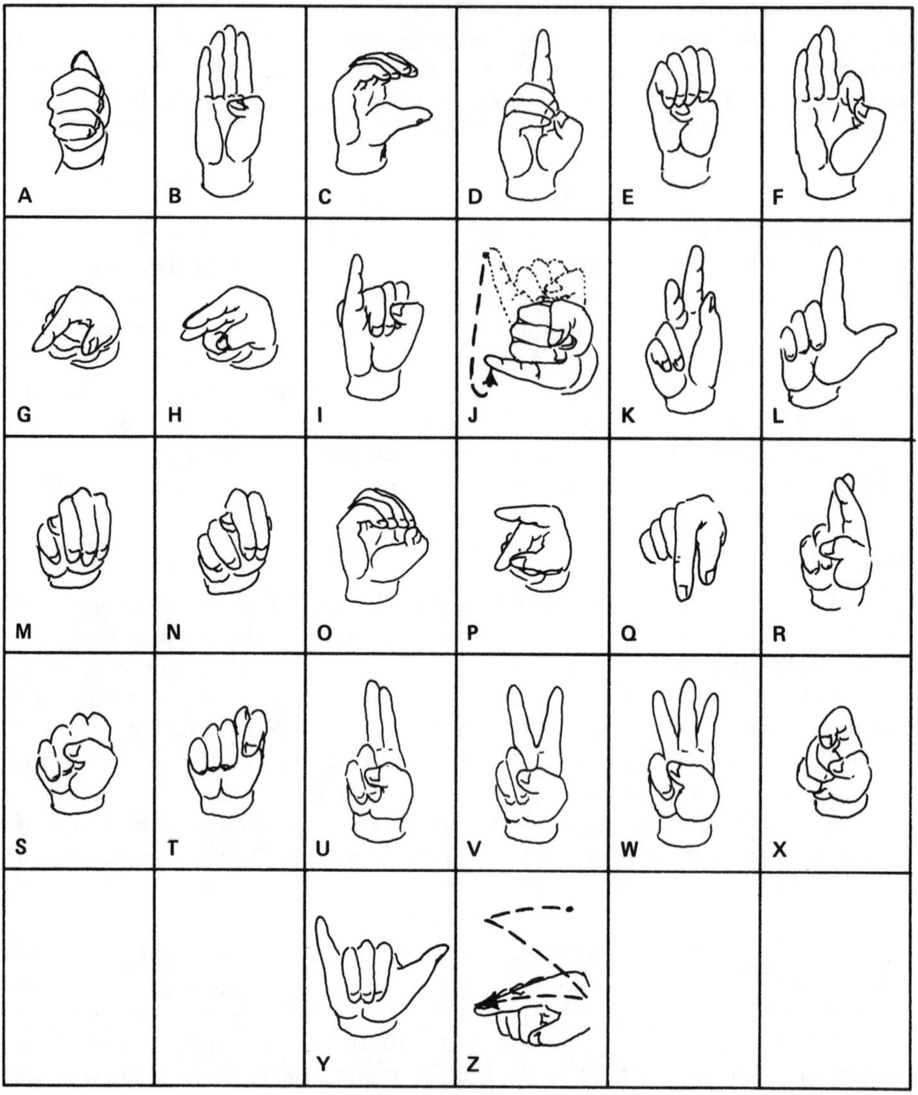

A	B	C	D	E	F
G	H	I	J	K	L
M	N	O	P	Q	R
S	T	U	V	W	X
		Y	Z		

Reprinted with permission from University Park Press (Christopher, 1976).

impaired subjects. The findings support use of fingerspelling to improve skills such as written language, reading, and speechreading.

Fingerspelling is also used widely by deaf persons as a link between sign language or sign systems and English. For example, proper nouns and words not represented in the sign language may be fingerspelled.

Fingerspelling is also relatively easy to learn by those who already know how to spell; in fact, it is a code learned by many adolescents to serve as a private communication system after they have outgrown "Pig Latin." Thus many adults working with the severely communication handicapped will already have learned the 26 basic handshapes, although extensive practice will be required to develop fluency in the system.

Since it can be readily learned by clients with good motoric and spelling capabilities (e.g., laryngectomees), fingerspelling could be an excellent choice for an interim system (e.g., while learning esophageal speech) or as a back-up system (e.g., on days when the client has a cold).

Although literature reports have not documented this, it is also feasible to use fingerspelling as a supplemental system. Beukelman and Yorkston (1977) had their dysarthric clients point to the first letter of each word they uttered on an alphabet-numbered board. The same procedure could be used with fingerspelling; that is, a client having intelligibility problems could fingerspell the first letter of every word spoken, or of those words which were unclear to the listener. This could also result in a slightly reduced speech rate, which might further facilitate intelligibility.

Who. Fingerspelling has several basic requirements for input and/or output:
1. *Good motoric control of one hand*—it requires small, rapid movements with a considerably greater degree of motoric coordination than signing (Wilbur 1979);
2. *Ability to spell*—the client must encode and decode words that have not been memorized;
3. *Good visual discrimination skills*—letters are often blurred together during production;
4. *High level of cognitive development*—cognitive stages range from late preoperations to early concrete operations (Chapman and Miller 1980).

Moores (1980) reports that fingerspelling is widely used with deaf children in the Soviet Union but employed in only a handful of programs in the United States. Reports of successful use of fingerspelling with other non-vocal populations are rare, although Chen (1971) did use a manual alphabet combined with manual sign gestures for several clients, including aphasics, dysarthrics, and laryngectomees. Potential candidates, in addition to the deaf, would seem to be those who had developed good language and spelling skills and had normal use of at least one hand. Potential audiences can learn the basic code quickly; however, as Wilbur (1979) points out, it is difficult to perceive and read fingerspelling produced at a fast rate. It may be necessary for the client to fingerspell very slowly, which could interfere with the communication process.

When. Wilbur (1979) suggests that, "Although a child may combine two or three signs into an utterance at about 18 months, fingerspelling does not emerge until much later" (p. 223). This is not surprising since spelling skills are used in fingerspelling. Thus fingerspelling would generally not be introduced, at least as an output system, until the client has developed or demonstrates a readiness to develop spelling skills.

How. Since fingerspelling is typically introduced at a higher cognitive stage than signing, it may be feasible to use a second language approach utilizing formal training with emphasis on drill and practice. Materials and guidelines for teaching in this manner are presented in Babbini (1974a and b). As an input mode fingerspelling may be introduced in a more natural manner, paired with speech.

Where. Materials for learning or teaching fingerspelling are available through the Gallaudet College Bookstore and the National Association of the Deaf (see Appendix C).

Discussion and summary. Fingerspelling may be considered a deceptively simple system. Thus, while it is easy for the unimpaired to learn the 26 handshapes, they may be quite difficult for those with poor motoric control. The difficulty in receiving messages transmitted at high rates of speed may also be a problem, as the normal flow of speech and intonation are interrupted. However, for non-vocal clients (who are not attempting to speak and fingerspell simultaneously) this may not be as much of a problem. If the major goal is communication of basic wants and needs, a fairly slow rate may be sufficient. To summarize, fingerspelling may have a limited population of potential users due to the motoric and spelling capabilities required. However, for those clients who can learn it fingerspelling may be extremely useful. It may serve them as a communication system or, more likely, as a supplemental system to be used with a specific audience or under certain conditions.

Gestural Morse Code

Silverman (1980) suggests that the dots and dashes of the Morse Code, which represent letters and numbers, can be signalled gesturally. For example, the code can be signalled by " . . . producing a single gesture at two durations (e.g., a brief eye blink for a dot and one approximately twice as long for a dash)" (p. 80). This system could be adapted to meet the needs of the severely physically handicapped client who is basically intact cognitively. Silverman notes that this system would be especially appropriate for clients who had learned Morse Code prior to the onset of their condition (e.g., a client with myasthenia gravis who was an amateur radio operator).

Cued Speech

What. Cued Speech was developed for use with and among the hearing-impaired. In this system one hand is used to supplement the information visible on the lips to make a spoken message clearly understood by the speechreader. Eight handshapes and four hand positions are used in synchronization with natural speech as illustrated in Figure 8-3. The intended result is a visually different pattern for each syllable of the spoken language. Thus "Syllables which look alike on the lips look different on the hand. Syllables which look alike on the hand look different on the lips" (Henegar and Cornett 1971, p. 14). It is the combination of cues and lip (oral) patterns that allows the decoder to gain meaning, as " . . . the hand serves only to identify a group of three or four sounds that are clearly different from each other on the lips" (Henegar and Cornett, p. 14). For example, one handshape allows the decoder to narrow the choice of consonants to /h/, /s/

Figure 8-3
Handshapes and hand positions for Cued Speech
(Henegar and Cornett 1971)

CHART I: Cues for English Vowels

	Group I (base position)	Group II (larynx)	Group III (chin)	Group IV (mouth)
open	[aː] (fäther) (gŏt)	[a] (thăt)	[ɔː] (fôr) (ought)	
flattened-relaxed	[ʌ] (but) [ð] (the)	[i] (ĭs)	[e] (gĕt)	[iː] (fēet) (meat)
rounded	[ou] (nōte) (boat)	[u] (gŏŏd) (put)	[uː] (blue) (fōōd)	[ə] (ûrn) (hĕr)

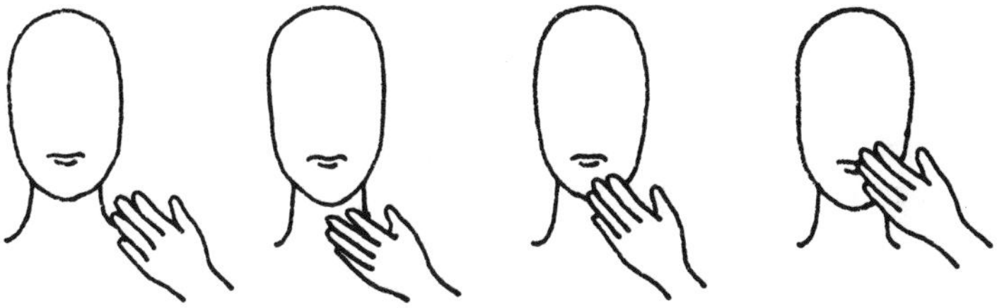

CHART III: Cues for English Consonants

T Group*	H Group	D Group	ng Group	L Group	K Group	N Group	G Group
t	h	d	(ng)	l	k	n	g
m	s	p	y (you)	sh	v	b	j
f	r	zh	ch	w	th (the)	hw	th (thin)

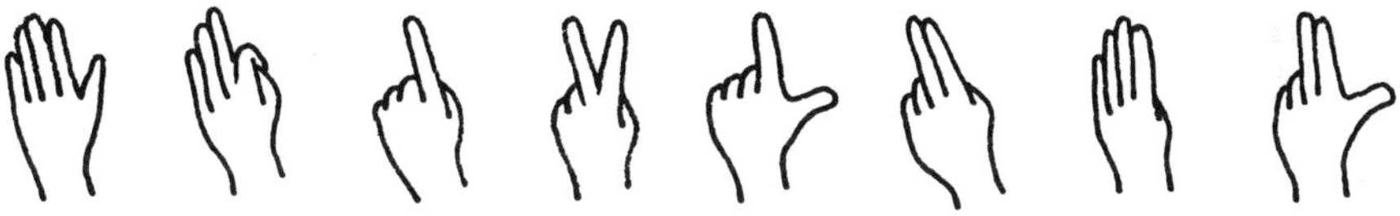

*Note: The T group cue is also used with an isolated vowel—that is, an initial vowel not run in with a final consonant from the preceding syllable.

and /r/. Observing the speaker's oral patterns will enable the decoder to determine which of those three consonants is actually being produced. Vowels are cued by hand positions plus information at the lips. Thus consonant-vowel pairs (e.g., "ma") may be represented by superimposing the consonant hand shape on the vowel hand position, resulting in increased efficiency of movement. Another example of efficiency in the system is its capability of indicating intonation to some extent through altering the inclination or orientation of the hand forming the cue. Similarly, increased stress can be indicated by increased emphasis of the hand movement while making the cue for the stressed syllable. All of these factors should combine to yield a higher rate of speed than fingerspelling. In addition, silent letters are not cued and digraphs such as "ch" (chair), "sh" (share), and "ph" (phone), which must be spelled out in fingerspelling, are represented by a single cue in Cued Speech. For example, production of the word "telephone" requires nine configurations in fingerspelling (T-E-L-E-P-H-O-N-E), but only four (te-lu-foe-n) in Cued Speech. Thus Cornett asserts that

> The simultaneous use of hand positions for vowel cues and hand configurations as consonant cues results in a speed theoretically twice that of fingerspelling for words such as *banana*, in which each vowel phoneme is preceded by a single consonant. For words with consecutive (sounded) consonants, such as *tremble*, the theoretical speed is somewhere between one and two times that of fingerspelling (1967, p. 6).

However, as Moores (1969) points out, fingerspelling requires only the hand configuration, as the hand stays in one position, with little or no movement. For Cued Speech the configuration and position change, and movement is required to get from one position to another. This could somewhat reduce the assumed speed advantage of Cued Speech over fingerspelling. The reduction would likely be slight, as the four positions for cuing are in a concentrated area near the mouth. Consequently, very little time would elapse in moving from one cue position to another. In summary, the various methods of achieving efficiency in Cued Speech should yield a greater speed for Cued Speech than for fingerspelling. This issue, we hope, will be resolved by research in the near future.

It should be noted that *cues* are not the equivalent of *signs*, as cues do not have meaning in isolation. With regard to sign language, Cornett (1974; 1979) notes that Cued Speech is not a replacement for sign language among the deaf. He suggests that deaf persons learn sign language (ASL) before puberty, if possible, because it still appears to be the most natural method of communication within the deaf community.

An Autocuer[11] is currently under development, sponsored by the National Aeronautics and Space Administration (NASA) and supported by the Veterans Administration (Prosthetics Research Unit) [Beadles and Brown 1979]. It is a device designed to provide the wearer with the equivalent of cues of manually Cued Speech. Thus the speaker would not need to learn Cued Speech. The device operates automatically from the sound of the speaker's voice. Cues are then seen as a visual image in the air, approximately four feet in front of the wearer. By positioning his or her head, the wearer can "place" the cues on the face of the speaker near the lips. Although many technical difficulties remain, preliminary field testing appears promising (Autocuer Feasibility Study 1979).

To summarize, Cued Speech is a method of making a spoken language (English, French, Italian) visible. Thus it is a tool not a language or a sign system.

Why. The primary purpose of Cued Speech is to aid in verbal language development (Cornett 1975) through providing a method of clear communi-

---

11. Contact the Cued Speech Program, Gallaudet College.

cation. Since Cued Speech parallels spoken English, with words cued as they are spoken, the potential for learning English is great. It is also suggested that Cued Speech will help the hearing-impaired child to acquire an accurate mental model of the spoken language, which should assist in the future development of speechreading skills (Cornett 1975). Cornett (1978) also asserts that Cued Speech will aid in providing a background for reading and writing, through development of a language base and, theoretically, the same coded word attack skills that a hearing child possesses. Finally, Cued Speech may be helpful in speech production training. The client may be instructed, through use of Cued Speech, where to place sounds that have been learned in articulation training. Thus the client's errors would be errors of execution, not of intention (Cornett, personal communication, as quoted from Alexander Graham Bell). That is, the client would know where sounds should be placed, even if he or she were unable to produce those sounds correctly. Thus Cued Speech may also be useful in clarifying pronunciation of difficult words.

Cued Speech may serve a variety of purposes, depending on the needs of the client. Cornett (1975) suggests that it is a self-limiting system. For example, hearing-impaired clients who have intelligible speech would not need to cue to hearing communication partners but could continue to receive Cued Speech, particularly for transmission of new or difficult information. Similarly, hard-of-hearing children would ignore those cues that they did not need. On the other hand, hearing clients with voice production disorders would need the system for output only. Thus a continuum of use can be envisioned regarding both production and comprehension of Cued Speech.

Who. As noted, Cued Speech was designed for use with the hearing-impaired and has been used primarily with that population. Requirements for application of Cued Speech with the hearing-impaired and other populations, as an input and output system, would include the following:

1. *Moderate motoric control of at least one hand,* sufficient to produce basic handshapes in one of four positions;
2. *Good visual acuity and discrimination,* for decoding the cues and lip information, if it is to be used as an input system;
3. *Good oral-motor control,* as production requires cues plus information at the lips;
4. *Cognitive development of at least sensorimotor Stage 5 or 6.*

Each of these requirements should be considered in view of the client's ultimate, not present, capabilities. For example, use of Cued Speech should not be negated because the client is currently not producing sounds in appropriate sequences or at appropriate places of articulation. However, the client should have assumed oral-motor capacity to accomplish the sounds after training. Therefore, Cued Speech would not be recommended for dysarthric or apraxic clients.

It is not clear yet what cognitive level is required, as use of the system has been reported thus far only with clients having essentially normal intelligence. It appears that this system would require higher level cognitive skills than, for example, a sign system. In sign systems the gesture (sign) can be related directly to the referent, while in Cued Speech a single gesture (cue) may be used for several different referents (e.g., "ham," "roof," and "sit" are cued the same), and the client must pair the cue with the oral pattern to obtain a label for the referent. Thus Cued Speech may initially be more difficult than a sign system, which may be introduced via a small number of highly iconic signs. Case studies document the use of Cued Speech with infants as young as seven months (Cornett, personal communication). However, since cues must be combined with information on the lips, it is impossible to determine at what point and to what extent these infants were reponding to the added information of the cues.

Based on these requirements, several populations would appear to be potential targets for use of Cued Speech. The hearing-impaired and deaf would be the most likely candidates, as discussed earlier. Several research studies involving hearing-impaired clients (Clarke and Ling 1976; Nicholls 1979; Rupert 1969) have demonstrated success in terms of skills such as increased comprehension of sentences and key words within sentences. In addition, the prolonged use of Cued Speech did not prevent or depress the development of auditory or auditory/visual (speechreading) skills. Other populations that could theoretically benefit from use of Cued Speech for output include those in which clients possess the requirements listed earlier but lack normal voicing. This would include, for example, laryngectomees and others with aphonia, spastic dysphonics, and clients with progressive disorders such as myasthenia gravis, yielding a very weak voice. Cued Speech might also be helpful, at least as an input mode, for those rare clients who exhibit difficulty in perceiving speech sounds, labeled acoustic agnosia.

When. Ideally, Cued Speech should be initiated as soon as the handicapping condition (e.g., deafness, laryngectomy) occurs or is diagnosed. Thus parents and teachers may begin cuing to young infants. However, infants or pre-schoolers would not be expected or required to begin cuing initially. Henegar and Cornett (1971) note that ". . .usually, a child spends several months in the initial receptive stage before he reacts expressively, even after he demonstrates a great deal of receptive understanding" (p. 75).

How. As indicated throughout the preceding sections, Cued Speech can be used as an input or output system, although it is designed to serve primarily as input with hearing-impaired children. For the client developing language, especially the young child, the initial focus will be on input. Henegar and Cornett stress that Cued Speech should not be *taught* to young deaf children; rather, they should be exposed to it naturally, much as young hearing children are exposed to spoken language in conjunction with meaningful events and actions. It is recommended that brief work sessions be carried out in addition to a variety of activities such as puppetry, games, and so forth.

For the deaf client who is older when Cued Speech is introduced, a two-way approach is recommended. Cued Speech should be used for communication and taught as a system. Henegar and Cornett suggest that Cued Speech be taught as much as possible through the language system the client is already using, whether that is sign language, written language, a picture language, or oral language. However, for the older child with a limited grasp of written language and speech sounds, it may be necessary to follow the suggestions for the preschool child, adjusting activities to the age level of the client.

Hearing parents, teachers, and hearing clients who possess an intact language system (e.g., laryngectomees) could also use a systematic training approach composed of drills and exercises. The length of time it takes to learn Cued Speech in this way naturally depends to some extent on factors such as motivation and amount of practice. It is suggested that a background in phonics might decrease learning time (Henegar and Cornett 1971). The number of cues that must be learned is quite small—only eight hand shapes and four hand positions. These can be learned in a matter of hours, but learning to use and comprehend them takes considerably longer. A general assertion is that "Most parents who use CS consistently (no matter what their cuing speed at first) find that within 6–10 months they are able to cue at the speed at which they speak to the deaf child" (*Cued Speech News* 1979, p. 5).

It is important to note that, like other systems which represent letters or sounds (such as fingerspelling, braille, Morse Code), Cued Speech has limited usefulness until the entire system is learned. That is, one cannot select a core vocabulary of five much needed cues and teach the client to use them to gain basic needs, as can be done with signs. This would seem to negate use of this system with the severely retarded. However, it is possible to have a limited utilization of the system, at least for input purposes. For example, Cornett (1967) suggests that a deaf person could train hearing co-workers to cue vowels only in order to help clarify their input. This assumes that the client knows the entire system. Thus Cued Speech, while having its primary usefulness as a complete system, could have some limited applications.

Where. Further information about Cued Speech, or assistance in learning and using it, may be obtained through the Office of Cued Speech Programs (see Gallaudet College, Appendix C). Training materials and suggestions are provided in the following sources: *Cued Speech Handbook for Parents* (Henegar and Cornett 1971; see Appendix A) and *Cued Speech Handbook for Teachers* (Lykos 1971; see Appendices A and B).

Discussion and summary. Cued Speech is a relatively recent augmentative communication system (Cornett 1967). The information reviewed in this chapter appears to indicate its success in use with deaf clients. Moores (1969) and Wilbur (1976) raise several objections to the use of Cued Speech, each of which will be considered. The first objection is that Cornett fails to distinguish between *language* and *speech* and assumes that language is learned by imitation. However, in Henegar and Cornett (1971) language and speech, and their relationship to Cued Speech, are carefully delineated. In addition, the authors stress that children will not learn Cued Speech merely by imitating adult cuers. They assert that, in addition to cuing every word that is spoken, parents must help the child associate the visible language with the objects, ideas, and concepts that they are talking about.

The second set of objections relates to *phonetic problems* in the Cued Speech system. Wilbur (1976) notes that no guidelines are set for helping the adult cuer determine which phonetic distinctions are important and which are not. Further, it is suggested that since Cued Speech is intrinsically tied to the sound system, it will have little or no transfer to reading. Although several case studies purport to show that Cued Speech does aid in developing reading skills (Henegar and Cornett 1971), hard evidence of this result is currently lacking. It would appear that the lack of one-to-one correspondence between the phonetically-based cues and traditional orthography in written speech would be no more difficult a transition than that between spoken and written versions of words.

The question is raised about *facility with respect to phonetics*. Wilbur (1976) cautions that, given the difficulty of phonetic transcription, adult cuers may not be able to determine which phonetic distinctions are important and may not be able to accurately cue what is spoken. Again, research is needed to answer this question. This issue of phonetic competence would be important also with respect to speech synthesis, to be discussed in Chapter 9.

A final concern regarding Cued Speech expressed by Wilbur (1976) is its *effect on lipreading*. He cites a study by Børrild (1972) which reported that students trained in a Danish mouth-hand system were ". . .rather helpless when it comes to lipreading" (p. 237). Two points should be noted regarding this concern. First, Cued Speech does not follow the same principles as the Danish mouth-hand system. In the Danish system some sounds may be identified from the hand gesture alone, so that attention to the lips is not needed. Second, use of Cued Speech has not been found to prevent the development of auditory or auditory/visual (speechreading) cues, as demonstrated by Nicholls (1979).

In summary, though it has not been extensively used or researched, Cued Speech does appear to have promise with various hearing but handicapped populations (e.g., clients with voicing problems but normal intelligence) as well as with the hearing-impaired. It does not appear appropriate for severely cognitively impaired, dysarthric, or apraxic clients.

Other Gestural Communication Systems

A number of gestural systems do not fit into any of the categories described earlier. That is, they are not sign languages or sign systems nor do they gesturally code a language. These systems range from the informal use of pantomime or natural gestures to the more formal use of a codified gestural system such as Amer-Ind (Skelly and Schinsky 1979). Only two of these systems, Amer-Ind and pantomime, will be described in detail. The remainder of these systems will be covered briefly, along with suggestions regarding sources of further information.

A number of communication systems, such as the Tadoma Method and the Glove Method, have been developed primarily for use with the deaf-blind. These are not gestural systems in the sense that they have been described in this book. For example, the Tadoma Method involves having the deaf-blind person decode speech by placing one or both hands on the face of the speaker in a prescribed manner (Norton et al. 1977). Coverage of these systems is beyond the scope of this book. For those interested in further information, Jensema (1979) describes a number of communication systems for the deaf-blind.

Natural gestures and pointing

Hamre-Nietupski et al. (1977) note that most nonhandicapped persons use body movements in communication. Many of these are generally understood gestures such as shaking the head from side to side to indicate "no." These are referred to in this section as *natural gestures*. Hamre-Nietupski et al. (1977) list three major advantages of using natural gestures:

1. Gestures are usually understood by teachers, parents, or other persons *without any specialized training* who wish to communicate with the student;
2. Gestures often involve gross motor movements, which can be important when selecting a non-verbal mediator for use with severely motorically and/or visually impaired students;
3. Since the communicator primarily uses his/her own body to communicate with generally understood gestures, extra equipment is unnecessary (p. 100).

Natural gestures are limited in comparison to standard sign languages or systems, but they may be useful as an interim system or as a supplement to another communication mode. For example, a severely dysarthric child might utilize natural gestures to establish context when a communication breakdown occurs by motioning for a person to come and remove an obstacle in front of his or her wheelchair. Natural gestures could also serve as an introduction to sign training.

Hamre-Nietupski et al. provide a list of more than 160 generally understood gestures plus curricular strategies for teaching production and comprehension of those gestures.

Pantomime (Mime)

What. Mime is an art form based on the technique of conveying information or ideas through pantomime. In this chapter we will refer to the technique used with the severely handicapped as *pantomime* to distinguish it from the art form, *mime*. Silverman (1980) notes several major differences between pantomime and other gestural systems, such as ASL or Amer-Ind:

1. It uses the musculature of the entire body, not only that (or primarily that) of the upper extremities;
2. The gestures tend to be dynamic rather than static;
3. More gestures usually are needed to convey a message than with the manual systems;
4. The gestures are an analogue of the message—that is, they are a dramatization of the message. (p. 72)

Another difference we have noted is the variety of ways that an event or object can be pantomimed. This is possible because pantomime is truly concept-based, unlike sign systems and gestural language codes.

Why. Pantomime is a basic form of communication. It may be used to reach clients who are not able to communicate through the auditory-vocal mode. Thus, pantomime could have great potential as an input system for some clients. It may also function as a primary or secondary output system. Many clients who lack capability for vocal communication may use mimetic communication attempts spontaneously, though perhaps not very effectively. The goal of the communication specialist in that case would be to improve the client's techniques while perhaps helping him or her to develop more flexible long-term modes of communication. Pantomime would probably not be selected as the primary long-term approach due to its relative inefficiency and limited scope.

Pantomime has also been demonstrated to be successful in facilitating language development (Balick, Spiegel, and Greene 1976). Moreover, it has been noted that pantomime may be very rewarding as an augmentative approach for clients who must communicate through an external aid such as a word board. For example, one severely physically handicapped child reported that her portrayal of a cat during a mime workshop was the first time she had experienced success in communicating directly rather than through a communication aid.[12]

Who. It would appear that there are many legitimate instances of the use of pantomime as therapy, either directly, with mimes holding workshops or training sessions with handicapped persons, or indirectly, with mimes training professionals who work with the handicapped (special educators, speech-language pathologists). However, there are few reports of projects in which pantomime has been used in an on-going format as part of a comprehensive communication program. Literature reports demonstrate use of pantomime with clients in the following disability groups: mentally retarded (Balick et al. 1976), aphasic (Dalgaard, Newhoff, and Barnes 1979; Schlanger 1976; Schlanger, Geffner, and DiCarrado 1974), and cerebral palsied (Levett 1969, 1971). Pantomime has also been used, though perhaps less formally, with other populations, including mentally retarded adults, hearing-impaired children, and multi-handicapped children.[13]

The requirements for pantomime as a communication medium are more basic than those for many of the other gestural systems presented in this chapter. They include the following:

1. *Voluntary control over gross musculature,* in order to execute the necessary movements; less precise motoric control would be needed for conveying a message in pantomime than for most other gestural systems;
2. *Cognitive development at about the Stage 5 sensorimotor level;* however, for exploiting of pantomime in portraying sequences of behavior and abstract concepts, a higher level of cognitive development would be necessary;

---

12. Personal communication, Avner Eisenberg, professional old world clown and mime and instructor of workshops for handicapped children and their teachers.
13. Personal communication, Keith Clemens, Avner Eisenberg, Ronlin Foreman, Dr. E. Reid Gilbert, Jean St. John, professional mimes.

3. *A rich experimental background,* in order to have experiences to draw from; this is important if the client is to initiate topics for which pantomimic routines have not been taught.

Thus pantomime appears to have potential application across a broad age and disability range. It would seem especially appropriate for meeting the needs of clients with symbolic deficits, such as aphasics or the mentally retarded.

The audience for a client using pantomime would theoretically be unlimited. Most older children and adults could be expected to correctly interpret well-executed pantomime without training. The key words here are are *well-executed,* since the production of effective pantomime depends on cognitive, experiential, and physical factors discussed earlier. However, the focus would be primarily on training the client for better execution rather than training those in the environment to interpret.

When. Some basic mimetic routines could be taught to very young children, perhaps as young as one year of age. Pantomime could also be used as input with very young children. It would also seem possible to introduce pantomime to adventitiously non-vocal clients as soon as they become medically able to participate.

How. A variety of approaches have been used with the art of pantomiming. As always, the goals will dictate the training methods to some extent. If the goal is to have the client use pantomime as a communication system, either primary or supplementary, direct tactics may be used, such as teaching specific routines and aiding clients to develop and perfect their routines. Eisenberg (personal communication), who has had considerable experience in using mime with handicapped children, suggests that teaching be preceded by a performance by a professional mime; this will demonstrate to the client that mime (pantomime) can be effectively used to communicate information. It may also help motivate the client to learn and use pantomime. Although traditional techniques such as imitation and physical prompting would be useful in training for the use of pantomime, the emphasis would be on a more dynamic process, including movement sequences and coordination of body movements. It should also be helpful to teach clients how to use alternative strategies when initial pantomime routines are unsuccessful. This is especially useful with pantomime since there are a number of possible ways to convey information.

Strategies for using pantomime as a facilitator of language may differ somewhat from strategies focused on pantomime as a communication system. Pantomime may be used to facilitate areas of language development such as concepts (e.g., spatial relationships and time concepts), expressive language (e.g., having the client verbalize what the mime is doing or what he or she is pantomiming), and receptive language (e.g., moving from pantomime + picture + verbalization to recognition of picture from auditory label alone) [Balick et al. 1976; Dalgaard et al. 1979; Eisenberg, personal communication].

Although special training may not be needed to interpret pantomime, it is necessary to teach it effectively. Since pantomime involves the whole body, and is a dynamic process, learning it from a two-dimensional source such as a book is extremely difficult. It is recommended that a professional mime and a communication specialist work together in developing intervention programs, if possible. A number of courses and workshops in beginning mime are available through colleges, universities, and mime studios (see the *where* section).

Where. For addresses of mimes, mime classes, and mime workshops, the reader is directed to *The Mime Directory, Volume 1* (1977)[14], which is cross-referenced alphabetically and by region. Several addresses of mime workshops are also listed in Appendix C of this book (see Mime Workshops). For a listing of books, articles, and films on mime, the major source is *The Mime Directory, Volume 2* (1978). Several books on mime and related arts may be helpful as references: *The Other Side of the Elephant: Theatre Activities for Classroom Learning* (Allen 1977), *Mime: A Playbook of Silent Fantasy* (Hamblin 1978), and *The Mime Book* (Kipnis 1976). Those references (with the exception of Allen) focus on the pure art form of mime; applications of the art form for therapeutic use must be made by the individual communication specialist. One reference which provides a specific protocol for use of pantomime as a facilitative technique in therapy is Dalgaard et al. (1979). That paper presents ". . .an auditory and verbal task continuum for a pantomime-centered aphasia intervention program" (p. 1). Descriptions and ordering information for the preceding references may be found in Appendix A.

Limited hospital or center-based systems

Several limited gestural systems have been developed at various hospitals, nursing homes, or residential centers throughout the country. These provide users with a small number of gestures for basic needs such as COME HERE, I'M HOT, OR I HAVE PAIN. Silverman (1980) describes several of these gestural systems. Typically, the systems require only moderate control of one hand. Since the number of gestures is limited (often less than 20), persons in the environment can learn them quickly. A chart illustrating the gestures may be displayed in a prominent place, such as over a patient's bed. These limited systems may be very useful as interim systems, for example, for a client who is too ill to learn or use a full communication system. They may also be useful as supplements to other systems, such as symbolic systems. That is, these gestures could be used when the communication aid is temporarily unavailable. For further information on these systems, the reader is referred to Fristoe (1975) or Silverman (1980).

Amer-Ind Gestural Code

As the name implies, Amer-Ind is neither a language nor a sign system. It does not have a linguistic base, but is, rather, a code or a signal system. It is based on universal American Indian Hand Talk, which was used by a variety of Indian tribes to accommodate their large number of spoken languages.

---

14. The two volumes of *The Mime Directory* are currently out of print. We recommend obtaining them through interlibrary loan.

Recently, Hand Talk has been adapted to serve the needs of non-vocal clients, resulting in the development of Amer-Ind. American Indian Hand Talk has been authenticated, to the extent that this is possible, through records written by non-Indians in limited contact with American Indian cultures (Clark 1885; Mallery 1881) and through the memories of still-living Hand Talk users around the country. Dr. Madge Skelly and her associates have also modernized the code, eliminating signals which are no longer applicable and adding signals needed to accommodate the changes of twentieth-century life. The new signals have been developed on the same principles as the ancient signals, such as concrete reference and ease of interpretation, and they have been submitted to one or more tribal elders for approval. Skelly is credited with being the primary force in developing Amer-Ind. She is part American Indian and was taught Hand Talk as a child by her Iroquois relatives.

Skelly and Schinsky (1979) describe several primary characteristics of Amer-Ind:

1. It is *nonlinguistic*; thus, it should not be interpreted by exact translation;
2. It is *concept-oriented*, yielding what is described as "kinetic photographs of ideas" (p. 110);
3. It is *action-oriented* rather than nominally organized, although clarifying signals can be used if necessary to indicate an object or person;
4. It is *reality-oriented* and conveys messages through a string of related signaled concepts;
5. It is *telegraphic*, using the fewest possible signals for encoding.

Since signals represent concepts rather than words, Amer-Ind signals are discussed in terms of a *repertoire* instead of a vocabulary. The current clinically tested signal repertoire includes 250 concept labels.[15] Each concept embraces several English words since Amer-Ind does not follow signal-for-word translation. For example, the concept label QUIET, made by holding the index finger of the hand to the lips, has the following synonyms: calm, dormant, hush, low [noise], mute, noiseless, serene, silence, silent, still, tranquil. The intended meaning is determined through context. Therefore, the repertoire has an English vocabulary equivalent to approximately 2500 words. In addition, this vocabulary equivalent may be extended through the process of *agglutination*, to be described later. It should be noted that, just as there is no one correct word which translates a signal, a specific concept can be indicated through use of one of several signals. For example, while NO can be interpreted as denial, disagreement, negation, or refusal, the basic concept of negation can be coded by signals with the following concept labels: NO, REJECT, STOP, or DEFY (Skelly and Schinsky).

Eighty percent of the clinical repertoire can be executed using only one hand. Most of the remainder can be adapted for one-handed execution, using suggestions provided by Skelly and Schinsky. For the eleven signals which cannot be readily adapted, Skelly and Schinsky suggest use of alternative signals.

---

15. This text follows the convention of printing Amer-Ind concept labels in capital letters, with the series of synonyms for each label printed in lower-case letters.

Skelly and Schinsky also describe several features of transmitting Amer-Ind:

1. *Transposition*, the process of encoding in signals;
2. *Clarification*, the methods designed to assist signalers having difficulty in transmitting messages; for example, a flat hand thrust can distinguish object from action, and the user may use the signal for PAST or FUTURE to indicate that action is not in the present; several other methods are suggested, including slowing the rate, adding information, and trying an alternative signal;
3. *Agglutination*, the principle which allows invention of new ways to express a concept for which a definite signal does not exist; typically, a string of signals is used, beginning with the most general and adding further information; examples are:

    teacher   = PERSON + GIVES + KNOWLEDGE (know)
    insane   = BRAIN + REJECT, or
                   BRAIN + FLY + DISTANT
    ambulance = DRIVE + PAIN + SHELTER + FAST

4. *Execution*, the way in which the signals are produced; signals may be static (the hand position is held, such as HIGH), kinetic (a specific movement is required, such as FISH), or repetitive (a specified movement is repeated three times, such as SMART); in addition, there are three criteria for effective signaling: precision, consistency, and completion.

In summary, Amer-Ind is a gestural code based on American Indian Hand Talk and intended for use with non-vocal clients of various etiologies.

Why. Amer-Ind appears appropriate for a variety of purposes relative to severely handicapped clients. Skelly and Schinsky assert that:

> The American Indian Code's low symbolic level, ease of acquisition, flexibility, speed, lack of grammatical structure and rules, and use of concrete, demonstrable referents, which enable the viewer to interpret without formal instruction, make it acceptable to the use of many patients who are unable to speak (p. 7)

It would appear to be an especially appropriate system for clients who are unable to learn other gestural systems or who are uninterested in other systems due to the limited audiences they permit. Amer-Ind seems especially useful as an interim communication system due to the transparency of signals and the relative ease of acquisition. Also, the conceptual base of Amer-Ind and the process of agglutination give the user, after learning a small number of signals (250 or less), the equivalent of a more extensive English vocabulary than most other gestural systems. These aspects, plus its action-oriented base, also make Amer-Ind useful as an input system. Finally, there is some evidence that use of Amer-Ind serves to facilitate both language and speech (Skelly and Schinsky, pp. 30–37). Thus Amer-Ind has the potential of serving a variety of functions for severely handicapped clients. Some of the potential limitations of the system will be considered in the discussion and summary section.

Who. Skelly and Schinsky list several prerequisite skills for introduction of

Amer-Ind: eye contact, attending, physical imitation, pointing, and shaping skills. Other requirements for use of Amer-Ind include:

1. *Moderate degree of motor control of one hand,* to allow execution of a limited number of hand configurations;
2. *Good range of motion in one arm,* for executing signals at various locations and with various movements;
3. *Sensorimotor Stage 5 or 6 intelligence.*

Amer-Ind has been used with varying degrees of success by persons having a wide range of disorders, including severe dysphonia, severe dysarthria, oral-verbal apraxia, severe and profound mental retardation, surgical deficits such as total glossectomy, total laryngectomy, and laryngectomized total glossectomy, and aphasia.[16] Skelly and Schinsky suggest that Amer-Ind may be used appropriately with clients from any of these populations. However, treatment approaches would differ, depending on the individual client's capacity for auditory reception of language and other factors. Their division yields three main groupings:

1. *Intact auditory comprehension of language,* in which the client retains skills such as normal symbolism; examples of client populations which might fall into this category are those having severe dysphonia, severe dysarthria, oral-verbal apraxia, surgical deficits such as glossectomy or laryngectomy, and aphasia with adequate auditory reception of language;
2. *Impaired auditory reception of language,* in which the client has problems of symbolization and/or conceptualization; examples of clients in this group are moderate to severe adult aphasics and mildly to moderately mentally retarded;
3. *Developmental impairment,* particularly characterized by concept deficits; examples of clients include the severely and profoundly mentally retarded.

For many of these clients the use of Amer-Ind will be temporary. For example, Skelly and Schinsky report use of Amer-Ind as an interim system for dysphonics during voice rest and for other clients, such as glossectomies and oral-verbal apraxics, while speech and/or language skills are being improved. In addition, it may serve as a supplemental system for many clients, either when communication breakdowns occur (e.g., with aphasic or dysarthric clients) or when speech is temporarily unusable due to physical problems (e.g., at the end of the day for clients with myasthenia gravis).

It is also important to determine who can interpret Amer-Ind. Nine research projects involving signal transmission are reported by Skelly and Schinsky. Briefly, the general findings are listed below:

1. Untrained viewers (of videotapes depicting execution of signals) were able to correctly interpret at least 80 percent of the signal concepts;
2. Instruction generally adds only a slight percentage increment; how-

---

16. See Skelly and Schinsky (1979) for reviews of 10 projects, by a number of researchers, dealing with acquisition of Amer-Ind across a wide range of populations.

ever, those who had initial difficulty in interpreting signals (as judged by low pre-test scores) may benefit greatly from training;

3. Very brief professional video orientation for a patient-related population (wives, relatives, friends) increased performance of all but one participant to the 90 to 100 decile;

4. The use of kinesis (manual execution of the signal) may help in learning signal meaning.

Thus, it appears that brief signal training sessions, while perhaps not necessary, may be desirable in increasing signal comprehension abilities of potential communication partners.

How. A natural language approach, as used for example with American Sign Language, is not recommended for Amer-Ind. Skelly and Schinsky present three treatment programs designed for the three client groupings listed earlier. Treatment Program A is intended for clients with *intact auditory comprehension of language.* The overall goal of this program is "use of signals at a level equivalent to propositional speech" (p. 138). The client's knowledge and understanding of English (or Spanish or Russian) is employed in training sessions, with frequent explanations of aspects such as the rationale and processes. Modifications are suggested for use with oral-verbal apraxics since those clients are often hemiplegic and may require a slower treatment pace. Oral facilitation procedures are also suggested.

Treatment Program B is a nonverbal, nonlinguistic approach designed for clients having *impaired auditory reception of language.* Amer-Ind may be used as an input mode as well as an output mode for these clients. Sessions in this program are more structured and content is more repetitive. Repeated demonstrations using real-life objects in naturally-structured situations are used in place of artificially-structured drills. The basic goal for Program B is to establish the use of 50 signals for basic social and need (e.g., self-care) situations, plus 10 habituated signals (e.g., HELLO), in 12 to 24 weeks.

Treatment Program C is intended for use with *developmentally impaired* clients. The goal of this program is "communication of basic needs in Amer-Ind with approximately fifty signals acquired over a period of one year" (p. 174). Again the trainer communicates with the client only in signals. Programmed segments of five weeks each are used for training groups of five signals. However, the objective is different for each week of a segment. The progression of objectives is as follows: first week, imitation with necessary assistance; second week, unassisted imitation; third week, replication of the signal after the model is removed; fourth week, retrieval from memory; and fifth week, initiation of signals.

In summary, training approaches used with Amer-Ind are quite different from those used with sign systems, primarily because Amer-Ind, being a nonlinguistic code, differs widely from most sign systems. The high degree of transparency of signals in Amer-Ind and its action-oriented basis also affect the training methods used.

Skelly and Schinsky note that ". . . because Amer-Ind has been easily interpreted by untrained viewers, many persons have concluded that it may be just as easily acquired and executed by the uninstructed signaler" (p. 114).

They stress that this assumption is false, and that communication specialists planning to teach or do research projects on Amer-Ind must learn the system fully. They recommend that Amer-Ind be learned from an experienced, knowledgeable signaler.

When. This system has been widely used with adventitiously non-vocal clients such as oral-verbal apraxics, aphasics, and laryngectomees. For these clients Amer-Ind training would likely be initiated as soon as the need becomes evident (e.g., the client's prognosis for usable vocal language is poor) and a physician's approval is obtained. Skelly and Schinsky recommend delaying direct training until the prerequisite skills listed earlier have been mastered.

Where. The two primary references for this system are a text, *Amer-Ind Gestural Code Based on Universal American Hand Talk* (Skelly and Schinsky 1979; see Appendix B); and the video-tape *Amer-Ind Gestural Repertoire*, a 1979 updating of the *Amer-Ind Video Dictionary* and *American Indian Sign* (Veterans Administration Hospital, St. Louis, Missouri, 1975).

Discussion and summary. Amer-Ind is different from most of the gestural systems presented in this chapter because it is not linguistically based. However, its signals are also different from natural gestures since it is codified and allows extension through agglutination. The basic features of Amer-Ind, such as its low symbolic level, flexibility, and lack of grammatical structure, make Amer-Ind especially suitable for some clients but restricts its application with others. As Skelly and Schinsky (1979) point out, Amer-Ind is particularly useful for clients with symbol deficits. On the other hand, clients who have developed a high level of linguistic competence, but have lost (or never had) the physical capability for vocal production may elect not to use Amer-Ind because it does not have a linguistic base, lacks grammatical structure, and so forth. Perhaps the major advantage of Amer-Ind for many non-vocal clients would be its high degree of transparency. No other gestural system can be expected to achieve such high levels of propositional discourse which can be interpreted by the untrained viewer. This feature would make Amer-Ind especially appropriate as an augmentative system, for use while vocal skills are being improved or in conjunction with vocal language or even another non-verbal system. For example, the client with a structural deficit such as total laryngectomy plus total glossectomy may choose to learn Cued Speech for communicating with those who are willing to learn that system. However, the same individual might also wish to learn Amer-Ind for communicating with the large number of other people in the environment who do not know Cued Speech. Thus, just as Amer-Ind is a very flexible code, its use with non-vocal clients may be equally flexible.

Discussion and Summary

The preceding sections have focused on more than a dozen gestural communication systems. It may be difficult to select a single system to best meet the special needs of a particular client. In fact, it may not be necessary or desirable to choose a single system, either gestural or symbolic. As Alpert (1980) suggests, it might be useful to carry out trial therapy with two systems to determine which is optimal. Also, it is likely that, as Harris and Vanderheiden (1980) point out, a non-vocal client may require more than one system, with each to be used in different situations. Finally, a single system may not be sufficiently flexible to grow with a client. For example, natural gestures may be useful as an initial system but would be quite limiting to the client with highly developed receptive language skills.

Each of the gestural systems discussed included consideration of basic client capabilities and suggested target populations. In addition, potential target audiences were also described. Several other factors, such as motoric requirements and vocabulary size, are listed in table 8-1 for each of the major systems covered. Matching those system features to client capabilities and needs and environmental support should aid in selecting the optimal system(s) for an individual client.

Selecting Content

A number of strategies may be used in choosing the initial content for gestural communication programs. Fristoe and Lloyd (1979) compiled a list of 850 words which appeared in two or more sign manuals. They note that the signs with the highest frequency of occurrence (CHAIR/SIT, BED/SLEEP, GOOD, STOP, and TOILET/BATHROOM/POTTY) ". . .would seem to be taught more for the convenience of the trainers in controlling the client than for their interest value for the client" (p. 366). There are certainly a number of other strategies which should be considered in choosing the gestures to be included in a training program.

To some extent selection may be determined by the type of gestural system or gestural program to be used. For example, initial gestures for teaching Cued Speech are recommended in the training materials for that approach (Henegar and Cornett 1971; Lykos 1971), and Skelly and Schinsky (1979) suggest initial Amer-Ind concepts. A number of the general strategies (such as student preference and frequency of occurrence) discussed in Chapter 3 will be useful in selecting initial gestures. Several modifications or additional strategies will be presented in this section.

Fristoe and Lloyd (1980) suggest a *core lexicon* of signs which should be consulted in selecting initial content. This lexicon is presented in the content and form format suggested by Lahey and Bloom (1977; see table 3-2 in this book). The communication specialist might find it helpful to use this lexicon as a starting point in determining optimal gestures for a client.

A second general strategy which can be adapted for gestures is *ease of production*. This depends to some extent on the client's motoric capabilities, but normal motor development sequences can also be consulted. A physical or occupational therapist should be consulted if possible. For example, the following general suggestions are provided by a development occupational therapist (Dunn 1979). First, one should consider the *relationship of movement to the body*. In this regard Dunn suggests several factors which might affect ease of learning:

Table 8-1
Primary features of gestural communication systems.

Gestural Systems	Cognitive			Motoric					Interpretation			Linguistic Structure			Vocabulary Size		
	SensoriMotor	Early Pre-operations	Late Pre-Operations to concrete Operations	Gross	Moderate	Fine	One Hand	Two Hands	Transparent	Translucent	Opaque	Primarily English	Own Structure	Relatively Un-structured	Small (Under 1000)	Large (Over 1000)	Unlimited
American Sign Language	X				*	X		X	*	X	*		X			X	o
Signed English	X				*	X		X	*	X	*	X				X	o
Signing Exact English	X				*	X		X	*	X	*	X				X	o
Duffy's System	X			X				X	*	X				X	X		o
Fingerspelling			X		*	X	X			*	X	X					X
Cued Speech			X		*	X	X				X	X					X
Amer-Ind	X				X		*	X	X	*			X		X		
Natural gestures	X			X	*		*	X	X					X		X	
Pantomine	X			X	*		*	X	X					X	X		

X = indicates that the system primarily falls into this category.
* = indicates that the system has a large component or may be adapted to fit in this category.
o = indicates that a large vocabulary is available with the use of fingerspelling.
Transparent indicates that the gesture may be readily guessed (e.g., it is iconic).
Translucent indicates that the gesture may be understood once the basis or meaning is explained.
Opaque indicates that the gesture is arbitrary.

1. *Hand-mouth pattern*—this is basic and is practiced often (EAT)[17];

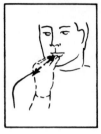

EAT

2. *Movement toward midline*—this is generally easier than movement away from midline (SHOE vs. FREE);

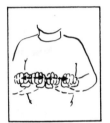

SHOE   FREE

3. *Touch signs are generally easier than non-touch signs*—Dunn (1979) suggests that for clients having difficulty non-touch signs may initially be modified to form touch signs, by the client's using the other hand as a base (AIRPLANE);

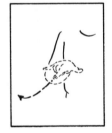

AIRPLANE

4. *Signs within vision are easier*—this is due to the relative lack of proprioceptive development in some young or handicapped clients (SUMMER may be difficult as the hand is at the forehead, out of vision);

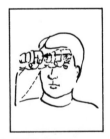

SUMMER

---

17. Signs are reprinted with permission from Christopher (1976), published by University Park Press.

5. *Palm orientation*—supinated forearm signs, with palm up, are more difficult than signs with palm down (WANT is more difficult than WONDERFUL).

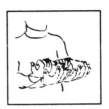 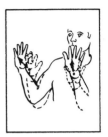

WANT   WONDERFUL

Dunn also suggests that *hand usage patterns* be considered in selecting early signs. The sequence of development for patterns relative to signing is as follows (from least to most difficult):

1. *Unilateral hand usage*—Dunn notes that there is some controversy regarding whether one-handed or two-handed signs are easier (EAT, GIVE); one-handed signs are assumed to be easier;

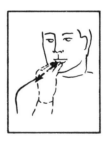 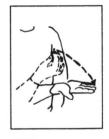

EAT   GIVE

2. *Bilateral hand usage*—this involves the same movement of both hands (WANT,SAD);

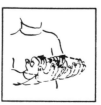 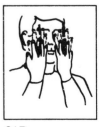

WANT   SAD

3. *Dominant-assistor pattern*—one hand stabilizes and the other acts (JUMP, WASH);

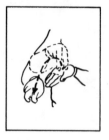 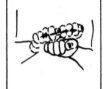

JUMP   WASH

4. *Reciprocal pattern*—the hands do opposite movements (BICYCLE); clients often turn this into a bilateral or dominant-assistor pattern.

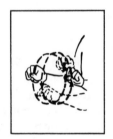

BICYCLE

A third motor component to be considered is the *handshape*. Again, Dunn suggests a sequence of development from simple to complex:

1. *Whole hand*—all digits perform the same action (EAT);

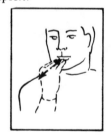

EAT

2. *Thumb isolation*—the thumb alone is differentiated (B,C);

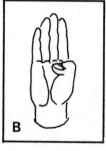 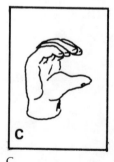

B   C

3. *Index-finger isolation*—the index finger alone is differentiated (PAIN);

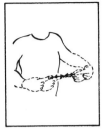

PAIN

4. *Little-finger isolation* (I)/*index-middle finger* (TWO)/*thumb-index-middle finger* (PEOPLE)—Dunn notes that the exact sequence of these is not clear;

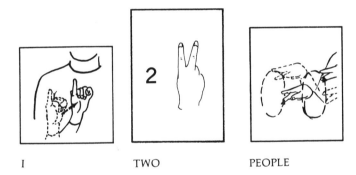

I   TWO   PEOPLE

5. *Complex*—for these handshapes it makes a difference what every finger is doing (I LOVE YOU).

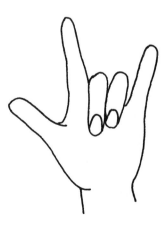

I LOVE YOU

It should be noted that most of these suggestions are not supported by research data. For example, Snyder-McLean (1978) did not find the touch aspect to be consistently related to the rate of sign acquisition. However, the suggestions are based on normal development data and clinical observations and may be used as a starting point, especially when planning the lexicon for young children.

The factor of *iconicity* is often mentioned as a strategy in selecting early signs (Fristoe and Lloyd 1980; Hamre-Nietupski et al. 1977). The research on this area is somewhat equivocal. Snyder-McLean (1978) reports that consistent training differences in rate of acquisition favored iconic signs over noniconic signs. However, the iconic signs were found to extinguish more quickly in several instances. The few instances of incidental learning of untrained signs also favored the acquisition of iconic signs. Konstantareas, Oxman, and Webster (1978) found that iconic signs were learned better than noniconic signs across all tasks—reproductive, receptive, and elicited signing. This was especially true for iconic verbs and adjectives. Thus it appears that the strategy of choosing initial signs based on their iconicity has some research support.

Several authors suggest that initial signs be *topographically dissimilar* (Hamre-Nietupski et al. 1977; Snyder-McLean 1978). Error analyses in the studies by Snyder-McLean (1978) suggested that similar topography of two signs was a major source of confusion and errors. Thus she recommends that trainers avoid grouping signs with very similar topographies in the same training set. An example of two similar signs would be AM and EAT.

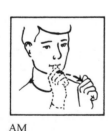

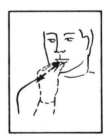

AM　　　　　　　EAT

In summary, Snyder-McLean (1978) noted that there was considerable variability between subjects in the studies she reported. Those studies dealt with factors such as iconicity and client preference. Thus the strategies suggested in this section are merely guidelines which must be modified to meet the needs of individual clients.

Methods of Teaching Gestural Communication

The general training methods will be determined by several factors, such as the gestural system selected, the capabilities and background of the client, and the intended function(s) of the system. The client variability regarding rate of acquisition (Skelly and Schinsky 1979; Snyder-McLean 1978) suggests that gestural training programs must be individualized.

Several gestural systems are accompanied by training materials and/or programs (e.g., Amer-Ind, Cued Speech, Signed English). In each case, however, flexibility is suggested. With the growing use of systems designed for one population applied to other populations, flexibility must be stressed. For example, use of Signed English with adults and with mentally retarded or autistic clients requires somewhat different strategies than those employed for using the system with the preschool deaf for whom it was intended. Further, some systems (e.g., American Sign Language, Cued Speech, Signed English) were not intended to be directly *taught* to their target population, the deaf. That is, environmental learning, rather than classroom or therapy instruction, was intended. However, with application to a wider range of populations this concept may have to be changed also. The capabilities and background of the client enter into this decision of type of training approach and methodology. For example, for the client who has already developed motor imitation skills, training strategies will likely capitalize on this skill. Similarly, clients who have acquired language competency will probably be taught through a modification of a second language approach rather than a natural language approach. The intended function(s) of the gestural system will also affect the training strategies to some extent. For example, if the intent is to have a language facilitation system, the focus will be on factors such as language concepts. If the intent is for a primary communication system, the execution of gestures will likely be emphasized at some point in the intervention process, as well as the client's success in transmitting messages. If the system is to serve primarily as an input mode (e.g., Cued Speech for a deaf child), the emphasis will be on the client's reception of the message.

Thus these major features should be considered in designing or selecting a program for training the use of gestures. Programs and strategies specific to individual systems have been suggested throughout this chapter. The present discussion will center on general training strategies for use with gestural systems.

Teaching Gestural Communication

Mayberry (1976) reports the use of three major methods in teaching gesture production:

1. *Molding*, or placing the client's hand(s) around an object; this may be used for teaching gestures which take the shape of the object they represent (CUP, BALL);
2. *Shaping or handshaping*, in which the trainer shapes the client's hand(s) into the desired position(s);
3. *Imitation*, in which the trainer (or another model) makes the sign and the client reproduces it.

It is not necessary to choose only one procedure. All three will likely be used in the course of training. Several authors have opted to use a naturally-structured format for training in gestural communication (Hamre-Nietupski et al. 1977; Jaffe, Blackstone, and Hanna 1980; Lykos 1971; Robbins 1978; and Skelly and Schinsky 1979). While each of the programs developed by those authors focuses on specific targets in any one session, interactive, conversational techniques are used, as opposed to rote learning and drills. This is especially true for clients learning a gestural system as a first language. However, Skelly and Schinsky (1979) also use a naturally-structured, reality approach, with emphasis on use of objects and activities of daily living for clients having normal linguistic competence (e.g., laryngectomees). The procedures for applying a naturally-structured approach may differ somewhat according to the basic factors listed earlier, but the basic premise of teaching communication in a naturally-structured situation remains. Another basic principle is that the client needs to receive training in gestural communication throughout the day, not just at designated "therapy" periods (Bonvillian and Nelson 1978; Kopchick and Lloyd 1976; Wilson, Goodman, and Wood 1975). Bonvillian and Nelson note that most studies reviewed indicate that clients received relatively low exposure to fluent sign language communication. The lack of frequent exposure and the lack of exposure to fluent users of the gesture system could severely limit the rate of acquisition and the level obtained. Both factors need to be considered in designing a gestural communication program.

Several examples of application of a naturally-structured approach in various situations are as follows:

1. For clients with *adult linguistic competence* (e.g., glossectomy) gestural commands may be given as a natural occurrence during a therapy session rather than as part of a drill (Skelly and Schinsky 1979); Example: client picks up a box of candy and trainer signals GIVE ME ONE; trainer and client enter a room, trainer looks at client, then at door and signals SHUT;

2. For the client learning a gestural system as a *first communication system* (e.g., deaf, multihandicapped) the trainer can contrive activities and wait for production of the appropriate sign (Jaffee et al. 1980; Robbins 1978); Example: the client is engaged in a favorite activity, such as tickling, which is stopped while the trainer waits for the production of TICKLE, MORE, or another appropriate sign;

3. For the client learning *receptive use of signs* the parent could contrive a need for the client to get a specific object which is not within view; Example: father is diapering infant, asks older deaf daughter to get bottle in the kitchen by making the signs BOTTLE, KITCHEN.

None of these examples is particularly innovative. The point is that all are examples of natural situations which have been contrived to elicit target behaviors. While naturally-structured, reality-based procedures may require more planning time, at least initially, they need not be inefficient in terms of rate of acquisition. It is feasible and desirable to keep data on this type of session, although it may be necessary to have an assistant keep data if several clients are working on different goals. If this procedure is not realistic, perhaps periodic probes can be carried out to document progress.

Several authors use a more direct artificially-structured approach to training (Kimble 1975; Stremel-Campbell et al. 1977; Wilson, Goodman, and Wood 1975). This approach, which generally follows a pre-planned ante-cedent-behavior-response pattern, is actually not radically different from the naturally-based approach except in the assumed *communicative intent*. In the naturally-structured approach communicative intent is usually assumed, while this may not be so for the artificially-structured approach. Recent researchers in the field of communication and communication disorders have stressed the importance of factors such as contextual support and communi-cative intent (Bates 1976; Bloom and Lahey 1978). These may be especially applicable to persons not having functional language systems.

It may be possible to combine the two approaches. For example, the treatment programs outlined by Skelly and Schinsky (1979) specify antece-dent events, client responses, and potential consequences. However, ante-cedent events are usually based on reality situations (e.g., presentation of a bar of soap to elicit WASH). Client behavior may be equally tied to reality, such as signalling WASH and washing hands. Whenever possible, consequences should be natural, as in fulfilling a client's request. If drills are deemed necessary, procedures can be designed to increase the interactional nature by contriving context or communicative intent. For example, the question "What is that?" can become meaningful, rather than a request for display of knowledge, if the client can see the referent (e.g., a picture of a baby) while the trainer cannot see it.

A number of gestural programs follow the general pattern of training in the following levels: reception, imitation, and production of gestures (Jaffe et al. 1980; Skelly and Schinsky 1979; Wilson et al. 1975). However, in some cases additional training levels are used within or at the end of those more traditional levels. For example, Skelly and Schinsky (1979) use the following hierarchy: recognition, imitation, replication (after the model has been removed), retrieval (from memory), transition to use, initiation, spontaneous conversation, equivalence to propositional speech. This training hierarchy underlines the need for generalization and self-regulation so that the client progresses beyond the retrieval stage. Most of the generalization strategies presented in Chapter 3 would be applicable to generalizing gestures to new situations, new people, and so forth. In addition, some of the gestural communication programs contain suggestions for generalization specific to the system being taught. One special problem relating to generalization is that the client may not receive the needed practice, feedback, or reinforce-ment from a verbal environment. This problem may be reduced by training parents, staff, and others to receive the gestural system or by selecting a system which is fairly transparent.

Several preliminary research findings also relate to methods of training gestural communication:

1. It appears that *manipulative responding*, in which the client actually manipulates objects, facilitates learning (Snyder-McLean 1978); thus it is recommended that real objects be used in training;
2. Production training was found to be equally effective for both the *nomination* (naming, as in "What is this?" CUP) and the *regulatory/instru-*

mental function (CUP, meaning "I want cup," or "Give me cup"); thus both functions should be represented in training (ibid);

3. It may be necessary to provide *over-training,* as signs acquired by minimal training (including some iconic signs) may not be retained as well as those acquired through extensive training (ibid);

4. *A simultaneous training approach* (signs plus speech) was found to be superior to a visual-only approach (signs plus mouthing of speech) for autistic children (Konstantareas and Leibovitz 1977); this was especially true for receptive language training, suggesting that a total communication type of approach will not interfere and may even facilitate sign acquisition.

For suggestions regarding training of nonmanual aspects of gestural communication, we recommend consulting one of the many texts on nonverbal communication. For example, *Nonverbal Communication Systems* (Leathers 1976) covers aspects such as kinesic communication systems (e.g., facial communication, including a facial meaning sensitivity test) and proxemics. Methods of observing, classifying, and measuring the quality of nonverbal communication are suggested.

Evaluating the Gestural Communication System

It is necessary to provide ongoing evaluation of client progress to determine the appropriateness of the gestural system, the content, and the intervention procedures and to determine goals for further intervention. Montgomery (1980a) suggests six points to consider in evaluating the effectiveness of communication aid use. Those six points are discussed in Chapter 9 of this book. By adapting these points to evaluate gestural systems the trainer would:

1. establish meaningful exit criteria;
2. determine how frequently conversation is initiated;
3. count the number of peer interactions;
4. assess the degree to which the system serves as a learning tool;
5. decide whether there is a need for a more complex system;
6. note how the client uses the system for various communication functions.

These general areas should be considered in using a gestural system. For example, exit criteria for an adult laryngectomee using Amer-Ind might be the equivalence of propositional use of English. Gestural systems are typically more *open* than symbolic systems; that is, the client may draw from a potentially large vocabulary, as compared to the limited content available to many communication aid users. In addition, gestures may be more open to interpretation than symbols on a communication aid, as they are more dependent on factors of client execution, such as precision, consistency, and completeness (Skelly and Schinsky 1979). Therefore, a criterion regarding execution of gestures and successful message transmission should be added. Execution of gestures should be evaluated in context as well as in citation form. For example, partners with whom the client typically communicates could converse with the client, judging each gesture or each gestural string as acceptable (e.g., correctly interpreted on first trial) or unacceptable. The client's response to communication breakdowns would also be important to assess.

Many of the more detailed suggestions regarding evaluation of effectiveness presented in Chapter 9 could apply to gestural communication systems as well. The gestural system used, the client's facility of use, and the appropriateness of interaction with those in the environment must all be periodically assessed.

Involvement of Staff and Family in Gestural Communication Training

It is essential to involve the client's parents (or other caregivers) and others in developing any communication system. This may be more difficult when introducing a gestural mode since gaining support will generally necessitate training potential communication partners in the use of a new mode. This will be an even greater problem for the client using a gestural system as an input mode since normal vocal input (adults talking, television) will be of much less benefit to the client. As Alpert (1980) stresses, "When the intervention mode is a nonspeech system, there is no doubt that parents *must* be included in the therapy process" (p. 416). A review of the literature on gestural training with the severely handicapped indicates that very few programs report direct training of parents, and several do not mention training of staff. This is quite surprising and indicates a need for the development of such parent programs.

For programs which do advocate training, group training is often suggested, due in part to the logistics but also to the personal support provided by sharing experiences. Skelly and Schinsky (1979) suggest scheduling these training sessions during therapy time for relatives of clients seen on an out-patient basis. They also recommend having family members and friends share in the transporting of the client so that a large number of persons may participate in training. It is noted that this training could be provided via videocassette for single viewers or small groups. Skelly and Schinsky (1979) also note that execution of gestures seems to facilitate learning even if the only goal is for the relatives to learn to receive the gestures. Thus training should involve gesture production as well as gesture reception. These approaches are highly suited to training in the use of Amer-Ind. However, for more extensive, less transparent systems, occasional training would likely not be sufficient. Some of the parent strategies suggested in Chapter 5, such as having parents write contracts, could help to establish parent participation. For example, parents could make a commitment to learn 10 new signs per week. Another goal for home practice would be to present each new sign at least one time per day at home. The same type of technique could be used for staff members, with data sheets posted on the bulletin board. For example, all aides could be taught the new sign(s) for a client, and each sign would be charted as shown in figure 8-4. Staff members

Figure 8-4

Sign training program: Staff involvement chart.

Client	Sign(s)	Level	MH					SB					RA					Weekly Total
			M	T	W	T	F	M	T	W	T	F	M	T	W	T	F	
Kate	CUP	(R)	+	+	T	C	+	+	+	+	C	+			+	C	+	+= 19
			+	+			+	+	−	+		+			+		+	−= 1
	EAT	(R)	+	+	T	C	+	+	+	−	C	+	+			C	+	+= 18
			+	+			+	+	+	+		+	+				+	−= 2
	WANT	(R)*	−	−	T	C	+	−	−	−	C	−			+	C	+	+= 11
			+	+			+	+	+	+		+			+		+	−= 8
Karen	EAT	(I)*	−	−	T	−	−	−	−	−	−	+	−	−	−	−	−	+= 6
			−	−		+	+	−	−	−	+	+	−	−	−	+	+	−= 22
James	ALL-GONE	(I)	+	+	T	+	+	+	+	+	+	+	+	+	+	+	+	+= 28
			+	+		+	+	+	+	+	+	+	+	+	+	+	+	−= 0
Jenny	PLAY	(I)	+	+	T	+	+	+	+	+	+	+	+		+		+	+= 24
			+	+		+	+	+	+	+	+	+			+		+	−= 0
	GO	(P)*	−	−	T	+	+	−	−	+	+	+	−	+	−	+	+	+= 13
			−	−		+	+	−	+	+	+	+	−	+	+		+	−= 13

Sign Level Code
R = reception
I = imitation
P = production
* = first week at new level

Scoring Code
+ = presented trial, successful
− = presented trial, unsuccessful
C = client absent
T = trainer absent

would then check off naturally occurring or contrived instances of sign presentation. This will ensure that training is spread throughout the day, with trials presented by several trainers. A procedure such as this would help prompt staff members to present training or generalization trials. This procedure also would indicate when training was neglected for a particular client or when one trainer consistently failed to carry out trials. This is only one example of a method for ensuring staff involvement.

Training siblings and peers of gesture users should also be considered. This can be accomplished through training sessions for older children and game-type formats for younger children. Again, it might be helpful to set specific targets, such as the "sign-for-the-day," to encourage use of the gestures introduced. Children seem to be tuned in to gestures, as can be seen in their enthusiastic response to songs involving gestures. Thus teaching target gestures through simple songs or sayings (preferably songs or sayings the children already know) may be another useful approach. For example, we have found that preschoolers readily pick up the signs for the saying "See you later, alligator." While ALLIGATOR may not be a very functional sign, the other three signs may be quite useful. We have also had great success in using the book, *Sesame Street Sign Language Fun* (Bove, 1980) with preschoolers. In this book, Sesame Street characters are illustrated engaging in activities and Linda Bove, the deaf actress who often appears on the *Sesame Street* television program, is pictured demonstrating signs. More than 200 signs are included, grouped into 20 categories, such as: "the family", "school days", "summer", and "the way you feel." Particular advantages of this book with young children are: the motivational value, the clarity of photographs (as opposed to the line drawings used in most sign language texts), and the illustrations which provide context, so that non-readers can learn signs without the aid of an adult. With the current emphasis on mainstreaming and normalization, severely handicapped clients will be using their new skills with increasingly wider audiences. It will be necessary to provide those audiences with the skills required for receiving and transmitting messages. For further information on applications of gestural systems to specific populations such as deaf-blind or autistic children, the following references are suggested: Bonvillian and Nelson (1978), Kapisovsky (1978), Stuckey, Kaehler, and Minihane (1977), and Wilbur (1979).

Chapter 9: Symbolic Communication Strategies

Introduction

Symbolic communication systems have become more widely used and more sophisticated over the last decade. One reason for their wide application is that they may be used even with the very severely physically handicapped. There is great diversity in the types of symbolic communication systems and in the methods of activating those systems. This chapter focuses on a number of symbolic communication systems and issues involving those systems such as assessment and methods of training. The major areas to be covered are included in the decision process model in figure 9-1.

Assessment of Use of a Symbolic Communication System

A number of professionals will likely be involved in the assessment process, including an occupational therapist, speech-language pathologist, physical therapist, and special educator (Harris-Vanderheiden, McNaughton, and MacDonald 1976). Other professionals (e.g., engineer) may need to be consulted, and the input of clients, parents, and/or other care-takers will, of course be vital. Careful assessment of the client prior to and during training will insure that the communication mode which has been selected is appropriate. Some questions that must be answered are the following:

1. How can the client respond?
2. What type of interface (e.g., input switch) is needed, if any?
3. What modes of output should be selected?
4. What type(s) of symbols will be utilized?
5. What will be the content of the communication board (e.g., how many symbols will be included and what level of language will they represent)?
6. How will the communication board be organized (e.g., what will be the spacing, size, and boldness of the symbols, and what type of display will be used)?
7. What methods of training are most appropriate for this client?

Harris-Vanderheiden and Vanderheiden (1977) recommend that assessment for use of any non-vocal system include consideration of *why* (the rationale); *what* (specific areas to be assessed); *who* (persons who will carry out the assessment); and *how* (methods of assessment). The seven questions posed above relate to the *why*. The *who* consideration includes the client, his or her parents, and professionals listed earlier. It is assumed that readers can develop methods to meet the *how* condition for each individual client, although some specific suggestions are presented in this chapter and in Appendix D. The sources listed and annotated in Appendix A contain suggestions for methods of assessment. We believe that the assessment model presented by Myers et al. (1980) is especially comprehensive and practical.

This chapter gives primary consideration to the *what* aspect of assessment through discussion of topics such as means of indicating, symbol

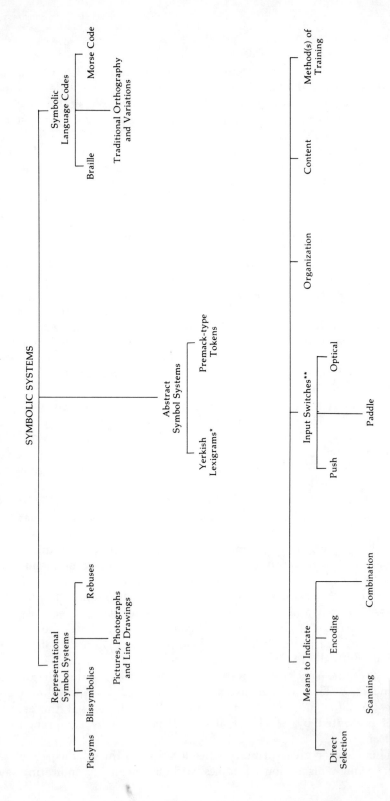

Figure 9-1
The Decision Process Model: Symbolic systems.

*Indicates communication systems which are not covered in depth in this book.
**Indicates that entries are merely examples of possible entries.

148

systems, and methods of training. For example, the entry level requirements are listed for each symbol system covered in depth. This indicates areas that must be assessed, such as cognitive level and visual discrimination skills.

Accessing the System:
Communication Techniques, Aids, and Options

Symbolic systems, by our definition, involve the use of symbols that are external to the body and are located on some type of communication device. The client must have some way to gain access to this communication device. Three major areas involving access are the input switches, the means of indicating, and the level of implementation, each of which will be covered briefly.

Input Switches

Input switches are " . . . switches which can be used as interfaces between severely handicapped individuals and special communication and control aids" (Holt, Buelow, and Vanderheiden 1978, p. 1). These switches enable the client to use whatever physical abilities he or she has to gain access to the vocabulary on the communication aid. A wide variety of input switches are available, to be matched with the client's needs and capabilities (Holt et al. 1978):

1. Push switches, such as push buttons and push plates;
2. Paddle switches;
3. Joystick and wobblestick switches;
4. Sliding or trolly switches;
5. Tip or tilt switches;
6. Pneumatic switches, such as sip and puff switches or air pillows;
7. Zero pressure switches;
8. Moisture switches;
9. Proximity switches;
10. Motion-detecting switches;
11. Eye controller switches;
12. Optical switches;
13. Sound-controlled switches, such as whistle or voice switches;
14. Bio-electric switches, such as myo-electric (EMG) or electro-enceph-alographic (EEG) switches;
15. Special switches for a specific body part, such as the eyebrow or tongue.

Many of these switches can be operated by more than one body part. For example, Silverman (1980, tables 7-1 and 7-2) suggests that a push plate switch could be activated by movements as diverse as elbow extension, wrist flexion, wrist extension, and neck flexion (using a headstick). Similarly, a single muscular gesture could often be used to activate a variety of input switches. For example, Silverman (1980, table 7-1) indicates that the muscle gesture of wrist flexion could be used to operate at least the following input switches: push plate, paddle, pillow, pad, squeeze bulb, and touch switch.

Simple, sophisticated switches are being developed for use by clients who have severe motor disabilities. For example, an ocular transducer is currently under study for the severely disabled non-vocal client (Rinard and Rugg 1977, 1978).\This device, which is attached to a pair of eyeglasses, detects the corneal reflection of an infrared source. The ocular transducer has been successfully interfaced with a number of aids, including an electric wheelchair, video games, a television terminal, and a modified ETRAN[a]* Eye Signaling System (Eichler 1975). When it is interfaced with a modified television terminal the user can "type" messages by using eye movements and slight teeth clicks; however, this device is difficult to control for individuals who have poor or spastic head movements. When it is interfaced with the modified ETRAN display, the user can print messages using eye control only, even if he or she does not have good head control.

Commercial information, descriptions, and illustrations of the various switches may be found in Holt et al. (1978), Silverman (1980), Silverman et al. (1978), and Vanderheiden and Grilley (1976). Holt et al. (1978) also provide a comprehensive overview of commercial switches currently available, including features such as: physical description, switch operation, pressure needed, features and comments, price, and delivery time.

Means of Indicating

This section will cover various techniques of indicating desired entries. Communication aids using the various techniques will be briefly described to serve as examples. Input switches enable the client to indicate an entry on the communication aid by one of several means. Direct access to the aid, such as pointing, or use of eye gaze, a headstick, or a mouthstick may also be used in indicating by clients who do not need special switches. There are three basic means of indicating: direct selection, scanning, and encoding (Holt, Buelow, and Vanderheiden 1978). Combinations of these methods may also be used.

Direct selection

The classic definition for direct selection is:

> Any technique or aid where the user directly indicates the desired message elements. Only one non-time dependent pointing motion is required to indicate each message element.
>
> Fothergill et al. (1978, p. ii).

Direct selection can involve the use of an unaided body part; for example, the client could focus his or her eyes on a desired entry or point with one finger or with the fist, elbow, or toes. A number of appliances are available to assist in pointing, such as headsticks, handsticks, and mouthpieces.

A number of communication devices are available for use with the direct selection technique; for example, traditional communication boards, book-

---

*Small letters refer to endnotes which list addresses of manufacturers or organizations. These endnotes are found at the end of this chapter.

lets, and typewriters. Devices may be adapted to serve the needs of the client. For example, a typewriter may be fitted with a keyguard to assist the client in achieving accuracy.

In summary, because of its simplicity direction selection is appropriate as an initial technique and as a technique for clients with low cognitive levels (Harris and Vanderheiden 1980). Since direct selection is normative, it would be the preferred technique for a client with good control over the pointing technique. It is potentially a very rapid means of indicating. However, the technique requires that the client have the necessary physical capability, generally including a wide range motion and control of fine motor skills (Harris and Vanderheiden).

Scanning
Scanning involves:

> . . . any technique or aid where the message elements (or groups of message elements) are presented to the individual sequentially. When the desired message element is presented, the user indicates it by signalling with a pre-arranged signal or switch. (Some scanning techniques also allow the user to control the order in which the items are presented—as in directed scanning techniques).
>
> Fothergill (1978, p. ii)

Scanning techniques include simple ones such as the "twenty questions" approach in which the message receiver asks a variety of questions until the client indicates "yes" by using a pre-arranged signal such as raising an arm or blinking the eyes. More complex approaches may also be used.

Harris and Vanderheiden describe two basic types of scanning. In *linear scanning*, entries are presented one at a time until the desired entry is reached. A rotary scanner, in which a pointer indicates entries placed like numbers on a clock face, is an example of an aid using linear scanning (See figure 9-2). Another is a simple communication board in which the communication partner points to each entry in turn until the client signals the desired entry.

Group-item scanning involves arranging entries in groups or rows. The entire group or row is scanned until the client signals, at which time each entry in that group or row is scanned to determine the exact entry. An example of this method is row-column scanning, in which a row is scanned until the column containing the entry is reached. Each column entry is then scanned until the desired entry is reached. This procedure is illustrated in figure 9-2.

Silverman (1980) also describes a *directed scanning* approach, in which the path to the message entry may be vertical, horizontal, angular, or a combination of the three. The intent is to provide the shortest path to the desired message element. Thus linear scanning will be the slowest approach and directed scanning the quickest. Depending on physical and cognitive skills, either the message sender or the message receiver may control the scanning process, or both may use an input switch to activate the scanner on an electronic aid such as the *Zygo Model 16.*[b]

Scanning has the advantage of being useable even by clients who are

Figure 9-2
Schematics of Various Types of Scanning Approaches.

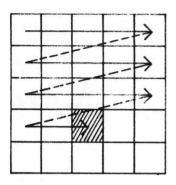

a. *Linear scanning*
   1) Communication board

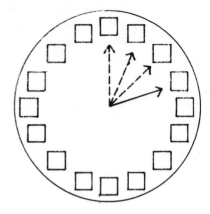

2) Rotary device

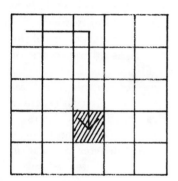

b. *Group-item scanning*
   1) Row column scanning

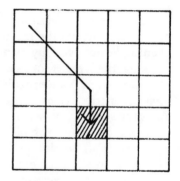

2) Directional scanning

Adapted from Harris and Vanderheiden (1980); Silverman (1980); and Vanderheiden (1976a).

very severely physically handicapped. The speed of scanning may be adjusted to meet the needs of the client. For example, some clients may find that a slower scanning pace is necessary as the day progresses, to compensate for increasing fatigue. Harris and Vanderheiden (1980) note that, while scanning is not as straightforward as direct selection, it can be an appropriate initial approach for the severely handicapped client. Also, if the client has a reliable physical gesture for operating an input switch, this technique may be faster and less fatiguing than direct selection, even for clients with gross pointing abilities.

Encoding

A definition for encoding is:

> Any technique or aid in which the desired message elements are indicated by a non-time dependent pattern or a series of input signals. (With an aid, any number of switches may be used. The code may involve activating the switches sequentially or simultaneously).
>
> Fothergill et al. (1978, p. ii)

The code for this technique may be memorized or placed on a chart for reference by those involved in the communication exchange. Harris and Vanderheiden suggest that this technique is useful for clients with some motor control but with poor range of motion. There are a variety of approaches to encoding. In *two-movement encoding* the client uses two-element combinations to indicate entries. The two-element combinations could consist of two numbers (e.g., 2,1) or a number plus color combination (e.g., 2, red). The combination may refer to a specific entry on a chart (e.g., 2,1 = entry 21 = the word "please") or may indicate the row and column numbers (e.g., 2,1 = row 2, column 1 = the picture for "milk"). These examples are illustrated in figure 9-3. Another example of encoding is the use of the Morse Code to indicate letters. Eye gaze is often used in encoding as well. For example, the client may look at numbers or colors for encoding. The ETRAN chart is an example of a communication device which uses eye gaze for encoding. The sender gazes at the general group in which the entry is located and then indicates its specific location in the group with a second eye gaze.

Figure 9-3
Schematics of Uses of Two-Number Encoding System.

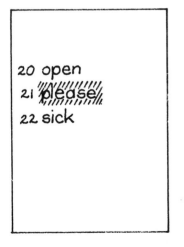
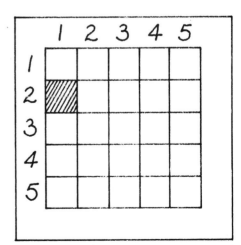

Adapted from Harris and Vanderheiden (1980).

In summary, encoding techniques may provide the client with access to a relatively large vocabulary while requiring only a limited range of motion. However, due to the relative sophistication of this technique, it may not be suitable for use as an initial technique or for use with the cognitively impaired.

Combination techniques

Two or more of these techniques may be combined to provide the optimum means of indicating for an individual client. For example, Harris and Vanderheiden suggest use of a *point and scan* technique, in which a client with gross pointing skills points toward the desired entry, and the communication partner scans that area, if necessary, to determine which specific entry was intended. For the client who is cognitively able to use the encoding technique, encoding may be used in combination with either direct selection or scanning in order to increase potential vocabulary. For example, the client could point to numbers to encode communication board entries which were too closely spaced for successful direct selection.

This brief review of basic techniques for indicating has illustrated the diversity of techniques and general aids available to the non-vocal client. The most appropriate means of indicating will be determined primarily through physical assessment of the client. However, the client's attitudes or attitudes of the parents toward a particular means of indicating should also be considered. For example, a client may intensely dislike the feel of a headstick and choose to use a scanning mode instead. It is likely that a client will need more than one technique as needs or situation changes. Thus the communication specialist should know the many approaches available and should continually reassess the client to determine the optimum means of indicating.

Modes of Output

A variety of output modes can be used with communication devices. This discussion will follow the framework suggested by Cohen, Montgomery, and Yoder (1979), in which output is described as auditory or visual. In addition, a third output mode, tactile, will be included within this section.

Auditory output

Two types of auditory output modes may be described. These are included under the generic label of *VOCAs* (Voice Output Communication Aids). The first type of VOCA uses *pre-recorded speech*, in which the client selects words, phrases, or sentences which have been pre-recorded. An example of a commercial aid using this type of output is FORM-A-PHRASE,[c] which uses vocabulary cartridges, each of which can be pre-programmed with utterances of one to five words spoken in a male, female, or child voice.

A second type of auditory output aid produces *synthesized speech*, in which segments of speech are blended to form words. An example of a speech synthesizer is the PHONIC MIRROR HandiVoice,[d] which blends phonemes to produce virtually any word in the English language.

Auditory output allows the user considerable flexability, as the aid may be used in telephone conversations, in addressing groups, and in conditions where the message receiver cannot attend to a visual or tactile display (e.g., while driving a car). If a permanent record is desired, the vocal output may be tape-recorded. While synthesized speech allows the user an unlimited vocabulary, higher cognitive and academic skills are required for sound blending than for use of pre-recorded speech. Montgomery (1979) recommends a minimum of second grade level spelling skills and capability to learn sound blending skills as two entry level skills for use of the synthetic speech communication aid. Goodrich (1979) notes that "... an alternative to requiring the user to master phonetic representation of speech is to provide a computer program which automatically converts from conventional orthography (spelling) to phonetics" (p. 6). He describes several commercial and experimental communication devices with this capability, including *Anglophone*,[e] which converts English text to the phonetic commands used by voice synthesizers. Further information on voice generation techniques, including additional communication devices, may be found in Goodrich or Vanderheiden (1976a).

Visual output

There are several types of output in which the communication partner attends to a visual display to receive the message. The first and most basic type is *direct viewing of entries*. This involves having the communication partner look at the communication device and note which entries the user indicates. Since this requires remembering entries until the message is completed, it might be helpful for the message receiver to verbalize each entry as it is indicated and/or to write down the message. Either of these procedures would also help to avoid misinterpretation and would be especially useful during the learning phase or for clients who make frequent errors in indicating entries. Direct viewing of entries can be an output choice with many aids and is a straightforward manner of presenting output.

A second type of visual output is *hard copy*, such as that provided by a strip or line printer or a typewriter. An example of a strip printer is the *Lapboard Strip Printer*,[f] which yields 1/10" characters on a ¼" wide tape, with characters visible to the user immediately following printing. An example of an adaptive typewriter is the *Dvorak One-Hand Typewriter*.[g] Teletypewriters also fall into this category. These aids print messages onto a continuous roll of paper and can print in response to coded electrical signals generated by a second teletypewriter or by a computer (Silverman 1980). Thus they have special usefulness for communicating over the telephone and in interfacing with computers. An example of a teletypewriter is the MCM/D,[h] which is compatible with all deaf tele-communications equipment. Silverman notes that a device may be added which permits the use of rolls of paper rather than sheets of paper, thus making the aid more appropriate for clients with limited control of the upper extremities.

A third type of visual output is the *cathode-ray tube or CRT display*. In this case messages are printed on a television screen, either character by character (e.g., letters, numbers, Blissymbols), or in larger units such as words. Silverman notes that these devices generally have an editing capability and can be adapted to almost any size television screen. An example of this is *SPLINK*[i] (Enderby and Hamilton 1979), which utilizes a standard television set.

A fourth type of visual display is a *light-emitting diode (LED) or liquid-crystal display (LCD)*. LED characters are formed by miniature transistors (diodes), such that the characters appear to be outlined by light, as on many electronic calculators. Characters on LCD panels are generally formed by short vertical and horizontal lines such as those seen on digital clocks (Silverman 1980). Silverman notes that LCDs use less current and can be made thinner than LED displays; thus they may provide more flexibility for the user. An example of a communication aid using the LED display is the *VIP Communicator,*[j] a highly portable communication aid with a "walking display," in which characters on the right side of the display move to the left as more are entered.

Tactile output

Communication aids may also yield tactile output, typically in the form of the raised dots of the braille system. These may be produced by use of a slate and stylus or a braille writer such as *SAGEM,*[k] which prints full-page braille in response to a variety of input (typewritten, braille-keyboard, etc.). Another aid, the *Optacon,*[k] offers independent access to print for many persons who cannot read visually. The output of the Optacon is raised, vibrating print which passes under the index finger of the hand resting on the tactile array.

The non-vocal individual may also need a signaling device as part of his or her available output. This could be a separate device, such as the *CALL SIGNAL.*[l] A signaling device may also be incorporated into an aid, such as the *ZYGO Model 100.*[m] This capability is especially important for communication aids which store a message, as the client can signal when the message is ready for transmission.

Summary

Several features of output modes should be considered in determining the optimal mode. These features may cut across the various types of output:

1. *Permanence of output*—this refers to the production of a permanent record, such as a hard copy or a tape of auditory output;
2. *Recall capability*—this refers to the retention of an entire message or portion of a message (e.g., 45 characters) for presentation as a unit when the client completes the message; this determines whether the message can be read subsequent to production or must be read simultaneous with production;
3. *Editing capability*—this refers to the ease of changing characters which have been entered; for example, CRT output is very amenable to editing.

Silverman (1980)

The type(s) of output selected for an individual also depends on a number of factors relating to that individual's needs and capabilities. Several of the major factors are considered here.

The *client's physical abilities* are very important. For example, a client who requires several minutes to complete a message will need an output with recall capability so that the message is not forgotten before it is completed. In addition, a permanent record may be desirable when receivers lack the time to wait for formulation of an entire message. Some clients with severe physical handicaps may also need editing capability to compensate for mistakes.

The *situations which the client frequently encounters* should also be considered. For example, a client in an academic situation will likely need a permanent record. One who needs access to telephone communication could use a vocal output communication aid (VOCA) or a teletypewriter. A client who participates in group situations could use a VOCA or a cathode-ray tube display on a large screen. The client who is ambulatory might benefit from a very portable output system such as an LED or LCD communication aid.

The *symbol system which the client uses* is another factor to consider. The potential types of output may be limited to some extent by the symbol system used by the client. The most flexible symbol system in this regard is traditional orthography. However, there is increasing capability to produce other types of symbol systems, notably Blissymbolics, having various output modes. Other symbol systems, such as braille and Morse Code, may be transformed into English orthography and then represented by various outputs such as hard copy.

As implied in the preceding discussion, a single output mode will rarely be sufficient as a long-term communication aid for a sophisticated user. A combination of output modes will often be required, though the client's primary communication may be in one mode.

Summary

The communication devices reviewed in this section all interact with each other and with client skills to determine the optimum communication techniques and aids for a single client. It should be noted that, while general categories have been described (e.g., push switch input, scanning technique), variations exist within these categories. Thus, while both the *Talking Brooch*[n] and the *VIP Communicator* are direct selection aids with light-emitting diode (LED) output displays, a number of design features are different. For example, with regard to the direct selection panel, the *Talking Brooch* utilizes an almost standard typewriter kepboard, while the *VIP Communicator* uses an alphabetically-arranged calculator-style keyboard. Regarding the LED output display, the *Talking Brooch* has a 5-character display, and the *VIP Communicator* has an 8-character display. There are other similarities and differences between the two aids. The point is that differences in design may make some aids more suited to the needs of individual clients. In some cases a single aid may have the necessary options to meet primary needs. For example, the

Versicom° allows use of scanning, encoding, direct selection, and combination approaches. A variety of input switches may be used; and LED, strip printing, voice synthesizer, electric typewriter, or cathode-ray tube displays may be used as output. A number of the commercial aids offer a wide range of options or can be adapted to use these options. Research and development of new equipment is ongoing at various laboratories and manufacturing firms, so that further advances may be expected.

This section has attempted to indicate what aids, techniques, and options to select. Although several communication aids have been presented as examples, a complete listing of available aids is beyond the scope of this book. The following resources, all described in Appendix A, include descriptions of devices and lists of commercial companies. These should help in selecting appropriate aids: Copeland (1974); Harris and Vanderheiden (1980); Howard (1979); Mallik (1977); Melichar (1977, 1978); Vanderheiden (1978); Vanderheiden and Grilley (1976). The following organizations or publications listed in Appendix C also offer information on various communication aids: Adaptive Systems Corporation; *Communication Outlook*; Swedish Institute for the Handicapped; Trace Research and Development Center.

Types of Symbolic Communication Systems

The symbolic communication systems to be covered in this section can be divided into three major categories:

1. *Representational symbol systems*—these systems primarily include symbols which suggest their meanings such as pictures, photographs, and line drawings; although Rebus and Blissymbolics use some abstract symbols and alphabetic characters, they are primarily representational systems.
2. *Abstract symbol systems*—in these systems the meaning of the symbol is not suggested by its appearance; examples are Yerkish lexigrams and Premack-type tokens, such as those is the Non-SLIP program (Carrier and Peak 1975);
3. *Symbolic language codes*—these are codes which represent the letters or sounds of a language such as English; examples are the alphabet, phonemes, words, alphabetic clusters, braille, and Morse Code.

Each of these symbolic systems will be reviewed in this chapter. Several systems will be covered in some detail, using the *what, why, who* format introduced in Chapter 8.

Representational Symbol Systems

In these systems, symbols represent their referents, either pictographically (e.g., an outline of a house to represent "house") or ideographically (e.g., a drawing of a heart to represent "emotion"). Often, pictographs and ideographs will be combined within a system, since it is difficult to represent abstract concepts through pictures. The representational systems to be covered in this chapter include: pictures, photographs, and line drawings; Picsyms , Blissymbolics; and Rebus.

Pictures, photographs, and line drawings
There is a great variety in the materials which may fall under this symbolic system. It may include black and white or color photographs, pictures cut from magazines, or hand-drawn or commercially prepared line drawings. For example, the *Picture Communication Symbols*[p] comprise a set of over 700 line drawings available in one-inch or two-inch sizes. These symbols include minimal detail and have the label printed above each symbol. Factors such as abstractness and complexity help determine which items are more appropriate for initial introduction. Silverman (1980) discusses *abstraction continuum*, in which photographs have a relatively low level of abstraction, while line drawings demonstrate a relatively high level of abstraction. The amounts of detail and the extent to which the foreground stands out from the background helps determine the complexity of a pictured item.

Williams and Fox (1977) recommend that tasks begin with real objects, people, and events, and progress to photographs with simple backgrounds, to more abstract materials such as line drawings, and then, to photographs with a complex background. Thus, they have combined factors such as abstraction and complexity in determining a general sequence. However, they stress that all clients will not need to follow all steps of this sequence.

Pictures are or can be used with a number of commercial communication prostheses (e.g., *Picture Communication Board*, [q] ZYGO Model 16). Printed words often accompany the pictures.

Why. Pictures, especially those that are very simple, may provide an intermediate step between real life objects, events, and people, and more abstract symbols such as Picsyms, Rebuses, or Blissymbols. They may be adapted to the needs of the individual by using photographs of people, objects, and events familiar to the client. Furthermore, speech-language pathologists and special education teachers frequently use pictures during therapy which may reinforce the entries on the communication board.

Who. Picture systems may be especially appropriate for clients who have low cognitive levels, including young children and older mentally retarded clients. Silverman (1980) also notes that clients with cortical damage, who suffer from an abstract-concrete imbalance as defined by Wepman (1951), may benefit from use of concrete pictures.

Entry-level requirements for introducing a picture system would include the following:

1. *Sensorimotor Stage 5* level of cognitive development (Chapman and Miller 1980);
2. *Average visual discrimination skills,* with the level of skill required depending on the abstractness and complexity of the pictures selected.

The potential audience for comprehending picture systems would be unlimited, as most pictures would be considered "transparent." Those pictures that were not transparent, such as pictures personalized for the client, could be labeled with words.

When. As noted, Chapman and Miller suggest a sensorimotor level of Stage 5 for the introduction of a pictorial communication system. This stage falls at approximately 12 to 18 months for nonhandicapped children; thus pictures can be the initial symbol system.

How. Several authors suggest procedures for teaching clients that pictures represent specified referents. In some cases, these training procedures could be modified for use with other symbol systems such as Blissymbolics. A basic procedure followed in many training programs is a *match-to-sample task*, in which the client matches the picture to an object, event, or person (Williams and Fox 1977). This may be preceded by match-to-sample tasks involving matching objects to objects. Several authors have presented special techniques for demonstrating that pictures represent real objects. For example, McDonald (1980) suggests that the trainer take an instant photograph of the referent (e.g., the toilet) and allow the client to watch it develop. For line-drawings, Liebergott (1980) recommends pointing to the referent, such as the child's hand, then placing it on a sheet of paper and tracing around it. In both of these examples, the picture is produced while the client is watching which should help him associate the picture and the referent.

If it is intended that the client use the pictorial symbol system to produce relatively complex syntactic structures, several English language programs are available (e.g., *Developmental Syntax Program,*[r] *Fokes Sentence Builder Kit*[s]).

Where. Pictures may be hand-drawn, cut from magazines, produced photographically, or ordered commercially. Reviews of communication devices are in Mallik (1977), Vanderheiden (1978), and Vanderheiden and Grilley (1976). Other sources for commercial picture sets include traditional speech-language pathology equipment firms. Vicker's book (1974b) is an especially good source of ideas for training use of communication boards. It also contains a packet of design samples and instructions for construction pictorial communication boards.

Picsyms

The Picsyms System will be discussed only briefly, as it is still under development at the Meyer Children's Rehabilitation Institute of the University of Nebraska. Picsyms is a graphic symbol system based on the language development of children (Carlson and James 1980). It was designed specifically as a communication system, unlike many other systems which have been adapted for this purpose (e.g., rebuses, Blissymbolics). The system is intended to meet the needs of non-speaking or language-disordered people. Symbols are based on semantics and follow logical principles of development. For example, arrows are used to indicate the direction of movement in those symbols which represent action verbs, while time and holiday symbols are enclosed in a square to indicate the calendar. Picsyms are reproducible and new symbols may be created using the logic of the system. Thus, the system is openended to meet the constant influx of vocabulary needed by children learning language. Picsyms have been used clinically with non-speaking or language-disordered children, and several studies involving the system are in progress. A dictionary of Picsyms is being prepared by Carlson and James. This dictionary will contain over 1800 symbol-words listed alphabetically and in categories. The dictionary will also include instructions for reproducing symbols and creating new symbols. Four examples from the Picsyms Dictionary are presented:*

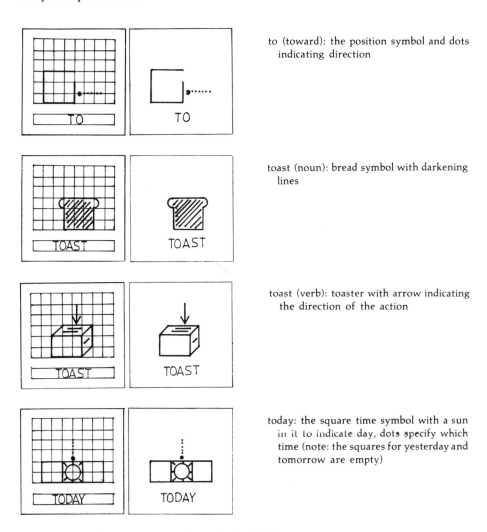

to (toward): the position symbol and dots indicating direction

toast (noun): bread symbol with darkening lines

toast (verb): toaster with arrow indicating the direction of the action

today: the square time symbol with a sun in it to indicate day, dots specify which time (note: the squares for yesterday and tomorrow are empty)

From *The Picsyms Dictionary*, © 1980 by Faith Carlson.

---

*Further information on the Picsyms System may be obtained from Faith Carlson or Cynthia A. James, Meyer Children's Rehabilitation Institute of the University of Nebraska Medical Center, Omaha, Nebraska, 68131.

Blissymbolics*

What. Blissymbolics is described by McNaughton and Kates (1980) as ". . . a graphic nonalphabet communication system" (p. 305). It was created by Charles K. Bliss over a period of more than 20 years, and was intended to serve as an international communication system. Bliss, an Austrian-born chemical engineer, conceived the idea in China, where he learned to read Chinese ideographic writing. Other precursors to the development of this system were his early introduction by his electrician (and optician) father to the logic of blueprints and the symbols they contain, and his later introduction to the logical languages expressed in chemical and mathematical symbols. Moreover, because he was born near the Russian border, Bliss was exposed to the frustration of multiple languages (Bliss and McNaughton 1975). The system he developed was termed "Semantography" (from Greek, "a meaningful writing"), and is extensively described in the book, *Semantography* (Bliss 1965). The first application of Blissymbolics as an augmentative communication system was in 1971 at the Ontario Crippled Children's Centre (Kates and McNaughton 1975).

Blissymbolics is a visual, semantically based system. Blissymbols can be categorized into four types (McNaughton and Kates 1980):

1. *Pictographic symbols*, which picture what they represent; these symbols are highly "transparent" or guessable:

| flower | house | chair | man | woman |

2. *Ideographic symbols*, which represent ideas about the referent; these symbols may be considered translucent, since they are readily understood and remembered once the meaning is explained:

| animal (four legs) | insect (six legs) | mind (outline of skull) | protection (roof) |

3. *Arbitrary symbols*, which are assigned meanings; these include two subcategories:

   a. *International symbols*, which were used before Blissymbolics was created; these are recognized and used throughout the world:

---

*Blissymbolics © used herein, Blissymbolics Communication Institute, 1981, Toronto, Canada.

***The Blissymbolics Institute recommends placing labels above the symbols so that labels are not covered up while the client is pointing.*

| addition | multiplication | question mark | forward (direction) | musical note |

b. *Arbitrary Blissymbols*, created by Bliss; these are generally opaque, and must be memorized:

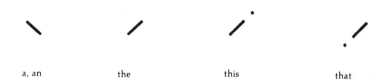

| a, an | the | this | that |

4. *Mixed symbols*, composed of pictographic [P], ideographic [I], and/or arbitrary [A] components; these may be transparent, translucent, or opaque, depending on the combination of components:

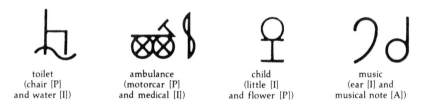

| toilet (chair [P] and water [I]) | ambulance (motorcar [P] and medical [I]) | child (little [I] and flower [P]) | music (ear [I] and musical note [A]) |

Meaning can be achieved by a number of modifications. Examples of these modifications are as follows:

1. *Size*

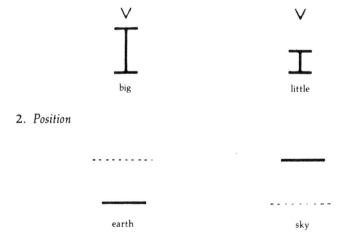

big   little

2. *Position*

earth   sky

3. Direction/orientation

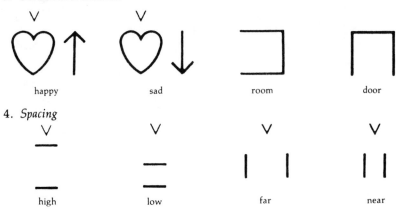

| happy | sad | room | door |

4. Spacing

| high | low | far | near |

5. Pointers

| leg | foot |

6. Positional references

| under | over | (to) forget | (to) understand |

Adapted from McNaughton and Kates (1980) and Silverman, McNaughton and Kates (1978)

There are two basic methods for extending the meaning of symbols, thus enlarging the available vocabulary. The first method is the use of *indicators*. Indicators that may be used with appropriate symbols include plural, thing, action (verb), description (evaluation), and tense indicators. Examples of use of several indicators are illustrated:

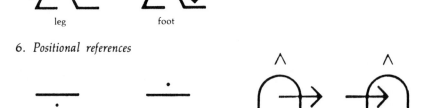

| drink | drinks | (to) drink | drank |

Strategies may also be used to expand the Blissymbol vocabulary, with strategy symbols typically placed one-quarter space before the symbol. Strategies are available to represent opposite meaning, "part (of)," metaphor, and intensity. Examples of the use of strategies are as follows:

branch
(part + tree)

lake
(much + water)

As seen in the preceding illustrations, many symbols are *compound symbols*, formed by two or more basic elements which may be sequenced or super-imposed. These symbols are groupings created by Bliss or accepted into the standard vocabulary. Examples of compound symbols are:

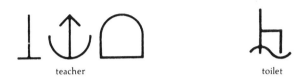

teacher   toilet

Where there is no standard symbol, the instructor or symbol user may create a new symbol for personal use. This is termed a *combined* symbol, and must be sequenced, using the *combine indicator* before and after the symbol grouping. Examples are:

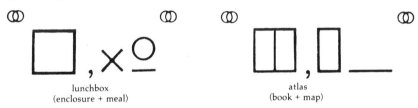

lunchbox
(enclosure + meal)

atlas
(book + map)

Examples from Silverman et al. (1978)

Mr. Bliss developed his own syntax but the production of syntax similar to English is possible through symbols representing content words (nouns, verbs, and adjectives) and function words (prepositions, articles, and conjunctions). However, in the sentence forms suggested by Bliss (*Semantography*, 1965, pp. 421–48) symbols for function words are omitted unless they are considered absolutely necessary. Silverman et al. suggest that the syntax used for a client will depend on the reason(s) why the system was chosen. This issue will be discussed further in the "how" section of this chapter.

Currently, several output options are available with Blissymbolics. Symbols can be viewed directly, as on direct selection, scanning, or encoding communication boards.[t] Blissymbols can be printed on tape, using the *Blissymbol Printer*,[u] a portable symbol printing aid (Silverman and Kelso 1977). It is also possible to portray Blissymbols on a home television set, using the *Blissymbol Terminal*[v] (Giddings et al. 1979).

To summarize, Blissymbolics, originally designed for the purpose of international communication, is currently being used with a wide range of non-vocal persons. It is a very logical, visual-graphic system, which is meaning-based, using symbols from a small number of basic components.

Why. The semantic base of Blissymbolics allows a small number of symbols to be combined into a large number of entries. The pictographic and ideographic nature of many of the symbols allows them, theoretically, to be easily learned and retained. This makes the system ideal for clients who are not ready for spelling, but who have the potential to learn large vocabularies. Thus, Blissymbolics may be appropriate as a primary communication system for many non-vocal clients. Since traditional orthography is paired with the symbols, extended use may enhance reading skills, as indicated by case reports (Silverman et al. 1978). However, it is noted that controlled research on this topic is needed.

McNaughton and Kates (1980) note that applications of Blissymbolics with the handicapped have greatly expanded from initial use as an augmentative system for the severely physically handicapped to a broad range of experimental uses. They report that (p. 313):

> Blissymbolics is being explored as an educational tool for blind, deaf, and autistic students; for pre-reading activities; for remedial reading programs; for visual-perception remediation; for second language teaching; for concept and language development; as an enrichment activity; and for communicating with students with severe behavioral and emotional problems.

They note that while some of these newer applications show promise, carefully developed research efforts are needed to demonstrate their use. In addition, Blissymbolics is not intended as a panacea for all clients and all problems. McNaughton and Kates (1980) list both advantages and disadvantages of the system, as well as positive and negative effects on symbol users.

Who. Blissymbols have been used successfully with clients in the following disability groups: physically handicapped (Kates and McNaughton 1975; Silverman et al. 1978; Waugh and Gibson 1979); mildly to severely mentally retarded (Harris-Vanderheiden 1976; Song 1979); multiply handicapped (Elder and Bergman 1978); deaf (Goddard 1977); and adult aphasics (Saya 1979).

McNaughton and Kates suggest that the following skills are required by the user:

1. *Good visual discrimination skills,* in order to distinguish between differences in features such as size, shape, and orientation of shapes;
2. *Cognitive skills at the late pre-operations or early concrete operations stage* (Chapman and Miller 1980); McNaughton and Kates (1980) note that the client " . . . must be able to comprehend that a visual symbolic representation can serve as a communication signal" (p. 318);
3. *Reliable means of indicating* symbol position, through electronic or non-electronic means;
4. *Moderate to good auditory comprehension and visual matching skills* appear to be necessary for use with adult aphasics (Saya 1979); these criteria may also apply to other populations.

For sophisticated use of the system, involving aspects such as creation of needed symbols through the combine indicator, the user should have a higher cognitive level (at least concrete operations) and a rich experiential background. This will enable the user to understand the logic of the system and its meaning-based symbols, rather than responding in rote manner to meaningless visual configurations.

Thus, while Blissymbolics is " . . . particularly valuable to physically handicapped persons whose physical limitations restrict them to a specific number of symbols" (McNaughton and Kates, p. 311), the system also has great potential for a variety of applications to a wide range of clients.

The audience for Blissymbol users includes, theoretically, persons who can read English. This may be somewhat misleading, however, since meaning in English cannot always be determined by reading the words under the symbols. For partners to be able to decode messages from sophisticated users, they must have some understanding of the basic logic of Blissymbolics. For example, understanding use of the metaphor strategy should help the partner understand that the symbol sequence GO TO GARAGE, preceded by the symbol for metaphor, can be translated as "get lost" (Silverman et al. 1978). The logical base of the system and the small number of basic components (e.g., wheel) which are used in numerous symbols (e.g., the component wheel is used in the symbols for car, bus, train, bicycle) should make this a relatively easy system for the non-impaired adult to learn.

When. McNaughton and Kates note that studies are needed to determine the earliest cognitive level at which Blissymbols can be used functionally. Blissymbols have been used successfully with preschool children as young as two years of age (Silverman et al. 1978; Waugh 1979). Interestingly, Saya (1979) found that aphasic clients who were more than two years post-onset (mean = 6.8 years) did better on acquisition of Blissymbols than those of recent onset (mean = 8.8 months). This may be explained in part by one of two factors. First, the late onset group was also younger (mean age = 53 years) than the early onset group (mean age = 68 years). Second, Saya (1979) suggests that the long-term aphasic patient " . . . has come to the realization that speech is a futile attempt and is willing to consider an alternate system of communication" (p. 7). Thus, it appears that motivation is one indicator of when Blissymbolics should be introduced to adult aphasics. Of course, if the client could perceive Blissymbolics as means of communication, rather than an alternative to vocal communication, he or she might be motivated at an earlier stage.

How. McNaughton and Kates (1980) note that there is no formal teaching methodology for Blissymbolics. The application will depend on the individual's goal(s). Silverman et al (1978) present an extensive section on assessment which should help the communication specialist determine the most appropriate goals and procedures for the client. A very slow learner who requires continuous drill and shows no interest in creating new symbols would require a different training approach than one who learns symbols quickly and readily attempts to create new symbols.

Although no single program of instruction is recommended, an Evaluation Study did help to identify three models for the application of Blissymbolics with the communication handicapped. These three models are in the formative stage and are recommended only as a framework for assessment and programming. In addition, they should not be considered as rigid or mutually exclusive (Silverman et al. 1978).

Model One consists of ". . . using Blissymbolics as an expressive language augmenting developed receptive native language" (McNaughton and Kates, p. 315). This model would be appropriate for interim use (e.g., a temporarily dysphonic client) or long-term use (e.g., a client with severe cerebral palsy). This client should use symbols for propositional conversation, master a large number of symbols, and create new symbols with the combine indicator. He or she could be taught the general logical basis of the system and a variety of strategies.

Model Two involves ". . . using Blissymbolics as an expressive language paralleling and contributing to the development of native language" (McNaugton and Kates, p. 315). This would allow a young child to interact with the environment while still in the early stages of language acquisition. This is viewed as a facilitative approach. The client would be taught in the normal sequence of language development, using principles from normal language development whenever possible. Silverman et al., (1978) suggest that this model could be applied to existing vocal language programs (e.g., Horstmeier and MacDonald, 1978; Miller and Yoder, 1972, 1974; MacDonald and Blott, 1974).

Model Three consists of "using Blissymbolics as a surface communication system" (McNaughton and Kates, p. 315). This involves a non-developmental approach to language learning, and assumes "limited learning potential and impaired language capability" (Silverman et al., p. 91). A small number of symbols would be presented for rote association of meaning and simple stereotyped sentences. More specific teaching strategies as well as materials (e.g., worksheets and games) are presented in *The Handbook of Blissymbolics* (Silverman et al. 1978; Appendix B of this book) and *Teaching and Using Blissymbolics* (McDonald 1980).

Where. A wide variety of texts, materials, and other information on Blissymbolics is available from the Blissymbolics Communication Institute (see Appendix C). Training sessions for potential teachers of Blissymbolics are also organized through the Institute.

Rebus
The term "rebus" comes from a Latin word meaning "thing" (Woodcock 1968). Rebuses are symbols which represent entire words or parts of words. It is not a closed symbolic system, as anyone may design rebus symbols. The rebuses described in this book will be taken from a published set included in the *Standard Rebus Glossary* (Clark, Davies, and Woodcock 1974; see Appendix A).

Rebus symbols may be classified into three basic categories, with combinations of the symbols yielding a fourth category:

1. *Concrete symbols*—these primarily depict objects or actions:

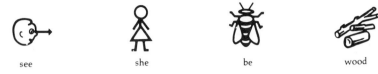

| see | she | be | wood |

2. *Relational symbols*—these primarily depict locations or directions:

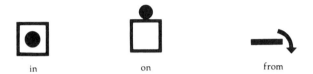

| in | on | from |

3. *Abstract symbols*—these are primarily arbitrary symbols, although some are ideographic:

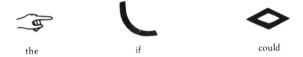

| the | if | could |

4. Combinations—
   a. *compound symbols* in which two or more rebuses are joined:

| into | somewhat |

   b. *combined symbol using affixes* in which a root word is joined to an affix such as present progressive "-ing", past tense "-ed", or plural "s":

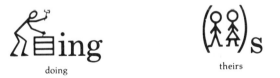

| doing | theirs |

   c. *combined symbols using letters* in which rebuses are joined with letters of the alphabet:

| son | sat | sand |

As indicated in the preceding examples, Rebus is to some extent a phonetically-based system. For example, the pictographs representing the words "be" and "would" are not semantically related to the meanings of their referents. Instead, a pictograph of a bee is used for the word "be," since the two words sound alike. This is true for a number of the rebuses, and especially for combinations involving the use of letters. Clark and Woodcock (1976) explain that " . . . the reader decoding words represented by the rebus principle is required to transfer the meaning of the pictographic symbols into sound chunks, then process the sound chunks into a new or second-order meaning" (p. 554).

Since letters may be added to rebuses as needed, any morphological inflections may be produced. Special rebuses are used for irregular verbs and nouns. The syntax of Rebus could therefore parallel English or another language.

Why. Rebus could be a useful system for non-readers. Rebuses have been demonstrated to be easier to learn than traditional orthography (Woodcock 1968; Clark et al. 1974). Another study (Clark 1977) found that rebuses were easier to learn than traditional orthography, Blissymbols, and Carrier-Peak symbols (converted to graphic form for this study). Subjects for the Clark study were non-handicapped, non-reading children (CA 4 yrs. 4 mos. to 5 yrs. 5 mos.). Rebuses have been standardized to some extent, and are available in rub-on form, thus increasing their usefulness on communication aids. They may also facilitate reading development.

Who. Rebuses have been used for different purposes with a variety of populations: the culturally disadvantaged (Woodcock 1968); hearing impaired (Clark et al. 1975); and mentally retarded (Apffel et al. 1975). They might not be accepted well by non-vocal adults, due to the childish nature of many of the rebuses.

Clients using Rebus as a symbolic communication system would need the following skills:

1. *Good visual discrimination skills,* in order to distinguish among the rebuses; however, Woodcock (1970) suggests that this is less crucial than for traditional orthography, since there is greater uniqueness among a set of rebuses than among a set of spelled words;
2. *Sensorimotor Stage 5 cognitive development,* for decoding the pictographic symbols; for symbols using letters, higher cognitive skills would be required;
3. *Skill in sound blending,* in order to decode combined symbols (unless they are to be learned by rote).

The audience for Rebus would be broad, as many symbols are iconic. In addition, they are usually displayed with the English word printed below the symbols, making them accessible to the English-reading community.

When. This could be used as an initial symbolic system, particularly if the concrete symbols were emphasized. As noted earlier, decoding pictographic symbols could be possible after the client has reached the Stage 5 level of sensorimotor development at approximately 12 to 18 months of age in the non-handicapped child.

How. A variety of materials and several programs are available for teaching the use of rebuses. The approach used would depend on the capabilities of the client and the goals. The *Minnesota Early Language Development Sequence* (MELDS) was developed to provide a receptive language program for young hearing-impaired children. This program contains 120 structured classroom lessons which are correlated with 120 parent lessons. The entry–vocabulary contains 393 items including a variety of signs, words, rebuses, and sentence patterns (Clark et al. 1975).

A reading program, *The Peabody Rebus Reading Program*, has also been developed (Woodcock, Clark and Davies 1969). In addition, a number of separate materials are available, such as a glossary, rebuses in rub-on form, and rebus glossary cards. These may be utilized in programs designed to meet the needs of the clients.

Where. Materials on the Rebus system are available from the American Guidance Service.[w] Primary sources of information include *The Standard Rebus Glossary* (Clark, Davies, and Woodcock 1974), the *MELDS Glossary of Rebuses and Signs* (Clark and Greco 1973), and *The Peabody Rebus Reading Program.*

Discussion and summary. Rebuses may be used as entries on communication aids, especially for children. The liberal use of traditional orthography in combined rebuses, and the lack of semantic basis for many symbols (e.g., would, be) may make it more difficult to learn the entire system than some other systems, such as Blissymbolics. More comparative research is needed to evaluate various systems.

Abstract Symbol Systems

The "abstract symbols" in this discussion are symbols that represent words. They are considered abstract because their form does not suggest their meaning. Two abstract symbol systems will be presented:

1. Premack-type tokens;
2. Yerkish lexigrams.

Premack-type tokens

What. The symbols used in this system are different plastic or masonite shapes, each of which represents a word. They are based on Premack's work with chimpanzees (Premack 1970). An example of the use of these shapes is the *Non-SLIP* symbols, developed for the Non-Speech Language Initiation Program (Carrier 1976; Carrier and Peak 1975). Each of the *Non-SLIP* symbols has a unique shape, is color-coded, and is keyed to indicate in which sequence of the program it is to be used. The English word is printed on each symbol. These symbols are manipulated by placing them in the appropriate sequence on a form board. Hollis and Carrier (1978) suggest several ways of making the system more accessible to severely physically handicapped children, such as mounting symbols on small blocks of wood to enable clients to grasp them or knocking them over to indicate selection. Deich and Hodges (1978) have attempted to develop the Premack-type symbols as a functional communication system (unlike the *Non-SLIP* system). Therefore, they modified the symbols to make them more iconic or representational.

Why. The *Non-SLIP* program is a language initiation program, which " . . . is viewed as a starting point for children who are not able to meet entry requirements for other more advanced programs . . . . the role of *Non-SLIP* is not so much one of teaching functional communication responses as it is one of teaching tactics for acquiring those responses" (Carrier 1976, p. 529). Thus, it may be viewed as a language facilitator. The plastic symbols could also be used as a symbolic system. Silverman (1980) notes several potential advantages of Premack-type symbols:

1. *They can be identified either by sight or by touch,* making them potentially useable by visually-impaired or blind clients;
2. *They place minimal demands on memory,* due to the manner of use, in which symbols forming a message are lined up in a visible display;
3. *They may be easier to learn and remember than other symbols,* since they may be recalled through vision or touch.

Thus, both the symbols and the training system (*Non-SLIP*) may be useful for some clients. However, the abstract nature of the symbols, the logistical difficulty of keeping numerous bulky symbols within reach, and the necessity to manipulate the symbols may make this system unuseable for many severely handicapped clients.

Who. The *Non-SLIP* approach was designed for training severely and profoundly retarded nonverbal children, but has been used with other populations, such as children diagnosed as autistic, psychotic, or emotionally disturbed. Carrier (1976) reports that this program seems to succeed with a large percentage (over 90% in available data) of children with previously low likelihood of success. Success is viewed as helping the clients begin the process of learning communication skills. Other researchers have used Premack-type symbols and similar programs with a variety of disability groups, such as: adult aphasics (Velletri-Glass et al. 1973; Gardner et al. 1975); autistic children (McLean and McLean 1974); and profoundly handicapped children (Deich and Hodges 1978). Each of these projects has reported some success.

Requirements for use of this system would include:

1. *Adequate gross motor skills,* in order to grasp and manipulate the symbols, or to knock them over to indicate selection;
2. *Sensorimotor Stage 5 or 6 intelligence,* according to Chapman and Miller (1980); however, Clark (1977) and Deich and Hodges (1978) found that initial learning of these abstract symbols was more difficult than learning more concrete or iconic symbols, raising the possibility that a higher level of intelligence may be necessary;
3. *Good visual discrimination skills,* including color discrimination, if the symbols are color-coded; however, these symbols are not as visually similar as some other symbolic systems (e.g., orthography, Blissym-

bols); this may be due to the small number of symbols currently available.

Carrier (1976) reports that the following groups of children have been least successful with the *Non-SLIP* approach to using these symbols:

1. Children with motor problems that interfere with the required responses; however, he suggests that the program may be modified to allow responses other than symbol manipulation (e.g., scanning);
2. Children with frequent and severe seizures, as they have difficulty retaining behaviors learned prior to the seizures; Carrier recommends use of retention programs (as in *Non-SLIP*) to overcome this problem;
3. Severely and profoundly retarded clients with clear emotional overlay, especially if they demonstrate resistance to learning.

Thus, with adaptations, this symbolic system appears useable with many severely handicapped clients. However, its selection will likely depend on the function it is intended to serve. Current research has demonstrated the usefulness of this system for facilitating language. Application of Premack-type symbols for use as a communication system, whether primary or supplemental, has not been adequately documented.

If words are printed on the symbols (as in *Non-SLIP*), the potential audience would be the reading community.

When. The timing of introduction of Premack-type symbols depends on the purpose of use. If they are intended as a language initiation system, as most researchers have used them, they could be introduced as soon as the client develops the readiness behaviors listed in the "who" section. However, using these symbols in a language initiation program constitutes an extensive training program for behaviors which are preliminary to functional communication. Therefore, this program might be considered when and if a client demonstrates failure or lack of readiness for other communication training approaches.

How. Two main procedures have been developed for application of Premack-type symbols. The first is the Non-Speech Language Initiation Program (Carrier and Peak 1975), which is reviewed in Appendix B of this book. It is a highly structured direct training program, which teaches clients the following basic behaviors: sequencing (several steps which lead to sequencing of symbols by color/number cues); labeling (in which the client matches symbols to pictures); and constituent selection (several steps which teach the client to use nouns, verbs, objects of prepositions, and prepositions meaningfully in the sequence). Upon completion of the program, the client can generate appropriate seven-word sentences (e.g., THE COW IS SITTING ON THE CAR), in response to pictured stimuli.

The second major application of Premack-type symbols is presented by Deich and Hodges (1978). The Appendix of their book provides information about the initial application of this program and subsequent modifications to make the symbols more concrete.

Where. Information about this symbolic system and its applications with severely handicapped clients may be found in the following sources: Carrier (1974, 1976); Carrier and Peak (1975); Deich and Hodges (1978); and Premack (1970).

Discussion and summary. It is difficult to separate the Premack-type symbols from their widely used application in the *Non-SLIP* approach. To date, Premack-type symbols have been used primarily for language facilitation, and difficulties have been encountered in using them for functional communication (Deich and Hodges 1978). Recall that *Non-SLIP* culminates in production of sentences such as THE HORSE IS PLAYING ON THE SIDEWALK. While these are clearly not highly functional responses, Carrier (1976) asserts that the clients have also learned a variety of behaviors necessary for using language to communicate. He reports the following examples: using symbols to represent picture stimuli; responding symbolically to parameters of a stimulus that cue verb [or preposition] selection; sequencing symbols in appropriate grammatical order (p. 536). It may be argued that these behaviors are not necessary for learning language to communicate. For example, it is possible to communicate quite effectively without ever using symbols to represent picture stimuli. However, the behaviors learned through *Non-SLIP* may serve as useful tactics in future language learning. For each client, the communication specialist must determine if it is appropriate to justify delaying functional communication training until the client has completed this language initiation program. We look forward to research which answers the question of whether initial use of a language initiation program such as *Non-SLIP* accelerates eventual progress in functional communication.

Yerkish lexigrams

Yerkish is a synthetic language designed for use in Project Lana, an ape-language research project. The correlational grammar for Yerkish was written by von Glassersfeld (1977). The symbols for this language are *lexigrams*, which are distinctive geometric figures that function as words. These lexigrams are composed of one or more of nine basic elements, such as a dot, a line, a diamond, and a circle. Word classes are potentially differentiated by the background color (Rumbaugh and Savage-Rumbaugh 1978). Examples of lexigrams are as follows:

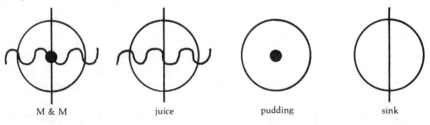

| M & M | juice | pudding | sink |

For Project Lana, lexigrams are used as keys on a board. Selecting and depressing those keys yields visual facsimiles, so the user and communication partner can see which symbols have been produced. A computer monitors all linguistic events, evaluates them grammatically, and records them. The computer used in Project Lana can honor correctly formed requests such as PLEASE MACHINE GIVE PIECE OF APPLE.

The design of both the Yerkish language and the lexigrams is based on several considerations which may influence use of the system as a primary communication mode in humans. For example, an important consideration was developing a grammar which could be comprehended by a relatively small computer (Rumbaugh and Savage-Rumbaugh). The resultant grammar is somewhat restricted compared to a language such as English; this could be an advantage or a limitation, depending on the client. The choice of design elements in the system also relates to the need for a system that can be easily produced by machine. This makes the system readily available for modification for use on a communication aid. In fact, a portable electronic conversation board using lexigrams has already been developed (Warner, Bell, and Brown 1977). The highly abstract nature of these symbols may make them difficult for some severely handicapped persons to learn. In addition, the combination of only nine design elements would seem to place high demands on the client's visual discrimination skills. Research and clinical experience will decide if this system can be applied to severely handicapped individuals. Rumbaugh (1978) reports some success in pilot work with six severely and profoundly retarded children in a residential center. He suggests that: "In all probability, it is the attractiveness of the lighted keyboard with its colorful array of keys, its prompt feedback of correctness and incorrectness, and all of the activities attendant to the system that creates motivation and excitement among our low-level subjects" (Rumbaugh 1978, p. 23).

For further information on the use of Yerkish lexigrams, the reader is referred to Rumbaugh (1977) or the Yerkes Primate Regional Research Center.[x]

Symbolic Language Codes

This category includes systems which represent a spoken or written language. The most common of these systems is the alphabet. Under this classification traditional orthography is used to represent a written language such as English. Phonemic alphabets may be used to represent spoken languages. There are numerous variations of both traditional orthography and phonemic alphabets, some of which are useful as symbol systems for non-vocal individuals. Finally, there are symbol systems which are designed to represent either traditional orthography or phonemic alphabets, similar to the gestural systems of fingerspelling, gestural Morse Code, and Cued Speech. The symbolic systems of Morse Code and braille are examples of systems which represent traditional orthography. Each of these major subcategories of symbolic language codes will be discussed separately.

Traditional orthography and variations

What. Traditional orthography refers to the written alphabet, such as the Roman alphabet used to represent English. In English there is often not a one-to-one correspondence between sounds and letters, due to the frequency of silent letters and letters which take different sounds in different words. There have been a number of attempts to give added clues to traditional orthography in order to aid the process of learning to read. Clark and Woodcock (1976) divide these into *controlled traditional orthography* and *elaborated traditional orthography*. The controlled approaches emphasize what is termed the linguistic aspect. Here the spelling patterns of traditional orthography are controlled, yielding sentences such as "A man ran a tan van" (p. 560). Several reading programs developed around this approach are described by Clark and Woodcock. They note that findings on the success of these programs are equivocal and that ". . . the value of learning to read words in isolation with a de-emphasis on reading for meaning has been questioned" (p. 562).

The elaborated approaches involve elaboration of symbols, but without altering the spelling (Clark and Woodcock). Programs based on this approach use strategies such as color coding of vowel phonemes (Bannatyne 1968); *Diacritical Marking System* (Fry 1964); and *Symbol Accentuation*, in which words are accentuated to represent meaning, such as adding stripes to the word "candy" (Miller 1968). Clark and Woodcock report that results of research on these systems are inconclusive, but that reading ability seems to be enhanced while the system is being learned. The enhancement diminishes as the system is removed.

Even if traditional orthography is not altered, it may be presented differently on communication aids. For example, many aids include the 26 letters of the alphabet, even if another symbol system, such as Blissymbols, is being used. Use of words requires the client only to decode traditional orthography or to read rather than to encode or spell. It also increases the speed of transmission since the client need only point to one entry, rather than a series, to produce a word. Traditional orthography may also be combined with other symbols to add meaning. For example, words could be printed on abstract symbols such as Premack-type tokens or printed below or above graphic symbols such as Blissymbols. Letters or letter combinations (e.g., prefixes) may also be added to symbols such as rebuses to change their meaning. Beukelman and Yorkston (1977) suggest use of an alphabet-number cuing board, with the client pointing to the initial letter of each word spoken.

Thus communication boards could potentially use as orthographic symbols the following: traditional orthography, alone or in conjunction with other symbols and in the form of letters, syllables, or words; elaborated traditional orthography, to help the client decode the entries. Controlled traditional orthography would not be useful as a symbol system but might be considered in training.

Why. Traditional orthography has the advantage of being a normative system and having a large audience of users. If the alphabet is used and the client spells out words, the potential vocabulary is unlimited. Traditional orthography also also has applications in combination with other symbol systems, and there is some evidence that written words may be learned without direct teaching, by pairing them with symbols such as Blissymbols (Silverman et al. 1978).

Who. Traditional orthography and variations have been used with a variety of disability groups such as the cerebral palsied (Vicker 1974a).

Entry level requirements for use of traditional orthography and its variations would include the following:

1. *Good visual discrimination skills,* in order to recognize small differences between characters;
2. *High level of cognitive development,* (Chapman and Miller [1980] suggest late preoperations to concrete operations), especially if the client is expected to encode words;
3. *Good spelling skills,* if the client is expected to use letters to encode words;
4. *Knowledge of the structure of language,* in order to pair written words with spoken words.

These requirements may be reduced somewhat if the client is expected only to decode words (read) and not to encode words (spell) as well. The use of elaborated traditional orthography, especially with accentuation of symbols, may further reduce the cognitive and linguistic requirements. For example, Clark and Woodcock report that the *Symbol Accentuation* system was originally designed for use with the severely retarded but has also been utilized with adult aphasics and deaf children, as well as other less handicapped populations.

Use of initial letter cuing, as suggested by Beukelman and Yorkston (1977) would be especially useful as a supplemental system for clients with intelligibility problems (e.g., dysarthria, apraxia). This method would have the advantages of: (1) decreasing rate of speech output, possibly further adding to intelligibility; and (2) placing minimal demands on spelling skills.

Thus traditional orthography and its variations may be useful for clients in a wide range of populations, from the retarded to the cognitively intact physically handicapped. The target audience would be all persons who read the language.

When. As noted in the entry requirements, a high level of cognitive development is required, at least for encoding with the use of traditional orthography. Even with elaborated systems it is unlikely that this would be an initial system for developmentally non-vocal clients. However, it might be combined with a primary system (e.g., pictures) with the intent of fading out that system when the client developed reading skills. For adventitiously non-vocal clients, such as laryngectomees, orthography often serves as an immediate communication system until another system (e.g., esophageal speech, Amer-Ind) can be established. The requirements in this case would be that the client was a reader/speller before onset and retained those abilities.

How. The procedures for teaching these systems would be those used for teaching reading and spelling. The approach chosen would depend on the system chosen (traditional orthography or one of the elaborated systems) and client characteristics such as cognitive level. For example, training procedures have been developed for teaching the use of various elaborated traditional orthography systems. Training programs have also been designed for teaching selected reading and spelling skills to severely handicapped clients: Nietupski et al. (no date); Snell (1978). Nietupski et al. found six sub-skills under the cluster of skills needed to determine the meaning of printed words:

1. verbal labelling skills;
2. whole word skills (labelling and determiing meaning);
3. whole sentence and story skills (gaining meaning from longer strings of words);
4. context skills (determining meaning through utilization of surrounding words and/or pictures);
5. phonics skills (using letter-sound associations);
6. spelling skills.

They review studies and present procedures for training severely handicapped clients in each of those sub-skills. The sub-skills chosen for teaching a particular client depend on the content of the communication aid. For example, if the aid will include a relatively small number of words, the whole word approach might be selected. This may be feasible in training for communication aid use since the number of entries may already be limited by the format of the display.

The area of teaching reading is primarily the realm of the special educator and reading specialist. The communication specialist should play a role in providing input regarding content, with the intention of transferring reading skills learned to use with a communication aid.

In summary, the question of how to teach may be answered in part by considering the type of symbols and the client's abilities. It is recommended tht a reading specialist with experience in training handicapped clients be consulted if possible.

Where. A number of reading approaches are available for teaching specific elaborated traditional orthography systems. Several such systems are described and sources are given in Clark and Woodcock (1976) and Snell (1978). The following present approaches for teaching reading and/or spelling skills to the severely handicapped: Nietupski et al. (no date); Nietupski, Williams, and York (no date); Snell (1978); Wulz and Hollis (1980).

Phonemic alphabet systems

What. A number of phonemic alphabets have been devised to represent spoken languages. This discussion will focus on phonemic alphabets which represent English, since the sound-grapheme correspondence between spoken and written English is poor. Clark and Woodcock (1976) report that these graphic systems "...provide a close sound-to-symbol relationship by increasing the number of alphabetic symbols (beyond that of 26) so that they more nearly match the number of English phonemes" (p. 567). Thus a sound typically has only one spelling, and silent sounds are not written in phonemic alphabet systems. Clark and Woodcock (1970) review a number of phonemic alphabet systems which have been used in teaching reading. They conclude that, similar to elaborative systems, phonemic alphabets accelerate initial reading acquisition when compared to programs using traditional orthography. However, this advantage tends to fade after transition is made to traditional orthography. Due to lack of research, it is not known whether there are any special benefits of these systems for use with handicapped persons.

The phonemic alphabets described by Clark and Woodcock were designed for use as teaching aids, not as entries on communication devices. However, several of these phonemic systems have been demonstrated to be successful as entries on communication devices. For example, Shane and Melrose (1975) utilized the *International Teaching Alphabet* (i.t.a.), which was developed to facilitate beginning reading. In this system, ". . . ostensibly, each i.t.a. character represents only one sound and each sound is represented by only one character" (Clark and Woodcock, p. 570). However, Clark and Woodcock note that there are a few exceptions to that rule. Shane points out that graphemes in i.t.a. ". . .have a logical resemblance to the letters contained in the Roman alphabet, a feature not always true of the IPA [*International Phonetic Alphabet*]" (p. 3). Shane also notes the efficiency of i.t.a. relative to traditional orthography; for example, eight different Roman alphabet configurations are required to represent the phoneme /u/, while only one i.t.a. symbol is needed. Shane taught a limited version of the i.t.a. (16 of the 44 symbols) to two severely physically handicapped, non-vocal clients. The results of testing indicated that both subjects were capable of using the i.t.a. symbols appropriately and were able to generalize this learning to some extent. Application of the entire 44-symbol i.t.a. system was found to be successful with a third client in a separate study (Carol Cohen, personal communication).

A modified version of the standard *International Phonetic Alphabet* (IPA) is used with the PHONIC MIRROR HandiVoice. The 45 phonemes available in that vocabulary include IPA symbols and variations of IPA designed for use in diphthong combinations or to indicate stress or durational differences (Cohen et al. 1979). These entries are used in generating synthesized speech. *International Phonetic Alphabet* or *International Teaching Alphabet* symbols may also be useful in phoneme cuing systems, similar to the letter cuing system suggested by Beukelman and Yorkston (1977). Instead of pointing to the initial letter of a word, the client would point to the symbol for the initial phoneme (Shane, personal communication).

Another adaptation of the phonemic alphabet is *SPEEC*[y] (Goodenough-Trepagnier and Prather, in press). A French version of SPEEC is *Par lē si la b.*[y] The entries for *SPEEC* are phoneme sequences which have a high frequency of occurrence in spoken English, plus a set of single phonemes. These are represented in a consistent, simplified orthography. This *syllabary*, as it is termed, is intended ". . .to provide an optimal middle ground between the alphabet and word lexicon" (Goodenough-Trepagnier 1978, p. 422). The *SPEEC* system is available in lapboard form, of 256 or 400 entries, with entries arranged in alphabetic order of frequency-alphabetic order and on encoded eye-gaze selection (ETRAN) charts.

Why. Phonemic alphabet systems have several advantages over traditional orthography. First, they are more efficient since silent letters are not indicated. The *SPEEC* system is especially efficient, as it uses phoneme sequences, or groups of sounds. Goodenough-Trepagnier and Prather (1980) calculated the number of letter selections and *SPEEC* unit selections (using *SPEEC*-400) in passages typed by a non-vocal person. The relative efficiency was 3.9 for letters and 1.6 for *SPEEC* units, indicating that *SPEEC* required 2.44 times fewer selection gestures than letter-by-letter spelling. This could be very significant for the severely motorically-impaired client. However, it must be compared against the larger number of units (256 or 400) from which the selection must be mde. Goodenough-Trepagnier and Deser (1980) compared rate of output in structured speech with a *SPEEC* board and a *Canon Communicator*, which uses an alphabetic symbol system. They found that while the client produced more entries per minute on the *Canon* (27.2) than the *SPEEC* (11.3), the resultant output in words per minute was lower for the *Canon* (4.8) than for the *SPEEC* (7.2). Thus, while the smaller entry-field of traditional orthography yielded more rapid selections, the larger entry-field using phoneme units ultimately resulted in more efficient communication for that client. The effect of fatigue could also be less for more efficient systems since fewer gestures would be required. The final determination of relative efficiency will have to be made on a client-by-client basis.

Both single phoneme and phoneme sequence units lend themselves well to vocal output. Vocal output is currently available with the modified International Phonetic Association Alphabet (*PHONIC MIRROR Handi Voice*) and will be avilable with the *SPEEC* unit system.

Who. Use of the phonemic alphabet systems described here has been reported primarily with the severely physically handicapped such as clients with cerebral palsy (Cohen et al. 1979; Goodenough-Trepagnier 1978).

Entry level requirements for the systems would be as follows:
1. *Good visual discrimination skills,* in order to recognize differences between phonemes or phoneme sequences;
2. *High level of cognitive development* (likely late preoperations to early concrete operations), to comprehend the relationship between abstract symbols and sounds;
3. *Good sound blending skills* or capability of developing them in the future.
Cohen et al. (1979)

Goodenough-Trepagnier and Prather (1980) suggest that clients who have not yet acquired English orthography may be able to master *SPEEC* since it does not involve the extremely complex set of rules and exceptions found in traditional orthography. However, there is currently not enough data to support this theory.

The audience for these systems would depend on the type of output. If the system were used on a vocal output communication aid, the audience would be unlimited. Goodenough-Trepagnier and Prather (1980) have demonstrated that visual output from the *SPEEC* system may be comprehended by reading adults with a low error rate after minimal training sessions (one half hour to 45 minutes).

When. As noted previously, it is not clear when phonemic alphabet systems can be introduced, although it appears that this may be somewhat earlier than for traditional orthography, if use in encoding messages is compared.

How. The phonemic alphabet systems described in this section are entries on commercial aids, and training procedures focus on training the system through use of the aid. Training may also relate to aspects of phonemic alphabet training such as sound blending.

Where. For information on the modified International Phonetic Alphabet used with the *PHONIC MIRROR HandiVoice*, contact HC Electronics, Inc. (see endnote d). Guidelines for training use of that system and aid combination are presented in a seminar manual distributed by that company (Cohen et al. 1979). Information regarding *SPEEC* and the *SPEEC* Manual and boards (Goodenough-Trepagnier and Prather 1979) is available from the Biomedical Engineering Center of Tufts-New England Medical Center (see endnote y).

Symbol systems which represent traditional orthography

What. This section will describe two widely used systems which represent traditional orthography. These are at a higher level than the language codes previously described because the user must understand that this code represents traditional orthography, while traditional orthography represents the intended referent. Thus, these systems are two steps removed from natural language. The two codes to be described are braille and Morse Code.

The *braille symbol system* is a tactile system invented for use with the blind. It consists of 63 characters, each of which is formed by a raised-dot pattern based on a six-cell matrix. In addition to the 26 letters of the alphabet and digits, punctuation marks, several frequently used words (e.g., *for*), and letter combinations (e.g., *er*) are included in the system (Silverman 1980). It may be used as an input or output system.

The *International Morse Code* is a system which encodes letters and digits, plus a few additional elements (e.g., punctuation, error signal) through a series of dots and dashes.

Both of these systems may be encoded by a client using adaptive devices. For example, many of the switches mentioned in the section on activating the symbol system could be used to encode Morse Code. The client could use two switches, one transmitting a dot, one a dash, or could use one switch in two ways (e.g., a long depression indicates a dash, while a short depression indicates a dot). An example of an aid which utilizes Morse Code as input is *Scriptonic II.*[z] Output is hard copy via an electric typewriter. An example of an aid which utilizes braille is SAGEM (see endnote k).

Why. These systems may be selected due to the client's disabilities (e.g., blindness). Morse Code appears to be a relatively efficient system for speed of message transmission; Newell (1974) reports that on the average fewer than three operations are required per letter typed. Since both of these systems represent traditional orthography, they would be especially useful to clients who learned how to read and spell before onset of their condition.

Who. Braille is designed for blind and blind-multihandicapped clients, while Morse Code has been adapted primarily for use with severely physically handicapped non-vocal clients. Some of the entry requirements would be the same for the two systems:

1. *High level of cognitive development* (Chapman and Miller [1980] suggest late preoperations to concrete operations), since the client must be able to understand and use the code;
2. *Good spelling skills* would be helpful since these codes are based primarily on traditional orthography.

In addition, use of braille requires *good tactile perceptual skills* since the client must be able to recognize and interpret the patterns of raised dots of the system. Use of Morse Code requires the *ability to produce two distinct signals*, for example by activating two switches or by activating one switch with two durations (e.g., sip or suck on an air tube).

If the output of the aid is the code, the audience must also learn the code. This should not be too difficult for non-handicapped reading adults since both codes represent traditional orthography. In many cases the communication aid will yield output which is in written form, so that the potential target audience is increased.

When. Since these codes are based on traditional orthography, they may be introduced readily to clients with spelling abilities (e.g., adventitiously non-vocal clients). However, for developmentally disabled clients, the systems may replace traditional orthography and may be introduced when spelling skills would normally be introduced.

How. Teaching braille is primarily the responsibility of the teacher of the visually impaired. Communication specialists may wish to learn to encode or decode braille to aid in their work with visually impaired clients. The optimum choice is to take a course in braille from a college or university. If that is not possible, correspondence courses are available through organizations such as the Hadley School for the Blind,[aa] which offers several levels of instruction in braille. Manuals are also available for teaching the sighted; an example is the one by Ashcroft and Henderson (1963; see Appendix A).

A number of resources are available to help interested persons learn Morse Code. The best alternative is to take a course from a licensed instructor. For the name of the nearest instructor, contact the American Radio Relay League (see Appendix C). There are also several resources which should aid in learning Morse Code. *Tune In the World with Ham Radio* is a self-teaching package which trains the reader to pass the requirements for the Federal Communications Commission Novice license. One area covered is Morse Code, which is taught by a 60-minute cassette tape. This course is designed to train the person to use code at five words per minute. Another set of materials, the *ARRL Code Kit*, is designed to increase code speed from five to 13 words per minute. It includes an illustrated guide to Morse Code, covering numerous suggestions, plus two cassette code tapes. Another resource is *Morse Code for the Radio Amateur*. Any of these resources can be used for independent learning, although training from a licensed instructor is highly recommended.

Once the trainer has developed some facility in sending and receiving Morse Code, he or she may begin training the non-vocal individual. If the client is also severely physically handicapped, it is likely that training procedures will have to be modified. For example, training a client to interface the transmitter by use of sip and suck would require different training procedures than for use of the standard Morse Code key.

Where. Further information about teaching and learning braille may be obtained from the following sources: American Foundation for the Blind, American Printing House for the Blind, and National Library Service for the Blind and Physically Handicapped (see Appendix C). The National Library Service offers a free reference circular, *Braille Instruction and Writing Equipment*, which lists manuals for teaching braille, braille correspondence courses, braille writing equipment, and a selected bibliography.

Information regarding Morse Code may be obtained from the American Radio Relay League (see Appendix C).

Discussion and Summary

Selecting the appropriate symbol system for a client will depend on factors inherent in the system, the client, and the client's environment. The goal(s) of the communication system will also influence this phase of the decision process. For example, if the system is intended to provide interim communication for a client learning a more permanent mode (e.g., a glossectomy in therapy to learn compensatory speech techniques), the system should be one that can be learned readily, preferably even one the client already knows, such as traditional orthography. As suggested earlier, consideration of these factors may indicate that a single system is not sufficient for a client. In addition, it is important to re-assess the symbol system periodically to ensure that it continues to meet the client's needs.

The preceding review of symbolic systems included consideration of basic client capabilities and suggested target populations. Potential target audiences were also described. Determination of symbol systems will also be related to decisions regarding input switches, means of indicating, and output mode. Some systems (e.g., Premack-type tokens) currently do not yield as many options as other systems (e.g., traditional orthography). Myers et al. (1980) offer numerous suggestions regarding demonstrations of device characteristics, some of which should be helpful in this regard. In addition to demonstrating device characteristics, several potential symbol systems could be demonstrated to the client, teacher, parents, and others to obtain their opinion. The client's range of motion and speed of indicating could affect the type of entry chosen (e.g., letters, phoneme sequences, words). Trial therapy with one or more potential systems may be helpful in selecting the optimal system. A number of system features, such as vocabulary size and cognitive level, are listed in table 9-1.

Selecting the Content

A number of commercially available communication prostheses include displays which are predetermined. That is, entries are the same for all clients using the prostheses. This may be appropriate for the sophisticated system user, as the selected entries are often based on research and field testing (e.g., SPLINK). However, the client just beginning to use a communication prosthesis may need a more personalized set of entries. This is especially true if the client is currently learning language or learning the symbol system as well. Thus many commercial aids will not provide appropriate initial content.

As with the gestural communication systems, content will be determined to a great extent by the system chosen. Some symbol systems have guidelines regarding symbols appropriate for initial content. For example, Silverman et al. (1978) recommend that, for Model Three application (Blissymbolics as a surface communication system with the severely retarded), initial symbols should be

1. Pictorial;
2. Visually dissimilar;
3. Related to concrete objects or persons in the immediate environment;
4. Immediately functional (e.g., symbol for "more").

These suggestions would be equally applicable to other symbol systems which include pictographic elements, such as Rebus and pictures. The final three suggestions would be helpful in determining initial content for abstract systems such as Yerkish lexigrams or Premack-type tokens. The strategies suggested in Chapter 3, such as client preference and frequency of occurrence, should also help in determining initial content for most symbol systems. However, several systems, because of their nature, must be learned in their entirety before they can be used functionally for communication. Examples of such systems are the alphabet, Morse Code, and braille (used for encoding). Thus, while some characters (e.g., the letter "0") might be easier to learn than others, they would achieve limited usefulness until they could be combined with other characters in the system.

For some symbol systems, such as traditional orthography and Rebus, the communication specialist must also determine whether to include inflectional markers (e.g., plural "-s", progressive "-ing") on the display. This would be determined by consideration of the client's physical, cognitive, and linguistic abilities and communicative needs. For example, a client with a very slow formulation rate might find that redundant aspects such as liberal use of inflectional markers were too limiting for speed of production. Another client, who used the communication aid for preparing more formal messages such as letters and homework, could opt for inclusion of a certain number of inflectional markers.

Due to the restricted vocabulary available with many communication

Table 9-1
Primary features of symbolic communication systems.

Symbolic Systems	Sensori/Motor	Pre-Operational	Late Preoperations or Concrete Operations	Pictographic	Ideographic	Abstract	Primarily English	Own Structure	Relatively Un-structured	Small (Under 1000)	Large (Over 1000)	Unlimited
	Cognitive			Interpretation				Structure		Vocabulary Size		
Pictures, Photographs, and Line Drawings	X			X	*				X	X		
Picsysms	X	*		X	*		X		X		X	
Blissymbolics	X	*	*	X	X	*	*	X			X	
Rebus	X	*	*	X	X	*	X				X	
Premack-type Tokens (Non-SLIP)	X					X	X			X		
Yerkish Lexigrams	X					X		X		X		
Traditional Orthography and Variations			X			X	X					X
Phonemic Alphabets			X			X	X					X
Braille			X			X	X					X
Morse Code			X			X	X					X

X = indicates that the system primarily falls into this category.
* = indicates that the system has a large component or may be adapted to fit in this category.

Pictographic symbols picture what they represent.
Ideographic symbols represent ideas about the referent.
Abstract symbols are arbitrary, with meaning assigned.

aids, the issue of content is particularly crucial. For a client with a very limited lexicon, due to physical limitations or developmental level, use of the core lexicon strategy, as suggested by Holland (1975) and Lahey and Bloom (1977), is recommended. A method for organizing an initial lexicon by content and by form is presented in Lahey and Bloom (1977) and reprinted in table 3-1 of this book.

If others in the environment are to be involved in using the device (e.g., pointing to entries for the client), instructions should be printed on it in a highly visible place. These instructions should indicate that the client uses the device to communicate and should describe exactly what the communication partner must do.

On devices with a limited number of entries and no spelling capability, the client should have some way to indicate that the desired message is not available. This could be accomplished by including a blank card on the symbol display panel.

In summary, the selection of initial content should receive considerable attention, as it may structure the client's initial communicative success to some extent. The early emphasis should be on functional content, with the understanding that content changes as the client progresses both developmentally and in relation to his or her communication aid.

Organizing the Content

Anderson (1980) asserts that ". . . communication aids sometimes seem to be built to conform more to the wheelchair tray or needs of observers than to the specific needs and abilities of their non-speaking users" (p. 41). This section will focus on organizing devices so that they meet *user* needs.

The organization of a communication device refers here to how the device is designed, how entries are arranged on it, and factors such as the size, spacing, and boldness of entries. For many commercial aids these questions may be determined in advance as the panels are pre-designed. This is true, for example, of most adaptive typewriters, which follow standard typewriter format. Even so, other organizational features may be altered; for example, the *PMV Keyboards,*[bb] which are part of the *PMV System,*[bb] come in four sizes depending on the client's physical abilities for direct selection (e.g., foot, elbow, hand, mouthstick, or handstick). These keyboards are used with an *IBM typewriter.*[cc]

Organization is particularly important in custom-designing a communication device such as a board or a booklet for a client. The general design of the communication board will differ according to the client's physical and communicative abilities. For example, a client who points only with his or her right arm will likely have no entries placed in the far left-hand corner. Several types of communication displays are available: single sheet display, multiple display, supplementary notebook(s), or a combination of these displays. Vicker (1974b) notes that the *single sheet display* is the easiest display for a client to use; thus it is often appropriate for initial use. Supplementary notebooks may be used in conjunction with this single sheet if the client requires a large vocabulary. Since the single sheet display allows access to very limited vocabulary, Vicker suggests use of *multiple displays*, which can be either sequential or simultaneous. A *multiple sequential display* consists of a combination of horizontal and vertical display areas. At the client's request the message receiver flips to a card with additional entries (see figure 9-4). Each card contains all or most of the categories used by the client. Vicker notes that use of this display may make it difficult for the client to produce sentences with good syntax; therefore, the client may conserve his or her energy by producing utterances which contain only content words (e.g., names, action words). A *multiple simultaneous display* allows nearly all linguistic categories to be exposed at the same time, but not all entries within each category are visible simultaneously (see figure 9-5). Vicker suggests that this type of display may help remind the client to include those relational words (e.g., auxiliaries, prepositions) which are frequently omitted when using other displays. *Supplemental notebooks* can be used in conjunction with either type of multiple display, though they would be less needed with the multiple simultaneous display. Supplemental notebooks often include words grouped into categories (e.g., food, animals, action verbs, colors). In this case the main display would contain the category heading such as "family." When the client indicated a category, the communication partner would make that category available to the client. This could be facilitated through use of color coding and/or index tabs indicating various categories.

Vicker (1974b) notes that, compared to single sheet displays, multiple displays require more difficult long-term vocabulary storage problems and longer utterance production time. A suggestion from Kladde (1974) may help the client handle the problem of long-term vocabulary storage, especially for the multiple sequential display. Kladde suggests that the top sheet(s) contain the most common entries for the category and an index to other entries. This would be most successful with noun categories; for example, cards containing toys, food, and so forth could be numbered and indexed. A *combination display* might help solve both the problem of vocabulary storage and production time by combining the features of a single sheet display with a multiple display (either simultaneous or sequential).

Another factor which must be considered in the general design of a communication board is the client's needs in various settings. It may be necessary to duplicate the board, making physical alterations as necessary to fit another frame (e.g., a stand-up box instead of a lap board). It may also be necessary to design a board with different entries and a different format to meet the needs of other settings. For example, a portable notebook which fits into a backpack or shoulder bag, or a wallet photo holder filled with communication cards may be developed for the use on field trips and family outings. Higgins and Mills (1978) suggest constructing "mini-communication boards," which are prepared around a limited theme. Entries on such a board could be pictures or words. For example, a board for use in a fast food hamburger restaurant would display several hamburger offerings, french

Figure 9-4
An example of a multiple sequential display*.

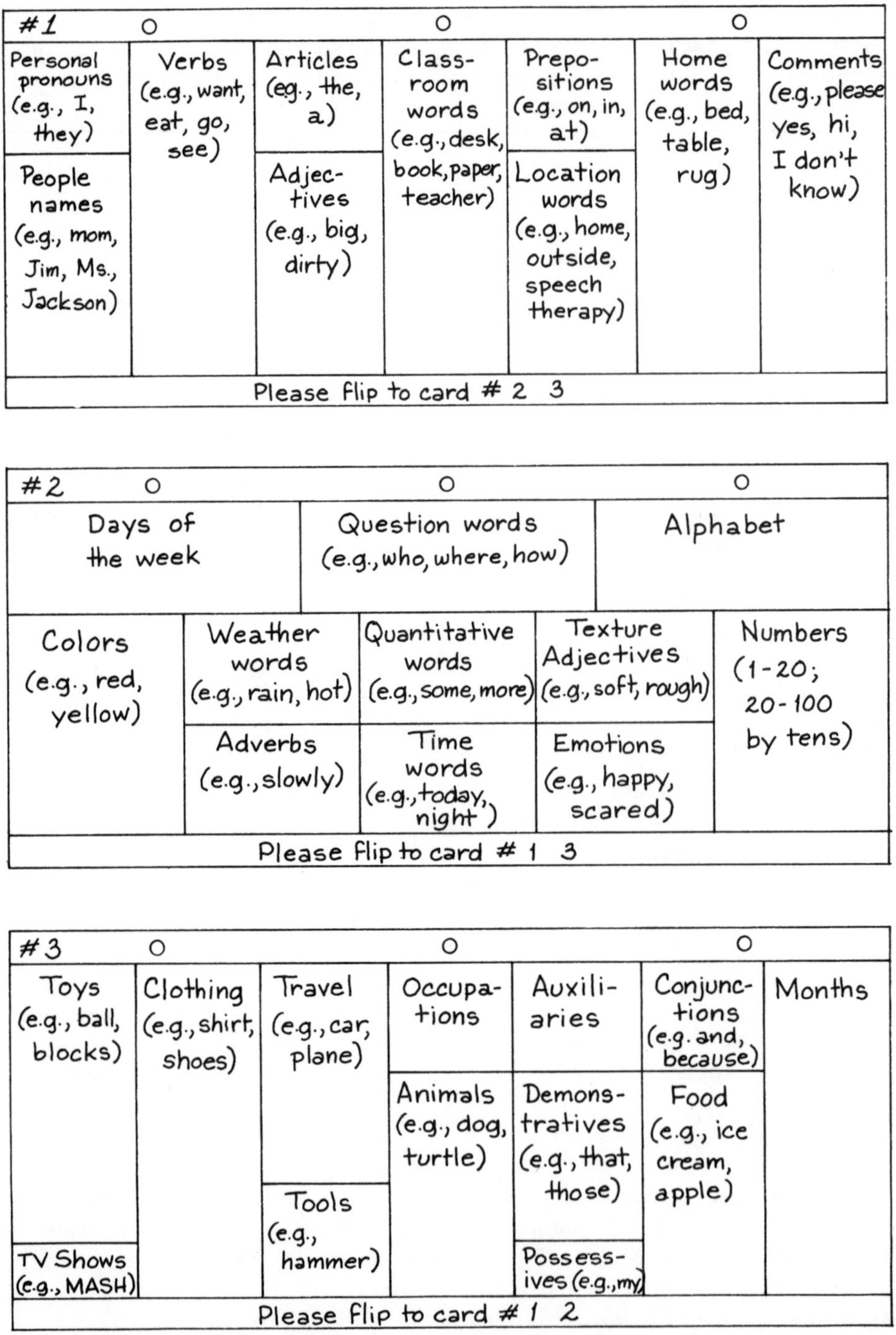

#1 ○			○		○	
Personal pronouns (e.g., I, they)	Verbs (e.g., want, eat, go, see)	Articles (eg., the, a)	Class-room words (e.g., desk, book, paper, teacher)	Prepo-sitions (e.g., on, in, at)	Home words (e.g., bed, table, rug)	Comments (e.g., please, yes, hi, I don't know)
People names (e.g., mom, Jim, Ms., Jackson)		Adjec-tives (e.g., big, dirty)		Location words (e.g., home, outside, speech therapy)		
Please flip to card # 2 3						

#2 ○			○		○	
Days of the week		Question words (e.g., who, where, how)			Alphabet	
Colors (e.g., red, yellow)	Weather words (e.g., rain, hot)	Quantitative words (e.g., some, more)	Texture Adjectives (e.g., soft, rough)		Numbers (1-20; 20-100 by tens)	
	Adverbs (e.g., slowly)	Time words (e.g., today, night)	Emotions (e.g., happy, scared)			
Please flip to card # 1 3						

#3 ○			○		○	
Toys (e.g., ball, blocks)	Clothing (e.g., shirt, shoes)	Travel (e.g., car, plane)	Occupa-tions	Auxili-aries	Conjunc-tions (e.g. and, because)	Months
			Animals (e.g., dog, turtle)	Demons-tratives (e.g., that, those)	Food (e.g., ice cream, apple)	
		Tools (e.g., hammer)				
TV Shows (e.g., MASH)				Possess-ives (e.g., my)		
Please flip to card # 1 2						

*These three cards would be arranged in a stack, with card #1 on top, card #3 on bottom.

Figure 9-5
An example of a multiple simultaneous display*.

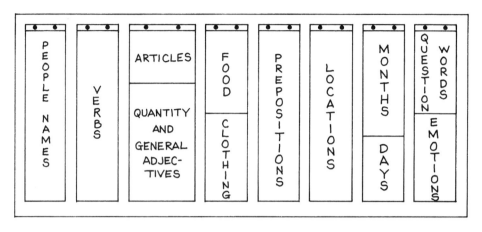

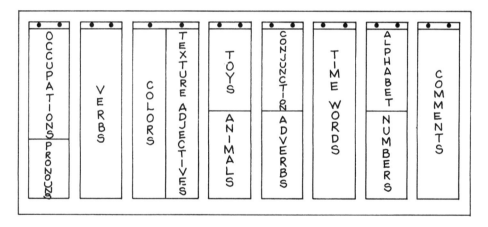

*This represents two "layers" of the display. For example, if the first column of the top page is turned from people names, it will reveal occupation names and pronouns.

fries, drinks, ketchup, a bathroom, and a general request for help. Schurman (1974), Silverman (1980), and Vanderheiden (1977) discuss the "how-to" aspects of designing and constructing a communication board or device. Appendices in Vicker's book present examples of communication display materials and frames.

After the general design of the board has been determined, the trainer must decide the most appropriate way to arrange entries on it. Many authors recommend use of a modified "Fitzgerald Key" (Kladde 1974; McDonald 1976, 1980; McDonald and Schultz 1973; Sayre 1963). This key, developed for use with hearing-impaired children, utilizes columns, with an appropriate heading at the top of each column to indicate the most common word order in English. Categories in an adapted version might include who, what, where, verbs, modifiers, when, and so forth. Kladde (1974) notes that, for persons knowing complex sentence structure, it is impossible to list words in all the locations where they might occur; for example, "who" or "what" words could occur as subjects, direct objects, and so forth. Therefore, she suggests that these words be placed in categories and locations where they are used most frequently by the individual. Several authors also suggest that category headings and entry labels be color-coded for non-readers (McDonald 1976; McDonald and Schultz 1973; Traub 1977).

A final step related to organization is determining the appropriate size, spacing, and boldness of each entry. These determinations are based on a number of factors, such as the client's motoric ability and visual skills, and the type of symbols to be used. Vicker suggests preparing sample display sheets with symbols appropriate for the client. These sheets should differ with regard to the size, spacing, and boldness of entries. Client capabilities and preferences could be evaluated using these sample displays.

In summary, organizational features must be considered whether purchasing a pre-designed communication aid or custom-designing a communication prosthesis for a client. In selecting a pre-designed aid, the communication specialist (and others involved in the decision process) must keep features such as placement, size, spacing, and boldness of entries in mind. For example, a laryngectomee who was a good typist before surgery might prefer a supplemental aid with a typewriter keyboard format, while a client who had not and does not expect to learn to type might choose an alphabetically-arranged keyboard. Organizational features are even easier to control in custom-designed devices, and they must not be ignored.

Methods of Teaching Symbolic Communication

Methods of training will likely be even more diverse for symbolic than for gestural communication, since in addition to learning the system, the client may also have to learn to operate an input mechanism and use it to indicate entries on the communication aid. There are an overwhelming array of tasks to be taught. Harris and Vanderheiden (1980) stress that they must not all be undertaken simultaneously. They suggest using intervention processes which are gradual and evolutionary. This is especially important for severely physically handicapped or multihandicapped clients, who will have to learn many skills in order to communicate more effectively.

Chapter 4 of this book presents preliminary skills usually trained before use of a symbolic communication system is initiated. Several areas relate to development of symbolic communication systems, such as tracking, scanning, and selection, attending, and cognitive development. It is our belief that many of these skills may be developed in the context of communication training rather than being trained in isolation, with progress to communication training contingent upon reaching pre-set criteria on preliminary skills.

Developing a Hand-Pointing Response

This section will give examples of procedures for training the child to use the hand-pointing system. This is a particularly desirable option because pointing is normative and therefore culturally acceptable. In addition, it is a universal gesture rather than an individualized gesture; therefore, it should be readily understood by others (Brown 1979). Reichle and Yoder (1979) distinguish two types of pointing: actually touching as with a communication board; and extended pointing, indicating objects that are out of reach. This discussion will focus primarily on the touching type of pointing. A number of components of pointing should be considered in designing a pointing program:

1. *Hand configuration*—will the client use the whole hand or one finger to point? If one finger (typically the index finger), will the other fingers be in a semi-curled or fisted position?
2. *Direction and distance*—will the client need to point in a vertical, horizontal, or diagonal direction? Will the objects or entries pointed to be within reach (actual touching) or out of reach (extended pointing)?
3. *Amount of pressure*—will slight, moderate, or heavy pressure be required to make the selection? This will depend on the communication prostheses used.
4. *Manipulation*—will any manipulation be required, such as pushing, sliding, or dialing?
5. *Need for appliances*—will any prosthetic devices be needed (such as T-shaped dowels secured to the hand or grapsed by the client?

Musselwhite and Thompson (1979)

These questions can be answered through physical evaluation of the client and through assessment of the needs imposed by the communication device selected. Several authors (Brown 1979; Schurman 1974) stress the importance of appropriate positioning for pointing. This should be determined in conjunction with the occupational and physical therapists.

It may be necessary to train some skills preliminary to teaching pointing as a means of indicating. However, this may be done in the context of communication training. Preliminary skills may include areas such as functional object use, tracking and scanning, and reaching (Brown 1979; Reichle and Yoder 1979). Reichle and Yoder noted that some clients do not readily learn reaching behavior. They suggest several strategies:

1. Match the direction of reaching with the orientation of the head;
2. Move an object toward a collision course with the client's face; the client will often reach up to bat the object away, and this reaching may be developed into a more functional reaching behavior (p. 208).

Brown suggests numerous pre-pointing activities such as giving and taking objects in a game, touching a great variety of objects, poking fingers in wet sand, soft clay, or toys with holes.

Target practice for pointing will involve consideration of the five components listed earlier. Numerous strategies are available, depending on the needs and capabilities of the client. For example, Dunn (1979) suggests that, in training the use of extended index finger, the trainer focus on the target finger, pulling the tip of the finger to extend it rather than attempting to curl the remaining fingers into a fist. Brown suggest using several tangible cues for training pointing. For example, she recommends using a small car taped to a child's hand, which can help the child gain proficiency in sliding the hand to the desired position before pointing. She also suggests having the client touch the trainer's finger, which is placed on the appropriate symbolic entry. These tactual cues would be faded as the client's accuracy improved.

The considerations and strategies previously described, while not intended to serve as a program for training a pointing response, should provide direction regarding primary areas of consideration.

Training Use of a Symbolic System and Communication Aid

This section will focus primarily on training in the use of a symbolic system for communication. Several systems (e.g., Blissymbolics, Rebus) are accompanied by guidelines for training. Similarly, for a number of communication aids and devices (e.g., PHONIC MIRROR HandiVoice, SPEEC, ZYGO Model 16C), training materials and suggestions may be obtained from the manufacturer. These materials will generally have to be adapted to meet the needs of the individual.

Several general training approaches are also available, to be used with a variety of symbolic systems (Elder 1978; Montgomery 1980b).

As with gestural systems, the purpose of the system will also influence training methods. If the purpose is to serve as a language facilitator, the conceptual base of the system (e.g., Blissymbolics) may be stressed. For the system intended to serve as a primary long-term communication system, training will also focus on factors such as clarity of message transmission, initiation of communication interactions, and use of the system in all situations. If the system is viewed as a supplemental system, for example to provide contextual support for a moderately dysarthric client, emphasis will be on recognizing communication breakdowns and using the system to clarify the message or establish context.

Thus general methods of training appear to depend on a number of factors, such as client capabilities, goals of the system, and features of the system. Since there is such a wide range of degree of complexity in these symbolic systems, training strategies would also differ greatly. General training strategies such as handshaping, used widely in gestural training programs, are less common in symbolic training approaches.

A number of toys and games may be used in training clients to use communication aids effectively. For example, the Basic Skill System[dd] has a display board containing a stimulus section and a response section. The client is required to match the lit stimulus cell with the matching target response cell, using a scanning light. Correct matching yields a pleasant tune, while incorrect matching results in a "raspberry" sound. Standard toys and battery-powered toys may also be used or modified in the training process. An example of a toy which can help train children in communication board use is Mattel's *See'n Say Talking-Learning System*, which includes 40 words, arranged like talking flash cards. Toys may be especially useful in teaching a child to activate an input switch. For example, the *Push-Button Farm* from Child Guidance demonstrates to the child that pushing a button produces an action, such as causing an animal to appear from behind a door. Descriptions of modified toys may be found in *Communication Outlook* (see Appendix C) and *Helping the Handicapped* (Howard 1979, see Appendix A). For information on modifying standard toys, contact the Telephone Pioneers of America (see Appendix C) or the Prentke-Romich Company.[ee]

As with gestural training approaches, symbolic training approaches seem to be either primarily artifically-structured or primarily naturally-structured. An example of a naturally-structured approach is the one described in the *Handbook of Blissymbolics* (Silverman et al. 1978), in which the symbols are used for communication immediately after they are introduced. For example, they assert that "Immediate opportunities should be provided to demonstrate and utilize purposefully new symbol learnings" (p. 143). They also recommend total immersion in Blissymbol communication, such that communication should be arranged with a wide range of persons in the environment and in all settings in which the client interacts with others. In addition, symbols should be incorporated into all play and learning situations. These naturally-structured strategies could be used also for other symbolic systems. Another component of the naturally-structured approach is that the trainer should initially communicate via the system to demonstrate its viability and usefulness (Jarrow and Northrup 1979). Once the client has learned basic use of the system, this modelling may be faded out. Modelling may also be used in training or demonstrating specific aspects, such as constructing questions.

Other approaches are primarily artificially-structured. The emphasis is on the client's correct behavior in response to antecedent events such as trainer-administrated stimuli. Examples of these programs include Elder (1978) and Hall et al. (1978). These approaches may be useful for clients who have failed to acquire or use a symbolic system following naturally-structured training. The small steps and specific procedures provided for clients experiencing difficulty may aid in introducing symbolic systems to severely handicapped clients. In addition, artificially-structured approaches may be useful for implementation by paraprofessionals. However, these approaches or programs, typically presented in individual training sessions, will likely not be sufficient in training the many skills the client must master to successfully utilize a symbolic communication system. Combination of the two approaches may prove both effective and efficient. For example, the artificially-structured approach could be used for problem areas, and the naturally-structured approach could serve as the all-day approach, designed to facilitate functional use and generalization of targets learned in artificially-structured sessions.

One area in which non-vocal clients might be trained, regardless of the system used, is communication interaction. Non-vocal persons need to learn strategies to maintain communication interaction. Several strategies should be considered:

1. *Eye contact*—although this may not be possible during message transmission, it may be feasible between messages and may help hold the attention of the communication partner;
2. *Facial expressions*—the client should be trained to be as expressive as is physically possible since much of the information transmitted through the voice (e.g., intonation, stress) is lost to non-vocal clients;
3. *Appropriate head and body movements*—for example, the client may provide feedback to the communication partner by nodding the head; he or she may also add information to a message through body movements such as leaning forward slightly when asking a question;
4. *Appropriate vocalizations*—the client who has voluntary control over vocalization may use this also as a method of feedback or enhancement of a message; for example, during an extended explanation by the comminication partner, the client may occasionally respond with an approximation of "uh-uh" to provide auditory feedback; this strategy would be especially important for communication that is not face-to-face, such as use of a vocal output aid on the telephone; vocalizations such as laughs may be used to emphasize a point made by either partner.

These strategies may be used alone or in combination, depending on the physical capabilities of the client. They are useful strategies both in terms of normalization and maintaining communication.

Cohen et al. (1979) point out that clients using a new symbol system or a new communication aid may need to be retrained to modify old habits and reinforce new behaviors. For example, a client moving from an approach in which other controlled the conversation (e.g., through "twenty questions" or operating a scanner for the client) may need to be trained to initiate conversation. Cohen et al. (1979) suggest strategies such as having the client practice initiating topics; provide second comments (in addition to "o.k." or "that's nice"); lengthen answers, then follow with a question; and incorporate humor into comments occasionally. Role playing may be a useful procedure for introducing some of these strategies, although they should be incorporated into natural situations as soon as possible. The opposite situation may occur for clients who have become used to vocal communication but have lost the ability to vocalize (e.g., due to myasthenia gravis). These clients may need to be trained to occasionally use shortcuts in communicating via symbol systems, in order to transmit a message in a reasonable amount of time.

Generalization and self-regulation skills are crucial to symbolic communication training. Use of a naturally-structured training approach may help facilitate generalization. In addition, some of the symbolic communication programs mentioned in this chapter and reviewed in Appendix B contain specific generalization strategies. This is an area that must receive attention in training if the client is to reach his or her potential as a communicator.

In summary, a few general and specific strategies for teaching use of a symbolic communication system have been presented. Several commercially available programs or approaches are reviewed in Appendix B of this book. Properly used, these resources may be combined to yield training approaches appropriate for individual clients.

Evaluating Effectiveness of Communication Aid Use

When the client has been trained in using a communication aid to employ a symbolic system, the communication specialist must measure the effectiveness of that aid and system. The following points to consider were developed by the staff at the Non-Oral Communication Center, Fountain Valley, California:

1. *Establish meaningful exit criteria*—How far do you *expect* a user to progress in what length of time? With what degree of speed or accuracy will he communicate? In what way or ways will he utilize the system?
2. *Initiation of conversation*—One of the highest levels of communication use is to generate or initiate discourse and not merely respond.
3. *Number of peer interactions*—The greatest amount of conversation or interaction time for all of us is that spent with peers. Using frequency counts or similar data, record the number of approaches or incidents of peer interaction. Pre- and post-system or comparison over time can be used.
4. *Serves as a learning tool*—We primarily use our language to solve problems, gain information, and exchange it with others. A child or adult who is using his non-speech system for learning is showing substantial efficiency.
5. *Need for a more complex system*—The need for a more sophisticated approach or an expanded vocabulary is a sign that the system has been successfully implemented.
6. *Expansion of purposeful use*—Can he use his system for any of these "purposes" of communication? (from Yoder and Riechle 1977):
   - giving information;
   - getting information;
   - describing events;
   - getting listeners to do something, believe something, feel something;
   - expressing one's own intentions, beliefs, feelings;
   - indicating desire for further communication;
   - entertainment;
   - learning new behavior;
   - rehearsal, reinforcement, feedback;
   - interaction;
   - personal gratification.

(Montgomery 1980a, pp. 1-3)

Beukelman and Yorkston (1980) suggest some data collection analysis procedures for evaluating the effectiveness of communication aids. They term this phase of assessment *performance evaluation*. They suggest that some aspects of this evaluation may be carried out in a clinic situation, such as rate and accuracy of message transmission. Other aspects, such as generalization to a number of environments and efficiency of use with a variety of communication partners, may best be evaluated in the client's environment. Beukelman and Yorkston performed both capability-need and performance evaluations on two non-vocal clients. They used tape recorders to gather 8-hour samples of communication and then analyzed these samples to obtain the following types of information:

1. Communication events per hour;
2. Communication partners per hour;
3. Different communication environments per hour;
4. Words per communication event;
5. Communication partner receiving rate (words per minute);
6. Message types (e.g., WH-questions, request information) in terms of percent of total events;
7. Modality used;
8. Resolution strategy for communication breakdowns (e.g., yes/no questions, multiple choice).

These analyses may help to answer questions such as which of two communication aids is more effective; which resolution strategies are most successful; and which communication partners interact more (or less) appropriately?

Summary

The diversity of communication aids, communication aid options, and symbolic systems, and the wide range of client capabilities necessitates flexibility in methods of training. The evaluation of the effectiveness of aids and client training in their use must be continually reassessed to determine future intervention procedures.

Involvement of Staff and Family in Symbolic Communication Training

It is crucial that those in the client's environment become involved in the symbolic communication training program since the non-vocal client's communication opportunities are already limited. Harris (1978) studied five children's use of their electronic communication aids in three school situations: free play, individualized instruction, and small group discussion. Aspects analyzed included the extent of participation in communication events, the communication modes utilized (e.g., gestural, vocal, symbolic), and the communicative functions expressed by the children. She found that these children generally appeared to be passive participants. They rarely initiated interactions and expressed a limited number of communicative functions. Ambiguous modes of interaction such as gestures and vocalizations were often used. Most communicative interaction was between teacher and child, with infrequent peer-to-peer interchange. Thus it appears that message receivers often assume responsibility for conversations with non-vocal clients. The goal of helping clients to initiate communication interchanges was discussed in the previous section on methods of training. It is also necessary to train communication partners regarding their roles in communicating with persons using symbolic systems. Cohen et al. (1979) also point out the need to train persons in the client's environment on appropriate means of interacting with the client.

DeHaven (1978) suggests that communication specialists should consider training a significant person in the non-vocal individual's environment. This person, often a family member, would provide support outside the therapeutic environment.

Several goals may be identified in training staff, family, and others working with symbolic system users:

1. *Training others to interpret the client's messages*—this may involve training in the symbolic system and/or the communication aid; for example, the logic and basic strategies of Blissymbolics may be explained, or procedures for decoding eye movements made in use of an encoding system such as *ETRAN* may be described; it will often help to let the trainees have hands-on experience with productive use of the symbolic system or communication aid;

2. *Teaching others to use appropriate interchange technqiues*—this may involve strategies such as having partners wait for the client to initiate a topic, asking the client more open-ended questions, and encouraging the client to clarify messages rather than interpreting for him or her (DePape 1980); appropriate interchange techniques will depend on factors such as the client's speed of message transmission and the capabilities of the symbolic system and the communication aid;

3. *Teaching others to serve as primary or secondary trainers for the client*—this could range from having the trainer administer a training program such as those reviewed in Appendix B to having him or her devise teaching games to play with the client;

4. *Training others to assist in generalization*—this could mean having siblings play symbol games which the client hs learned, having parents require and reinforce use of symbols learned in a training session, or having paraprofessionals make opportunities to use the client's aid to communicate throughout the day.

This brief discussion suggests several major areas of training for increasing the involvement of people concerned with the communication needs of symbolic system users. Training strategies could involve lecture, modelling, hands-on demonstration, role-playing, and question-and-answer sessions. Group and individual training sessions could be utilized. It is recommended that clients be involved in the training process so that they can provide input and become aware of expectations for themselves and others who communicate with them.

Summary

This chapter has addressed several of the primary uses regarding symbolic communication. A number of symbolic communication systems have been discussed, along with methods of achieving access to those systems, means of indicating, and modes of output. Implementation factors, which often interact, have been included. For example, some symbolic systems (e.g., Premack-type tokens) have limited modes of output, while others (e.g., traditional orthography, Blissymbolics) can provide several modes of output. Therefore, each of these areas must be considered in conjunction with others in programming for the severely communication-handicapped client. The goal(s) for use of the system must also be kept in mind throughout the decision process.

Endnotes

[a] Trace Research and Development Center, Waisman Center, 1500 Highland Avenue, University of Wisconsin-Madison, Madison, Wisconsin, 53706.

[b] ZYGO Industries, Inc., P. O. Box 1008, Portland, Oregon, 97207.

[c] SciTronics, Inc., 523 South Clewell Street, P. O. Box 5344, Bethlehem, Pennsylvania, 18015.

[d] HC Electronics, Inc., 250 Camino Alto, Mill Valley, California, 94941.

[e] Upper Case, 2011 Silver Court East, Urbana, Illinois, 61801.

[f] Prentke Romich Company, R.D. 2, Box 191, Shreve, Ohio, 44676.

[g] Typewriting Institute for the Handicapped, 3102 West Augusta Avenue, Phoenix, Arizona, 85021.

[h] Micon Industries, 252 Oak Street, Oakland, California.

[i] Medelec Limited, Manor Way, Old Woking, Surry, GU22,9JU, England.

[j] Prentke-Romich Company, R.D. 2, Box 191, Shreve, Ohio, 44676.

[k] Telesensory Systems, Inc., 3408 Hillview Avenue, P. O. Box 10099, Palo Alto, California, 94304.

[l] Prentke-Romich Company, R.D. 2, Box 191, Shreve, Ohio, 44676.

[m] ZYGO Industries, Inc., P. O. Box 1008, Portland, Oregon, 97207.

[n] Dr. V. Latham, Wolfson Industrial Unit, Department of Electronics, The University, Southampton, 5095NH, England.

[o] Trace Research and Development Center, Waisman Center, 1500 Highland Avenue, University of Wisconsin-Madison, Wisconsin, 53706.

[p] Mayer-Johnson Company, Box 393, Solana Beach, California, 92075.

[q] Cleo Living Aids, 3957 Mayfield Road, Cleveland, Ohio, 44121.

[r] Learning Concepts, 2501 North Lamar, Austin, Texas, 78705.

[s] Teaching Resources, 100 Boylston Street, Boston, Massachusetts, 02116.

[t] Prentke-Romich Company, R.D. 2, Box 191, Shreve, Ohio, 44676.

[u] Trace Research and Development Center, Waisman Center, 1500 Highland Avenue, University of Wisconsin-Madison, Madison, Wisconsin, 53706.

[v] NORPAK Industries; Contact Blissymbolics Communication Institute, 862 Eglinton Avenue East, Toronto, Ontario, Canada, M4G 2L1.

[w] American Guidance Service, Circle Pines, Minnesota, 55014.

[x] Yerkes Regional Primate Research Center, Emory University, Atlanta, Georgia, 30322.

[y] Biomedical Engineering Center, Tufts-New England Medical Center, 171 Harrison Avenue, Box 1014, Boston, Massachusetts, 02111.

[z]Irick Business Corporation, 2118 E. Desert Lane, Phoenix Arizona, 85040.

[aa]Hadley School for the Blind, 700 Elm Street, Winnetka, Illinois, 60093.

[bb]Medical Equipment Distributors, Inc., 1215 South Harlem Avenue, Forest Park, Illinois, 60730.

[cc]International Business Machines (IBM), International Headquarters, Armonk, New York.

[dd]Possum, Inc., 700 North Valley Street, Suite B, P. O. Box 4424, Anaheim, California, 92803.

[ee]Prentke-Romich Company, R.D. 2, Box 191, Shreve, Ohio, 44676.

Part Four: Appendices

Appendix A:
An Annotated Bibliography

Introduction

The following annotated bibliography is designed to acquaint the reader with recent literature in the area of communication programming for the severely handicapped. The entries represent communication theories, programs, and therapy techniques rather than reviews of technical research studies. The entries selected for inclusion in this bibliography are representative of available material in the area of communication programming for the severely handicapped and are not intended to be an exhaustive search of the literature.

The entries are listed alphabetically by authors. To assist the reader in locating entries related to specific communication modes and related topics an author index is included. The index is divided into seven sections. Some of the entries contain information which could be included in more than one section, and in those instances they are cross-referenced in the appropriate sections. Whenever possible, prices of texts and programs have been provided. The prices are current as of 1980.

A general description of each section is provided for ease of reference:

Assessment—Texts and articles presenting models of assessment and descriptions of a variety of devices (individual assessment devices are not included—see Appendix D for more information);

General—Texts and articles dealing with theoretical issues and background information on language development and language disorders;

Preliminary Training—Training and articles dealing with prelanguage or prerequisite skills such as attending and eliminating interfering behaviors;

Vocal Systems—Texts and articles dealing with programs and strategies for vocal communication;

Non-vocal Systems, General—Texts and articles dealing with gestural and symbolic communication modes;

Non-vocal Systems, Gestural—Texts and articles dealing with gestural communication systems such as American Sign Language and mime;

Non-vocal Systems, Symbolic—Texts and articles dealing with symbolic systems such as pictures, words, Blissymbols, and rebuses.

Assessment

Chapman, R.S. and Miller, J.F. (1980)
Darley, F.L. (1979)
Fiorentino, M.R. (1973)
Hutchinson, B.B., Hanson, M.L.,
 and Mecham, M.J. (1979)
Mallik, K. (1977)
McLean, J.E. and
 Snyder-McLean, L.K. (1978)

Meyers, L.S., Grows N.L.,
 Coleman, C.L., and Cook, A.M. (1980)
Nation, J.E. and Aram, D.M. (1977)
Shane H.C. (1980)
Silverman, H., McNaughton, S.,
 and Kates, B. (1978)
Tallal, P. (1980).

General

Adler, S. (1975)
Allen, K.E., Holm, V.A., and
 Schiefelbusch, R.L. (Eds.) (1978)
Baer, D.M. (1978)
Bloom, L. and Lahey, M. (1978)
Brown, L., Nietupski, J., Lyon, S.,
 Hamre-Nietupski, S., Crowner, J.,
 and Gruenewald, L. (1977)
Catalog of Federal Domestic Assistance (1979)
Chapman, R.S. and Miller, J.F. (1980)
Cohen, M.A., Gross, P.J., and
 Haring, N.G. (1978)
Finnie, N.R. (1974)
Haring, N.G. and Brown, L.J. (1976)
Haring, N.G. and Brown, L.J. (1977)
Holm, V.A. and McCartin, R.E. (1978)
LeBlanc, J.M., Etzel, B.C., and
 Domash, M.A. (1978)

Lillie, D.L. and Trohanis, P.L., (1976)
Lloyd, L. (1976)
Mallik, K.K. (1977)
McLean, J., Yoder, D., and
 Schiefelbusch, R. (1972)
Ruder, F. (1978)
Ruder, F. and Smith, M. (1974)
Schiefelbusch, R.L. (1978a)
Schiefelbusch, R.L. (1978b)
Schiefelbusch, R.L. (1980)
Schiefelbusch, R. and Lloyd, L.L. (1974)
Somerton, M.E. and Myers, D.G. (1976)
Sontag, E. (1977)
Tawney, J.W. (1977)
Thomas, M.A. (1976)
York, R.L. and Edgar, E. (1979).

Preliminary Training

Baer, D.M. (1978)
Brown, L., Nietupski, J., Lyon, S.,
 Hamre-Nietupski, S., Crowner, T.,
 and Gruenewald, L. (1977)
Fiorentino, M.R. (1973)
Gallender, D. (1979)
Horstmeier, D.S. and MacDonald, J.D.
 (1978)
Lyon, S., Baumgart, D., Stoll, A.,
 and Brown, L. (1977)
McCormack, J.E. and Chalmers, A.J.
 (1978)
McLean, J.E. and Snyder-McLean, L.K.
 (1978)

Nietupski, J., Stoll, A., Broome, D.,
 and Brown, L. (1977)
Popovich, D. (1977)
Scheuerman, N., Baumgart, D.,
 Sipmsa, K., and Brown, L. (1976)
Simmons, V. and Williams, I. (1976)
Soltman, S.F. and Rieke, A. (1977)
Sternat, J., Messina, R., Nietupski, J.,
 Lyon, S., and Brown, L. (1977)
Striefel, S. (1974)
Utley, B.L., Holvoet, J.F., and Barnes, K.
 (1977)
Woolman, D. H. (1980).

Vocal Systems

Bender, M., Valletutti, P.J., and
 Bender, R. (1976)
Bluma, S., Shearer, M., Frohman, A.,
 and Hillard, J. (1976)
Bricker, D., Dennison, L., Watson, L.,
 and Vincent-Smith, L. (1973)
Bricker, D., Ruder, K., and
 Vincent-Smith, L. (1976)

Bricker, W.A. and Bricker, D.D. (1974)
Cohen, M.A., Gross, P.J., and
 Haring, N.G. (1978)
Dunn, L.M. and Smith, J.O. (1966–1969)
Engelmann, S. and Osborn, J. (1976)
Fredericks, H.D., Baldwin, V.,
 Riggs, C., Furey, T., Grove, D.,
 Moore, W., McDonnell, J., Jordon, E.,

Hanson, W., Wadlow, M. (1976)
Fristoe, M. (1976)
Graham, W. (1976)
Gray, B. and Ryan, B. (1973)
Guess, D., Keogh, W., and Sailor, W. (1978)
Guess, D., Sailor, W., and Baer, D. (1974)
Guess, D., Sailor, W., and Baer, D. (1976)
Guess, D., Sailor, W., and Baer, D. (1977)
Guess, D., Sailor, W., and Baer, D. (1978)
Hart, B. and Rogers-Warren, A. (1978)
Hatten, J., Goman, T., and Lent, C. (1976)
Holland, A. (1975)
Horstmeier, D.S. and MacDonald, J.D. (1978)
Karnes, M.D. (1972)

Kent, L.R. (1974)
Lahey, M. and Bloom, L. (1977)
McLean, J.E. and Snyder-McLean, L.K. (1978)
Miller, J. (1977)
Murdock, J. and Hartmann, B. (1975)
Reichle, J.E. and Yoder, D.E. (1979)
Rieke, J., Lynch, L.L., and Soltman, S.F. (1977)
Schumaker, J.B. and Sherman, J.A. (1978)
Shane, H.C. (1979)
Siegel, G.M. and Spradlin, J.E. (1978)
Stremel, K. and Waryas, C. (1974)
Struck, R. (1977)
Swetlik, B. and Brown, L. (1977)
Waryas, C.L. and Stremel-Campbell, K. (1978)
Wetherby, B. and Striefel, S. (1978)
Worthley, W.J. (1978)
Yule, W. and Berger, M. (1976).

Non-Vocal Systems: General

Allen, J. (1977)
Alpert, C. (1980)
Bigge, J.L. (1977)
Bigge, J.L. and O'Donnell, P.A. (1977)
Hollis, J.H. and Carrier, J.K. (1978)

Moores, D.F. (1980a,b)
Shane, H.C. (1979)
Shane, H.C. (1980)
Wilber, R.D. (1980).

Non-Vocal Systems: Gestural

Allen, J. (1977)
Babbini, B.E. (1974)
Barnes, K.J., Murphy, M., Waldo, L., and Sailor, W. (1979)
Bornstein, H. (1973)
Bornstein, H., Hamilton, L.B., Saulnier, K.L., and Roy, H.L. (1975)
Christopher, D.A. (1976)
Crowner, T. (not dated)
Dalgaard, J., Newhoff, M., and Barnes, G. (1979)
Fristoe, M. (1976)
Fristoe, M. and Lloyd, L.L. (1977)
Golbin, A. (1977)
Goodman, L., Wilson, P.S., and Bornstein, H. (1978)
Gustason, G., Pfetzing, D., and Zawolkow, E. (1972)
Hamblin, K. (1978)
Hamre-Nietupski, S., Stoll, A., Holtz, K., Fullerton, P., Ryan-Flottum, M. and Brown, L. (1977)
Henegar, M.E. and Cornett, R.O. (1971)

Hopper, C. and Helmick, R. (1977)
Kent, L.R. (1974)
Kipnis, C. (1974)
Kohl, F., Fundakowski, G., Menchetti, B., and Coleman, S. (1977)
Kopchick, G.A., and Lloyd, L.L. (1976)
Kotkin, R. and Simpson, S. (1976)
Lykos, C.M. (1971)
Mallik, K. (1977)
Mayberry, R. (1976)
Moores, D.F. (1974)
Moores, D.F. (1980a)
Moores, D.F. (1980b)
O'Rourke, T.J. (1973)
Riekehof, L.L. (1978)
Schaeffer, B. (1980)
Siegel, G.M. and Spradlin, J.E. (1978)
Stokoe, W.C. (1980)
Stremel-Campbell, K., Cantrell, D., and Halle, J. (1977)
Struck, R. (1977)
Wilber, R.B. (1976)
Wilson, P.S., Goodman, L., and Wood, R.K. (1975).

Archer, L.A. (1977)
Ashcroft, S.C. and Henderson, F.H. (1963)
Bigge, J.L. (1977)
Bigge, J.L. and O'Donnell, P.A. (1977)
Carrier, J.K., Jr. (1976)
Carrier, J. and Peak, T. (1975)
Clark, C.R., Davies, C.O., and Woodcock, R.W. (1974)
Clark, C.R. and Woodstock, R.W. (1976)
Copeland, K. (1974)
Davis, G.A. (1973)
Elder, P. (1978)
Fristoe, M. (1976)
Golbin, A. (1977)
Goldberg, H. and Fenton, J. (not dated)
Hamre-Nietupski, S., Stoll, A., Holtz, K., Fullerton, P., Ryan-Flottum, M. and Brown, L. (1977)
Harris, D., Lippert, J.C., Yoder, D.E., and Vanderheiden, G.C. (1979)
Harris, D. and Vanderheiden, G.C. (1980a)
Harris, D. and Vanderheiden, G.C. (1980b)
Harris, S.L. (1975)
Harris, S.L. (1976)
Harris-Vanderheiden, D. (1976a)
Harris-Vanderheiden, D. (1976b)
Harris-Vanderheiden, D., McNaughton, S., and McDonald, E. (1976)
Harris-Vanderheiden, D. and Vanderheiden, G.C. (1977)

Holt, C. and Vanderheiden, G. (1976)
Horrocks, B.L. and Hollis, J.H. (1979)
Howard, G. (1979)
Kladde, A.G. (1974)
Mallik, K.K. (1977)
McDonald, E.T. (1976a)
McDonald, E.T. (1976b)
McDonald, E.T. (1980)
McDonald, E.T. and Schultz, A.R. (1973)
McNaughton, S. (1976a)
McNaughton, S. (1976b)
McNaughton, S. and Kates, B. (1980)
Melichar, J.F. (1977)
Melichar, J.F. (1978)
Nietupski, J. and Hamre-Nietupski, S. (1977)
Nugent, C.L. (1977)
Oakander, S.M. (1980)
Schurman, J.A. (1974)
Siegel, G.M. and Spradlin, J.E. (1978)
Silverman, F.H. (1980)
Silverman, H., McNaughton, S., and Kates, B. (1978)
Vanderheiden, G.C. (1976)
Vanderheiden, G.C. (1978)
Vanderheiden, G.C. and Harris-Vanderheiden, D. (1976)
Vanderheiden, G.C. and Grilley, K. (1976)
Vicker, B. (1974a)
Vicker, B. (1974b)
Vicker, B. (1974c)
Vicker, B. (1974d)
Woodcock, R. and Clark, C. (1969)
Wulz, S.V. and Hollis, J.H. (1980).

Adler, S. 1975. *The Non-Verbal child: An introduction to pediatric language pathology. 2nd ed.* Springfield, IL: Charles C. Thomas, 262 pp., $15.75.

This is a revision of Adler's (1964) book. It is intended for professionals in a wide variety of disciplines or for parents of non-verbal children. Therefore, it has a broad scope, but does not consider any topics in depth. The development and assessment of communication behaviors are reviewed briefly. Symptoms, testing, and causes are discussed relative to various dysfunctions, such as auditory, perceptual, and motor dysfunctions. A variety of different habilitation strategies are presented, with a few remediation suggestions for each (e.g., concept-formation training, music therapy). Appendices include source lists, a case history, and brief descriptions of general and specific programs developed by the author.

Allen, J. 1977. *"The other side of the elephant": Theatre activities for classroom learning.* Buffalo, NY: DOK Publishers, Inc., 56 pp., $3.50.

This workbook contains a number of theatre activities designed to be carried out in groups in a classroom setting. Some of the activities could be adapted to the needs of various handicapped populations (e.g., deaf, mentally retarded). Activities center on a variety of skills, such as imagination, memory, gestures, and this workbook contains a number of theatre activities designed to be carried out in groups in a classroom setting. Some of the activities could be adapted to the needs of various handicapped populations (e.g., deaf, mentally retarded). Information about each activity includes the following: title, objective, skills used, special equipment, time required, procedures (listed in step-by-step format), variations, and illustrations.

Allen, K. E., Holm, V. A., and Schiefelbusch, R. L., eds. 1978. *Early intervention—A team approach.* Baltimore, MD: University Park Press, 489 pp., $16.50.

This text explains and describes the services provided by the various members of an interdisciplinary team, and the activities of the team as a whole. Part I provides an introduction and overview of the team concept. Part II presents a philosophy that a behavioral analysis of trouble is required, regardless of the child's problem or the discipline(s) serving the child. Several behavioral intervention strategies, such as "timeout" are described, and a program for training imitative skills is included. Part III covers disciplinary contributions of potential team members, such as occupational and physical therapists and communication specialists. The role of each member is described, and a case study demonstrating their services is presented. One chapter also considers team issues and training in "interdisciplinariness." Part IV covers specific aspects of early intervention, such as a functional curriculum and ways to organize program implementation. Several of the book chapters are annotated in this bibliography.

Alpert, C. 1980. Procedures for determining the optimal nonspeech mode with the autistic child. In *Nonspeech language and communication: Analysis and intervention,* ed. R.L. Schiefelbusch. Baltimore, MD: University Park Press, 389–420, $24.95.

Alpert describes vocal and non-vocal aspects of communication in the autistic child, and notes potential problems in selecting a non-vocal training mode. A training/ assessment model is suggested for this population, with suggestions for applications to other populations. The model includes a method for determining the preferred non-vocal model and for planning short- and long-term training. The short-term training involves using two non-vocal modes, such as American Sign Language and Premack symbols, to determine the optimal mode for the individual client.

Archer, L.A. 1977. Blissymbolics—A nonverbal communication system. *J. Speech Hear. Dis.* 42: 568–79.

The author describes the Blissymbolics system, which was developed by Charles Bliss as an international language, and has been adapted for use with the handicapped (primarily the cerebral palsied and mentally retarded). Archer describes and gives examples of the three types of symbols which make up the system. She notes that by changing the position, the size, and the number of elements one can produce an infinite number of symbols; grammar and syntax may be indicated to some extent. She suggests criteria for selecting the candidates. Several general principles in teaching Blissymbols are provided. Advantages and disadvantages of the system are discussed.

Ashcroft, S.C. and Henderson, F.H. 1963. Programmed instruction in braille. Pittsburgh, PA: Stanwix House, Inc., 350 pp., $17.50.

This book is intended ". . .to provide an efficient means to attain mastery of braille and to develop strong positive attitudes toward it as a medium of communication" (p. viii). The book is organized into 10 units or "contracts," each of which is divided into "cycles." Each contract covers a specific topic (e.g. Contract 5: initial contractions), and the authors describe the concepts which are to be mastered for each cycle and contract. The contracts are in the form of programmed learning. Numerous exercises are presented for each cycle, combined with liberal use of facsimile (ink-printed) braille. Answers to exercises, summaries, and self-tests are also provided for each contract. Appendices for this book include braille proficiency self-test, general rules for the use of contractions, alphabetical index of braille signs, introduction to braille music notation, and a selected bibliography for additional reading.

Babbini, B.E. 1974. *Manual Communication: Fingerspelling and the language of signs. A course of study outline for instructors.* Urbana, IL: University of Illinois Press, 373 pp., $10.00.

This manual is designed for use by instructors of manual communication courses. It is intended for use in courses focusing on American Sign Lanugage and the American Manual Alphabet. The manual is divided into two main sections. The first section includes chapters covering general principles, general procedures, the use of video-taping equipment, and teaching fingerspelling. The second section presents an outline for a course of study which is divided into two levels: beginning (14 lesson plans) and intermediate (11 lesson plans). The material in each lesson is designed to be covered in a 2 or 3 hour class session. Each lesson includes information such as drill and practice materials, lists of signs to be taught, an outline format lesson plan, and tests to be administered. An annotated bibliography is provided including books, films, and teaching media relative to signs, fingerspelling, and deafness. A study workbook is available for $7.50.

Baer, D.M. 1978. The behavioral analysis of trouble. In *Early intervention—A team approach*, eds. K.E. Allen, V.A. Holm, and R.L. Schiefelbusch. Baltimore, MD: University Park Press, 57–93, $16.50.

This chapter proposes a behavioral analysis of the child's trouble, regardless of the underlying cause, or of the orientation of the professional. The author discusses the philosophy of reinforcing behavior and describes in some detail five reinforcement strategies, such as a token system and "time-out." An 18-step training program for teaching generalized imitative skill is included in the chapter. Ethical issues regarding behavior change are discussed briefly.

Barnes, K.J., Murphy, M., Waldo, L., and Sailor, W. 1979. Adaptive equipment for the severely multiply handicapped child. In *Teaching the severely handicapped, vol. IV*, eds. R.L. York and E. Edgar. Columbus, OH: Special Press, 108–52.

This chapter offers a valuable review of adaptive devices for the severely physically handicapped client. Descriptions, illustrations, and construction details are provided for a variety of special devices to meet specific needs in the following areas: positioning, development of lower extremities, development of upper extremities, fine motor development, self-help skill development, and communication (non-vocal).

Bender, M., Valletutti, P.J., and Bender, R. 1976. *Teaching the moderately and severely handicapped: vol. II Communication, socialization, safety and leisure skills*, Baltimore, MD: University Park Press, 420 pp., $16.50.

This volume contains a detailed section describing a practical method for assessing communication abilities and activities for training receptive and expressive language skills in the moderately and severely handicapped population. Although the major emphasis of this program is on eventual speech production, modification of proce-dures are suggested for the client who has severe motor coordination problems. See Appendix B in this book for a review of the program.

Bigge, J.L. 1977. Severe communication problems. In *Teaching individuals with physical and multiple disabilities*, eds. J.L. Bigge and P.A. O'Donnell. Columbus, OH: Charles E. Merrill Publishing Co., 108–36, $16.95.

This chapter outlines effectively 12 "'keys' for releasing communications 'locked' inside" severely physically impaired individuals. Establishing signals for "yes," "no," and "I don't know" are described as an initial goal. Recognizing "deadlock" situations which lead to much frustration for the client and person trying to communicate are discussed. A variety of communication devices including adaptive typewriters and tape recorders are illustrated.

Bigge, J.L. and O'Donnell, P.A., eds. 1977. *Teaching individuals with physical and multiple disabilities.* Columbus, OH: Charles E. Merrill Publishing Co., 279 pp., $16.95.

This book provides an overview of many physically handicapping conditions and offers suggestions for developing individualized training programs to meet specific needs (e.g., self-care, communication, leisure activities, work). The general framework for the book concerns using task analysis to carefully assess abilities and plan training procedures. Each chapter ends with "References" cited in the chapter and "Resources" which are sources of additional program suggestions.

Bloom, L. and Lahey, M. 1978. *Language development and language disorders.* New York: John Wiley & Sons, 685 pp., $21.95.

This book is divided into six main parts. Part 1 defines language and presents principles and procedures for describing language behavior. Part 2 contains seven chapters on the topic of normal language development from the perspective of an integration of content, form, and use. Part 3 comprises several chapters on deviant language development, including methods of identifying children who have language disorders and of describing deviant language. Part 4 presents four chapters relating to developing goals of language learning based on normal development. Part 5 reviews the correlates of language disorders from several viewpoints. The final part covers general and specific procedures for facilitating language learning. This book is based on considerable research by the authors and includes countless examples of their research data.

Bluma, S., Shearer, M., Frohman, A., and Hillard, J. 1976. *Portage guide to early education.* Cooperative Educational Services Agency 12, Box 564, Portage, WI. $32.00

The Portage Guide contains a detailed checklist of behavior for assessing and training severely handicapped individuals. The system has color coded cards each of which contain a training objective and activities that correspond to the assessment. Language development is one of the areas covered by this program. The objectives range from early awareness of sound to carrying on a conversation using complete sentences. Because this is a speech oriented program, alternative communication systems are not presented. See Appendix B in this book for a review of the program.

Bornstein, H. 1973. A description of some current sign systems designed to represent English. *Am. Ann. Deaf* 118: 454–63.

The author begins by describing the basic problems involved in modifying one language (American Sign Language) to represent another (English). A set of eight criteria is presented by which the user may judge a sign system. A brief history of sign systems is outlined and four recently developed systems are described: Seeing Essential English, Signing Exact English, Linguistics of Visual English, and Signed English. For each system, the following points are discussed: who the system was devised for; where and how the target vocabulary was developed; how a word is defined; how syntax is handled; what materials are needed; how signs are represented on paper; and what provisions are made for teaching the system.

Bornstein, H., Hamilton, L.B., Saulnier, K.L., and Roy, H.L., eds. 1975. *The Signed English Dictionary for preschool and elementary levels.* Washington, D.C.: Gallaudet College Press, 306 pp., $15.00.

This dictionary includes a short (6 pp.) introduction to Signed English. The purpose, nature, and use of Signed English are briefly discussed. The various teaching aids for Signed English such as story books and posters, are described. Dictionary entries are presented in alphabetic order. For each sign, the English gloss, an illustration, and a short description are provided. The dictionary includes gestures or signs used to represent the meaning of 2,500 English words used frequently by and with pre-school children. The American Manual Alphabet, numbers, and 14 sign markers (e.g., past regular "-ed", adjectives "-y") are also provided.

Bricker, W.A. and Bricker, D. D. 1974. An early language training strategy. In *Language perspectives: Acquisition, retardation, and intervention*, eds. R. Schiefelbusch and L. Lloyd. Baltimore, MD: University Park Press, 431–68, $16.50.

The authors begin by referring to several issues which they consider "pseudo issues in the processes of language development and language intervention" (e.g., language acquisition as an innate process); they suggest reasons why these pseudo issues may be set aside at least temporarily. An early language intervention system is recommended, "based on the sensorimotor lattice structure which indicates the primary sequential forms of behavior and the requisite behavior for each" (p. 445). A screening instrument designed for this purpose is described. The formal language training procedures and the assessment procedures related to each are discussed, including receptive, imitative, and syntactic processes.

Bricker, D., Dennison, L., Watson, L., and Vincent-Smith, L. 1973. *Language training program for young developmentally delayed children*, vol. 2, Institute on Mental Retardation and Intellectual Development Publications, Box 154, George Peabody College for Teachers, Nashville, TN. 37203, 81 pp., free.

This program consists of a three volume series "designed to span the training of language skills from infancy to the development of grammatically appropriate sentences." Volume 1 deals with the cognitive and linguistic prerequisites to a formal language system. Volume 2 focuses on training the basic actor-action-object proposition that serves as the basis for linguistic communication. Volume 3 is concerned with the modification of the kernel, declarative sentence with particular emphasis on training modifiers, prepositions, questions, and negation. All three volumes may be implemented within the classroom or the home by a teacher or parent. The program provides a model with suggested context and procedures to be modified by the trainer to meet the needs of the individual child. The major training areas of the program have been sequenced into a lattice which contains three aspects: (1) longitudinal programs (e.g., reinforcement program); (2) program steps (e.g., reinforcement); and (3) terminal states (e.g., reinforcement control established). Volume 2 "Training the basic actor-action-object preposition" follows a sequence of imitation/comprehension/ production for several targets (nouns, verbs, two-word phrases, and three-word phrases). Procedures for teaching verbal imitation from discrimination of speech sound production to shaping word production are presented. Each of the phases of this volume includes: objective, setting and words/objects, baseline and training probes, and generalization training. A lateralization program is also included to increase the child's vocabulary and help to generalize sounds to different sound combinations.

Brown, L., Nietupski, J., Lyon, S., Hamre-Nietupski, S., Crowner, T., and Gruene-wald, L. 1977. *Curricular strategies for teaching functional object use, nonverbal communication, problem solving, and mealtime skills to severely handicapped students*, vol. VII, part 1. Madison, WI: Department of Specialized Educational Services, Madison Metropolitan School District, 561 pp., $9.00.

This volume contains six entries. The papers include a discussion of issues regarding the least restrictive educational environment and a review of selected literature on nonverbal communication. The four curricula entries include strategies for teaching the following skills: functional object use, selected nonverbal communication use, selected problem solving skills, and selected mealtime skills. See individual entry annotations for additional information.

Bricker, D., Ruder, K., and Vincent-Smith, L. 1976. An intervention strategy for language deficient children. In *Teaching special children*, ed. N. Haring and R. Schiefelbusch. New York: McGraw Hill, $15.95.

This chapter describes a 43 phase language training program which is divided into two parts. Part I: Training of initial agent-action-object constructions begins with training functional object use and verbal imitation skills and proceeds through comprehension and production tasks from single words to three word constructions. Part II: Modification of agent-action-object constructions presents comprehension and production tasks that include use of pronouns, prepositions, the generation of questions, and use of negation. Each phase contains information such as setting and stimuli to be used, baseline probe, training procedures, and suggestions for generalization training. The need to use both concurrent and consecutive training procedures is discussed.

Carrier, J.K., Jr. 1976. Application of a nonspeech language system with the severely language handicapped. In *Communication assessment and intervention strategies*, ed. L.L. Lloyd. Baltimore, MD: University Park Press, 523–47, $16.50.

The author provides a background and rationale for a nonspeech language system (e.g., work with chimpanzees), then describes a child-oriented training program, the Non-Speech Language Initiation Program (Non-SLIP). Current applications of Non-SLIP (e.g., subjects with whom it has been used), and its current status (e.g., recommended use of programs) are discussed. See Appendix B in this book for a review of the Non-SLIP program.

Carrier, J. and Peak, T. 1975. *Non-SLIP Kit: Non-speech language initiation program*. H and H Enterprises, Inc., P.O. Box 3342 Lawrence, KS 66044, $238.00.

This program is designed "to give severely handicapped children (and some adults, including aphasics) some form of basic communication skill; it is essentially a language initiation program." The kit includes 59 symbols that represent words in the English language, a sentence tray, the manual covering rationale and procedures for the Non-SLIP programs, visual stimuli cards, and a set of step-by-step programs. See Appendix B in this book for a review of the program.

Catalog of Federal Domestic Assistance 1979. Superintendent of Documents, Government Printing Office, Washington, D.C. 20402, $20.00.

This document is issued yearly, and describes various government programs. It contains information regarding each program such as objectives, uses and restrictions, eligibility requirements, and information contacts. Several potential federal funding programs and the agencies that they fall under are:
1. Public Health Service I: Crippled Children's Services;
2. Health Care Financing Administration: Medicaid and Medicare;
3. Office of Human Development Services: Vocational Rehabilitation Services for Social Security Disability Beneficiaries; Rehabilitation Services and Facilities—Basic Support or Special Projects.

All of these programs fall under the Department of Health and Human Services (formerly the Department of Health, Education and Welfare), and information on them may be obtained by writing the appropriate agencies of that Department. This brief listing is not meant to be exhaustive but merely indicative of the various programs that may be consulted when seeking funds for projects or individuals.

Chapman, R.S. and Miller, J.F. 1980. Analyzing language and communication in the child. In *Nonspeech language and communication: Analysis and intervention*, ed. R.L. Schiefelbusch. Baltimore, MD: University Park Press, 159–96, $24.95.

This chapter addresses the issues of deciding which children are candidates for non-vocal systems and which systems are optimum for individual children. A developmental model is presented with descriptions of behaviors and appropriate programming strategies for each stage. Communicative characteristics, such as cognitive and linguistic prerequisites and limitations on meanings, are presented for each of 13 symbol sets (e.g., Blissymbols, American Sign Language). Five case examples are provided to demonstrate application of the developmental criteria suggested. Several tables and figures are used to clarify the model.

Christopher, D.A. 1976 *Manual communication*. Baltimore, MD: University Park Press, 530 pp., $14.50.

This is a programmed text and workbook designed to assist the beginning student professional (e.g., speech/language pathologists) learning the fundamentals of manual communication. Fingerspelling, number concepts, and Signed English using American Sign Language (ASL) signs are presented. Forty-eight lessons are included. The first 44 cover the American Manual Alphabet, number concepts, and the basic vocabulary needed to communicate in sign language. Each lesson covers 20 signs; the signs are not arranged in alphabetical order or in any functional grouping, such as categories. An illustration, a written description, and one English translation are provided for each sign. Exercises in encoding and decoding are included at the end of the lessons. The final four chapters involve application of the material learned for conducting speech, language, and hearing evaluations.

Clark, C.R., Davies, C.O., and Woodcock, R.W. 1974. *Standard Rebus glossary*. Circle Pines, MN: American Guidance Services, Inc., 95 pp. $4.70.

A standard set of rebus symbols, symbols that represent words or parts of words, are presented in this glossary. It includes over 800 different rebuses and several hundred combinations of rebuses or rebuses plus letters. Suggestions for use of rebuses in language instruction with non-vocal children and adults are described.

Clark, C.R. and Woodcock, R.W. 1976. Graphic system of communication. In *Communication assessment and intervention strategies*, ed. L.L. Lloyd. Baltimore, MD: University Park Press, 549–607, $26.50.

A detailed review of many graphic systems of communication are presented. Traditional orthography is compared with the alphabets of the Initial Teaching Alphabet (i.t.a.) and the International Phonetic Association (I.P.A.). Studies are cited to answer specific questions related to these systems. Blissymbols, rebuses (picture symbols), Signed English, and The Non-Speech Language Initiation Program (Non-SLIP) are also described. Implications of the use of each system with varied types of handicaps are presented.

Cohen, M.A., Gross, P.J., and Haring, N.G. 1978. Developmental pinpoints. In *Teaching the severely handicapped*, vol. I, eds. N.G. Haring and J.J. Brown. New York: Grune and Stratton, 35–110, $17.50.

This chapter suggests the use of normal development as a basis for identifying behaviors which should become the focus for training. Developmental "pinpoints", or measurable behaviors are included for several major areas, such as motor skills, communication (receptive and expressive language), and social interaction skills. These pinpoints are collated from 24 studies, screening batteries, and developmental checklists. Behaviors typically begin at about one month and progress to approximately 72 months. For each major developmental area, general discussion and selected references are included in addition to the developmental pinpoints.

Copeland, K., ed. 1975. *Aids for the severely handicapped.* New York: Grune and Stratton, 152 pp., $17.75.

The English editor has compiled a selective review of internationally available remote control devices and communication aids for the severely physically disabled. Technical descriptions of each device or system are provided. "One chapter records the special requirements and adaptations needed when children use these devices, and analyzes the solution of particular problems associated with the care of the young" (p. 10). Three appendices are provided: a list of references to papers and books; a list of institutions where the systems are being used or researched; and a list of international manufacturers of the aids. The format of the book, with major topic headings in the right hand margin, allows for quick and easy reference. The diagrams and photographs are excellent in illustrating the devices.

Crowner, T. n.d. *Signs for you: Communicating with sign language.* Madison, WI: MAZE Project, Madison Public Schools, 139 pp., $3.50.

This booklet begins with a brief discussion of how people in the client's environment can support learning and use of sign language. Seven general suggestions are covered, such as rewarding the student for communicating. Several considerations are presented for use in selecting the initial sign language vocabulary. The major section includes 130 American Sign Language Signs listed in alphabetical order. Each sign is presented on a separate page, and includes the following information: a large illustration, directions for producing the sign, suggested use of the sign, and a blank space for noting modifications.

Dalgaard, J., Newhoff, M., and Barnes, G. 1979. "Show me . . .": Enhancing receptive and expressive language through pantomime. A paper presented at the American Speech-Language-Hearing Association Convention, Atlanta, GA. Request copy from Jeannette Hoit-Dalgaard, Audiology/Speech Pathology Service, Veterans Administration Medical Center, 3350 La Jolla Village Drive, San Diego, CA 92161.

This paper describes and discusses a pantomime-oriented therapy designed and carried out with an aphasic client. The task continuum consists of eight levels. For each level, the following information is presented: a explanation; description of stimulus materials; description and example of procedures for each step of each level; and goals for each level. Results of the approach are described and the discussion section centers around possible reasons for success of the approach.

Darley, F.L., ed. 1979 *Evaluation of appraisal techniques in speech and language pathology.* Reading, MA: Addison-Wesley Publishing, $21.95.

Critical reviews of 87 published tests are presented in this book. It is designed to acquaint speech-language pathologists with a variety of tests available to assess abilities such as language, speech production, and auditory discrimination. Each test critique includes the following: identifying information; purpose; administration, scoring, and interpretation; evaluation of test adequacy; and a summary.

Davis, G.A. 1973. Linguistics and language therapy: The sentence construction board. *J. Speech Hear. Dis.* 38: 205–14.

A general description of the sentence construction board apparatus is given with therapy suggestions. This device is not specifically designed as a non-vocal aid, but as a technique to teach syntactical patterns to people with language disorders. The content of this article may be useful in designing a communication board for an advanced board user.

Dunn, L.M. and Smith, J.O., eds. 1965–69a. *Peabody language developmental kits*, Level P (1969), Level 1 (1965), Level 2 (1966), and Level 3 (1967). Circle Pines, MN: American Guidance Service, Inc., Level P — $235.00; Level 1 — $88.00; Level 2 — $106.00; Level 3 — $79.00.

These programs are based on a language stimulation-experience approach. Each kit contains 180 daily lessons plans designed for group administration. According to the manuals the activities at each level are appropriate for clients with mental ages in the following ranges: Level P, 3–5 years; Level 1, 4½–6½ years; Level 2, 6–8 years; Level 3, 7½–9½years. Each lesson provides a variety of activities requiring different skills (e.g., memory time, describing time, and pantomiming time). Each kit includes a detailed lesson plan manual, about 400 stimulus picture cards, 200–560 plastic color chips, large poster story pictures, prerecorded tapes with songs or stories, soft hand puppets and a variety of other materials. The programs have been used with disadvantaged, mentally retarded, and normally developing children.

Elder, P. 1978. *Visual symbol communication instruction, part I: Receptive instruction*, DESEMO Project, Center for Developmental and Learning Disorders, University of Alabama in Birmingham, P.O. Box 313, University Station, Birmingham, AL, 35294, 74 pp., $7.50.

This program provides an instruction/protocol which specifically teaches a visual symbol system (Blissymbols, rebuses, etc.) to non-vocal individuals, allowing a visual response by the severely physically handicapped person. The receptive instruction manual includes 25 sequential lesson plans which provide specific steps in teaching, reinforcement, and correction using a training device, the Visual Communication Display. Materials are described including a pictorial diagram and schematic of the Visual Communication Display. Program guidelines, record keeping, scoring, and retention testing are described and data sheets are provided for reproduction. See Appendix B in this book for further information.

Englemann, S. and Osborn, J. 1976. *Distar® Language I*. Chicago, IL: Science Research Associates, Inc., $185.00.

This program is designed to teach the language of general classroom instruction to preschool and early school age (through first grade) children. It has been used successfully with the educable mentally retarded, speech and language correction groups and to teach English as a second language. The language kit is packaged in a heavy cardboard box containing a teacher's guide, five teacher presentation books, a storybook, three take-home books, and colored group-progress markers. There are 160 daily lessons designed for 30 minute sessions with groups of five to ten students. The presentation books specify what the teacher is to say and to do as well as the expected responses from the children. An initial placement test is provided as well as individual tests to assure tasks are learned and maintained.

Finnie, N.R. 1974. *Handling the young cerebral palsied child at home*. 2nd ed. New York: E.P. Dutton, 337 pp., $4.95.

This book is intended for the parents of cerebral palsied children. It may also be used by teachers or therapists working with parents or parent groups. Topics addressed include general areas such as parents' problems, and more specific areas such as dressing, carrying, and teaching speech. There is a considerable amount of information on equipment, including chairs, wedges, and prone boards. The feeding and speech chapters were written by a speech pathologist. They provide brief introductions to normal development, common problems, and beginning intervention.

Fiorentino, M.R. 1973. *Reflex testing methods for evaluating C.N.S. development.* 2nd ed. Springfield, IL: Charles C Thomas, 57 pp., $10.00.

This text is intended to assist in the assessment of children through six years of age, and in the programming for neurophysiologically involved children. The focus for occupational, physical, and speech-language therapists is to determine the maturational level and abnormal reflexes for planning implementation procedures. Procedures are presented for testing reflexes at the spinal, brain stem, midbrain, and cortical levels. The test position, test stimulus, negative and positive reactions, and interpretation of findings are included for each reflex test. Photographs are provided to illustrate negative and positive reactions for each test.

Fredericks, H.D., Baldwin, V., Riggs, C., Furey, T., Grove, D., Moore, W., McDonnell, J., Jordon, E., Hanson, W., and Wadlow, M. 1976. *The teaching research motor development scale for moderately and severely retarded,* Springfield, IL: Charles C Thomas, 345 pp., $9.75.

This curriculum guide presents teaching objectives and suggested procedures for a wide variety of adaptive behaviors including areas such as motor development, socialization, and receptive and expressive language development. The main emphasis of the language areas is on comprehension and ultimate speech production as the primary means of communication. See Appendix B in this book for a review of the program.

Fristoe, M. 1976. Language intervention systems: Programs published in kit form. In *Communication assessment and intervention strategies,* ed. L.L. Lloyd. Baltimore, MD: University Park Press, 813–59, $16.50.

This appendix is based in part on information compiled in a national survey of language programs used with the retarded. For each of the 29 kits the following information is presented: target (population); level (of retardation); type (operant/nonoperant and stimulation/remediation); model (behavioral, cognitive, developmental, functional language, information processing, or other); emphasis (expressive, receptive, motor-imitation, and/or vocal); structure (high, moderate, slight, or unstructured); baselines (present or absent); users (professionals, teachers, aides); setting (individual therapy; group therapy, etc.); and cost. In addition, Fristoe's comments regarding each kit (e.g., special applications) are presented.

Fristoe, M. and Lloyd, L.L. 1977. Manual communication for the retarded and others with severe communication impairment: A resource list. *Ment. Retard.* 15(5): 18–21.

These authors have compiled an extensive list of articles and programs related to the use of manual communication systems. Some of these references pertain to the systems themselves (e.g., Signed English), while others describe the use of the systems with special populations (e.g., deaf, retarded). The authors indicate those items developed especially for use with mentally retarded, autistic, or multihandicapped populations.

Gallender, D. 1979. *Eating handicaps: Illustrated techniques for feeding disorders.* Springfield, IL: Charles C Thomas, 296 pp., $19.75.

This book contains two major sections related to the eating problems of handicapped persons. The first section covers the basic anatomy and physiology of structures involved in the eating process, such as muscles and nerves. The second section considers techniques and instructional materials for dealing with various eating problems. Over 200 techniques are suggested for decreasing abnormal behaviors such as the bite or gag reflex or enhancing normal behaviors such as jaw stability. Each chapter in this section begins with a narrative describing the general problem (e.g., rotary chewing), then presents several techniques, each consisting of several explanatory sentences. Techniques within chapters are typically not related or arranged in any order. Numerous pictures, diagrams, and illustrations are provided to clarify the text.

Golbin, A., ed. 1977. *Cerebral palsy and communication—What parents can do.* The George Washington University, Job Development Laboratory, 420 Ross Hall, 2300 Eye Street, N.W., Washington, D.C., 20037, $6.00.

This book offers five chapters dealing with communication needs of the cerebral palsied person. A glossary follows each chapter to aid parents in understanding professional words used frequently. Detailed descriptions of the speaking process and "mechanics for breathing" are presented with the caution that speech as a major means of communication may not be realistic for some people. Alternative communication systems are discussed including communication boards, electronic devices, and a special adaptation of manual signing for a client with cerebral palsy.

Goldberg, H. and Fenton, J., eds. n.d. *Aphonic communication for those with cerebral palsy: Guide for the development and use of a conversation board.* United Cerebral Palsy Associations of New York state, 220 West 42nd Street, New York, $1.25.

This handbook considers use of the communication board as a teaching tool, from the kindergarten level through the primary level and covers five conversation board levels. The kindergarten level board utilizes pictures with captions, while the five conversation boards include vocabulary words, letters of the alphabet, numbers, etc. Conversation board #1 consists of a basic 58 word sight vocabulary, while the adult board (#5) contains suffixes such as "-nt", and "-er", as well as more abstract vocabulary. Examples of each conversation device are presented. The authors include the Dolch List of Basic Words. Five case studies regarding use of these devices are included. Some suggestions of how to use the boards as classroom teaching aids are also presented.

Goodman, L., Wilson, P.S., and Bornstein, H. 1978. Results of a national survey of sign language programs in special education. *Ment. Retard.* 16(2): 104–6.

This report was prepared by a committee established by the Division of Speech Pathology and Audiology of the American Association of Mental Deficiency to obtain information on the use of signing with clients in special education programs. Two hundred questionnaires were sent to a total of 33 states, with results based on 127 questionnaires. Information was gathered on the following areas: (1) population characteristics, with the largest diagnostic group (79%) being the severely retarded; (2) program characteristics, including a consideration of why signing was chosen over other nonvocal systems, when programs had been initiated, who directed them, and ages of participants; (3) sign system characteristics, considering which signs, what systems of grammar, and what vocabulary was being taught; and (4) teaching procedures, including emphasis on comprehension of signs, articulation of signs, and non-language benefits.

Graham, W. 1976. Language programming and intervention. In *Communication assessment and intervention strategies,* ed. L.L. Lloyd. Baltimore, MD: University Park Press, 371–422, $16.50.

A variety of language approaches and programs are described. Four major approaches cited are developmental, nondevelopmental or remedial, manual, and aids for the nonvocal physically involved person. The importance of parent involvement in language programming is stressed. An extensive bibliography is included. An appendix provides information regarding commercial language program.

Gray, B. and Ryan, B. 1973. *A language program for the nonlanguage child.* Champaign, IL: Research Press, 181 pp., $6.95.

This book provides a description of the program commonly referred to as the "Monterey Language Program." Although this program was not designed for the mentally retarded, it is sometimes used with that population. The program includes 41 steps, with subjects' placement into the program being determined by a pretest. There are 13 core programs (from the identification of nouns to the use of "the"), 10 secondary programs (from plural nouns + the verb "are" to singular and plural past tense, using /t/ and /d/ endings), and 18 optional programs (was/were; an articulation program). Five speech models (combinations of immediate/delayed, complete/incomplete, and no model), use of branching, generalization steps, and a home carryover program are included in each step. New programs can be written as needed. It should be noted that the prospective trainer must be taught by a certified trainer before he/she can use the program. In addition to program description, this book contains a section on accountability which reports the results of this program with various groups (e.g., dysphasic, mentally retarded, English as a second language).

Guess, D., Keogh, W., and Sailor, W. 1978. Generalization of speech and language behavior. In *Bases of language intervention*, ed. R. Schiefelbusch. Baltimore, MD: University Park Press, 373–95, $14.50.

The authors discuss generalization of language skills in terms of stimulus generalization and response generalization. They review selected studies in each of those areas. Various methods of data collection (i.e., spontaneous speech probes, structured probes, and tests) are considered as they relate to generalization. Specific tactics for producing generalization are presented and described (e.g., "training sufficient exemplars").

Guess, D., Sailor, W., and Baer, D. 1977. A behavioral-remedial approach to language training for the severely handicapped. In *Educational programming for the severely and profoundly handicapped*, ed. E. Sontag. Reston, VA: Council for Exceptional Children, $14.95.

This article provides a description and rationale of the authors' *Functional Language Training Program for the Severely Handicapped* (Guess, Sailor, and Baer, 1976). They discuss the controversy concerning the use of remedial versus developmental logic, explaining why they have chosen the former as the basis of their program. The issue of the order of comprehension and production in a training sequence is also considered, with the authors opting to train both modalities simultaneously or in rapid succession, without expecting spontaneous transfer. The issue of generalization, described as a very crucial issue, is discussed. Their training program is also described. See Appendix B in this book for a review of the program.

Guess, D., Sailor, W., and Baer, D. 1974. To teach language to retarded children. In *Language perspectives: Acquisition, retardation, and intervention*, R. Schiefelbusch and L. Lloyd. Baltimore, MD: University Park Press, 529–63, $16.50.

The authors state that, "This chapter is meant to provide some review of past and current efforts, some argument about what may be lacking in these efforts, some guesses about where help could be found, and (consequently) a proposal for a different language training program" (p. 530). The review section briefly covers both normal speech and language development and studies which have used operant procedures to teach speech and language to children with speech and language defects. Deficiencies in the operant analysis are suggested. An experimental training program is proposed and described briefly, including consideration of the structure, logic, and context of the training program, and a description of the training steps. See Appendix B in this book for a review of the program.

Guess, D., Sailor, W., and Baer, D. 1976. *Functional speech and language for the severely handicapped*, Lawrence, KS: H and H Enterprises, Inc., $7.95 for each of 4 parts.

This program is divided into four parts: Part 1—Persons and Things, Steps 1-9 (93 pages); Part 2—Actions with Persons and Things, Steps 10-29 (84 pages); Part 3—Possession and Color, Steps 30-42 (85 pages); Part 4—Size, Relation, and Location, Steps 43-60 (85 pages). Each of the 60 steps in the complete program includes training goal, training item, instructions, summary forms, example trials, scoring forms, and programming for generalization. See the above annotation for more details. See Appendix B in this book for a review of the program.

Guess, D., Sailor, W., and Baer, D. 1978. Children with limited language. In *Language intervention strategies*, ed. R. Schiefelbusch. Baltimore, MD: University Park Press, 101-44, $15.75.

The authors present several issues concerning the designing of language curricula, particularly how curricula should be sequenced to establish language skills. They carefully define their view of developmental logic and remedial logic in designing curricula. The major emphasis for their language training program is a remedial approach with production skills taught before receptive skills are formally presented. The chapter contains a review of their program: *Functional speech and language training for the severely handicapped*. See listing for these authors in other entries in this bibliography and a full review of the program in Appendix B of this book for more information.

Gustason, G., Pfetzing, D., and Zawlokow, E. 1972. *Signing Exact English*. Order from National Association of the Deaf, 814 Thayer Avenue, Silver Spring, MD: 20910, 224 pp., $13.50.

This is basically a dictionary of Signing Exact English signs. A short introduction discusses the need for a sign system such as this one and presents the principles basic to developing and selecting signs. Signs are provided for the following: the alphabet, numbers, The Pledge of Allegiance, verbs "to be" and modals, pronouns, contractions, affixes, and vocabulary. Signs within each section are in alphabetical order. For each sign the authors include the English word, a brief description, an illustration of hand positions and movements, and where appropriate, a picture indicating why the sign is made as it is.

Hamblin, K. 1978. *Mime: A playbook of silent fantasy*. Garden City, NY: Dolphin Books, 192 pp., $6.95.

This book is an introduction to the art of mime. It covers techniques in five major sections: warmups (e.g., silence and marionnette); objects (e.g., creating or acting on objects such as balls, walls, and boxes); movements (e.g., various patterns of walking and climbing); characters (e.g., miming habits, using masks and props); and nuances (e.g., growing, singing). For each of these areas the author provides verbal explanations and numerous photographs. Suggestions for learning routines are also presented. Appendices include information on make-up, performance, teaching mime, and a bibliography of resources such as books, periodicals, and films.

Hamre-Nietupski, S., Stoll, A., Holtz, K., Fullerton, P., Ryan-Flottum, M., and Brown, L. 1977. Curricular strategies for teaching selected nonverbal communication skills to nonverbal and verbal severely handicapped students. In *Curricular strategies for teaching functional object use, nonverbal communication, problem solving, and mealtime skills to severely handicapped students*. vol. VII, part 1. Madison, WI: Department of Specialized Educational Services, Madison Metropolitan School District, 156 pp. $9.00.

This curriculum covers three non-vocal systems: communication boards and booklets, generally understood gestures, and standardized signs. Considerations in selecting the optimum system and initial communicative content are covered. Two sets of curricular strategies are presented, one for communication board/booklets and one for gestures/signs. Communication board use may be taught through concurrent or consecutive presentation strategies. Examples of instructional protocols, activities, and vocabulary lists are provided, with the bulk of the curricula consisting primarily of objectives. See Appendix B in this book for a more extensive review of this curriculum.

Haring, N.G. and Brown, L.J., eds. 1976. *Teaching the severely handicapped*, vol. I. New York: Grune and Stratton, 335 pp., $17.50.

This book comprises a collection of papers from a 1974 seminar on the severely handicapped. The first section presents an overview of comprehensive services and future directions in work with the severely handicapped. The second section addresses developmental sequence and curricula. Assessment and performance measurement strategies are described in the third section. The final section covers general intervention strategies for the severely handicapped, plus a chapter on language development programs for that population.

Haring, N.G. and Brown, L.J., eds. 1977. *Teaching the severely handicapped*, vol. II. New York: Grune and Stratton, 346 pp., $19.50.

This volume contains seven chapters written by participants at the second annual conference of the American Association of the Severely/Profoundly Handicapped held in Kansas City, Missouri in November 1975. The content of the chapters related to communication skills varies, including instruction in pronoun usage (Swetlik and Brown), and the use of telecommunications to educate severely handicapped children and their parents (Tawny). See individual chapter annotations for more information. The other five chapters cover the following topics, but are not annotated in this appendix: teaching rudimentary math skills, community transportation, work skill development, community vocational and workshop placement, and the need for adjunctive services.

Harris, D., Lippert, J.C., Yoder, D.E., and Vanderheiden, G.C. 1979. Blissymbolics: An augmentative symbol communication system for nonvocal severely handicapped children. In *Teaching the severely handicapped*, vol. IV, ed. R.L. York and E. Edgar. Columbus, OH: Special Press, 238–62, $24.50.

This chapter presents a brief introduction to Blissymbolics as a symbol system for use with non-vocal clients. Two research studies are presented describing the use of Blissymbols with severely physically impaired (cerebral palsied) children with normal or near normal intelligence and cerebral palsied children judged to be moderately to profoundly retarded. General guidelines for selecting the initial symbol vocabulary and general teaching procedures are listed.

Harris, D. and Vanderheiden, G.C. 1980a. Enhancing the development of communicative interaction. In *Nonspeech language and communication: Analysis and intervention*, ed. R.L. Schiefelbusch. Baltimore, MD: University Park Press, 227–57, $24.95.

This chapter begins with a discussion of several crucial issues in non-vocal communication, such as generic application of terms like "nonvocal". This chapter is addressed to the needs of the non-vocal severely handicapped persons. The importance of developing communication/interaction skills is stressed throughout the chapter. An evolutionary program approach is recommended, with six program aspects described in some detail (e.g., intervention entry point, program scope). Several general strategies are presented for developing communication/interaction skills. The chapter ends with a discussion of a number of critical research needs in the area of non-vocal communication techniques, such as the role of imitation.

Harris, D. and Vanderheiden, G.C. 1980b. Augmentative communication techniques. In *Nonspeech language and communication: analysis and intervention*, ed. R.L. Schiefelbusch. Baltimore, MD: University Park Press, 259–301, $24.95.

A variety of techniques and aids for the non-vocal severely handicapped are presented in this chapter. The authors recommend initial techniques such as direct selection and secondary techniques such as encoding. Communication aids are discussed in terms of complexity, with six levels of implementation, ranging from unaided techniques such as those using eye blinks to fully independent, portable aids. Advantages and limitations are suggested for each level. A partial survey is provided for scanning, direct selection, and encoding aids at various levels of complexity. Numerous diagrams and photographs are included to clarify the information presented.

Harris, S. L. 1976. *Managing behavior 8, Behavior modification: teaching speech to a nonverbal child*. H and H Enterprises, Inc., P.O. Box 3342, Lawrence, KS, 78 pp., $4.25.

This handbook is intended as a guide for parents and others interested in helping a handicapped child learn to talk. The author begins by identifying the target population ("the Silent Children") and briefly discusses research on teaching speech to nonverbal children. The basics of behavior modification and record keeping (e.g., defining behavior), are presented. Four stages are followed in teaching a child to use oral language: I-teaching attention; II-teaching nonverbal skills; III-teaching verbal imitation; and IV-teaching functional speech. Each stage includes a pretest and the training section with materials, procedure, data collection, reward, decision, and possible problems specified. Each section of the handbook contains examples from two children (one diagnosed as autistic, and the other as schizophrenic). Review questions are included at the end of each section, for which answers are provided. See Appendix B in this book for a review of the program.

Harris, S.L. 1976. Teaching language to nonverbal children—with emphasis on problems of generalization. *Psych. Bulletin* 82: 565–80.

The author reviews studies on language approaches for nonverbal children, focusing on the four stages often followed: (1) attention; (2) non-vocal imitation; (3) verbal imitation; and (4) functional language. She describes the procedures generally followed at each stage. Special consideration is given to the demonstration of generalization, either spontaneous or trained, at each stage. Suggestions are made for increasing generalization throughout the language training procedures. Prognostic indicators for success with verbal language programs are noted.

Harris-Vanderheiden, D. 1977a. Blissymbols and the mentally retarded. In *Non-vocal communication techniques and aids for the severely physically handicapped*, Baltimore, MD: University Park Press, 120–31, $12.50.

This article summarizes a study in which Blissymbols were used in a residential environment with five severely mentally retarded and physically handicapped children. Prerequisites for entry into the program were the skills of eye contact, object permanance, ability to attend to task and follow oral directions, and a demonstrated desire to communicate. No subjects were communicating functionally at the beginning of the project. The rationale for selecting Blissymbols as a communication system with this population is discussed. Simultaneous vocalization was encouraged, and was noted to increase during the project. The author describes how to involve the teachers and ward staff in the program (e.g., through use of a newsletter), and how to implement it with the children (e.g., by using symbol identification, symbol comprehension). Five case studies are presented and results of the 10-week program are discussed briefly.

Harris-Vanderheiden, D. 1976b. Field evaluation of the Auto-Com. In *Non-vocal Communication techniques and aids for the severely physically handicapped*, G. Vanderheiden and K. Grilley. Baltimore, MD: University Park Press, 114–51, $12.50.

This paper presents a description of the AutoCom (an aid for providing a visual display of the child's communication-board message), and a discussion of its use with seven physically handicapped students. Major findings were that use of the Auto-Com was found to enhance student's acquisition of basic skills, such as math, spelling, and sentence construction, as well as their personal and motivational development. Three primary features were shown to be significant for successful results: (1) the independence which the aid provided; (2) the ability to communicate through a visible correctable TV display; and (3) the ability to transport the aid to virtually any environment. The author suggests that many of the same results could have occurred with other similar aids.

Harris-Vanderheiden, D., McNaughton, S., and McDonald, E. 1976. Some remarks on assessment. In *Non-vocal communication techniques and aids for the severely physically handicapped*, eds. G. Vanderheiden, and K. Grilley. Baltimore, MD: Univeristy Park Press, 152–58, $12.50.

This chapter is divided into three sections. The first covers factors involved in an assessment, such as what is involved (physical, educational, communication, and language skills), who should conduct the assessment, what kinds of practical questions are to be answered, and what assessment tools (informal and formal) are currently available. The second section presents a description of assessment at Ontario Crippled Children's Center (OCCC). The role of each professional in an assessment and the type of recommendations made are discussed briefly. In the third section, informal assessment techniques are considered, including task analysis and diagnostic teaching; examples of each are presented.

Harris-Vanderheiden, D. and Vanderheiden, G. C. 1977. Basic considerations in the development of communicative and interactive skills for non-vocal severely handicapped children. In *Educational programming for the severely and profoundly handicapped*, ed. E. Sontag. Reston, VA: Council for Exceptional Children, $14.95.

This paper explores "some of the considerations and initial steps involved in developing augmentative non-vocal communication programs" for severely handicapped persons (p. 323). The authors stress the ongoing nature of decision-making, and considerations that must be made prior to, during, and subsequent to the selection of an aid or technique. Each of these considerations is described and discussed separately in five areas: (1) deciding which factors are to be evaluated and tracked (eight factors, such as the child's current communication needs and the professional and parent cooperation available); (2) selecting the aids and techniques (five factors, including the child's visual and auditory skills and his or her ability to associate, store, and retrieve meaning associated with pictures and events); (3) providing an effective augmentative physical response mode (direct selection, scanning, or encoding techniques); (4) selecting and developing a vocabulary system (five factors); and (5) evaluating the nonvocal system chosen (eight factors, including flexibility and transmission time).

Hart, B. and Rogers-Warren A. 1978. A milieu approach to teaching language. In *Language intervention strategies*, ed. R. Schiefelbusch. Baltimore, MD: University Park Press, 193–236, $15.75.

The concept of a milieu approach to language training is presented. As contrasted to individual language therapy, the milieu approach takes place during most of the day in the client's natural environment. "Its strategies involve making language functional by arranging situations in which the child works with language and by ensuring that the child's language works to produce attention, things and events" (p. 219). The approach stresses communication intent rather than grammatical forms. The basic concept of generalizing or maintaining new skills in the varied situations of the natural environment make this approach useful with a wide variety of handicapping conditions.

Hatten, J., Goman, T., and Lent, C. 1976. *Emerging language 2*. Tuscon, AZ: Communication Skill Builders, Inc., 58 pp., $5.95.

This volume is a revision of the authors' earlier work entitled *Emerging Language*. It is designed for speech clinicians and special educators as a program to help develop expressive language in "children ages 2-10 who have failed to acquire language through normal stimulation of the environment" (p. 1). The program is based on a developmental approach to language learning and is written in a series of 136 behavioral objectives. The program begins with single work utterances and progresses to multi-word responses including the generation of "wh" questions. A sample activity follows each objective as only a suggestion for a possible teaching technique. Two appendices are included: (a) negation development as an alternate teaching strategy to earlier objectives; and (b) materials. Selected objectives in the early stages of verbal language development section may be useful with the severely retarded.

Henegar, M.E. and Cornett, R.O. 1971. *Cued speech handbook for parents*. Cued Speech Program, Gallaudet College, Kendall Green, Washington, D.C., 20002, 217 pp, $3.00.

This book is intended for parents who have already learned the basics of Cued Speech and are beginning to use it with their child. The first eight chapters offer a background of information regarding Cued Speech, language, speechreading, and other related topics. The next six chapters deal specifically with the use of Cued Speech, including both narrative (e.g., "What to expect") and activities (e.g., "Finger Fun"). Additional issues such as the role of hearing siblings are covered in the remaining five chapters. The Appendix contains supplementary information, a basic vocabulary, practice materials, and a list of suggested materials that are available commercially.

Holland, A. 1975. Language therapy for children: Some thoughts on context and content. *J. Speech Hear. Dis.* 40: 514–23.

Although this article is not directed toward clinicians working with severely handicapped, many of the ideas presented will be useful with that population. The author focuses on context (interrelated environmental conditions) and content (words focused on in therapy). Five principles are discussed with regard to context; for example, item 2 presents the idea of "organicity," or the interrelatedness of the word, the activity, and the child. Concerning content, Holland demonstrates how to develop a 35-word lexicon, and includes a rationale for the selecting each word. She then applies this core vocabulary to a model of semantic relations, with examples provided in an appendix.

Hollis, J.H. and Carrier, J.K. 1975. Intervention strategies for nonspeech children. In *Language intervention strategies*, ed. R. Schiefelbusch. Baltimore, MD: University Park Press, 57–100, $15.75.

This chapter presents the framework of a basic communication system through consideration of several communication models. An intervention strategy for language deficiencies is then suggested, with several additional models presented. Symbol systems as response modes are "evaluated in terms of iconicity versus arbitrariness, the input and output modes used, permanence versus transitivity, complexity versus simplicity, time required for transmission, and degree to which presentation can be automated" (p. 96). Examples are provided to illustrate how the various symbol systems may be used to form a simple English sentence.

Holm, V.A. and McCartin, R.E. 1978. Interdisciplinary child development team: Team issues and training in interdisciplinariness. In *Early intervention—A team approach,* eds. K.E. Allen, V.A. Holm, and R.L. Schiefelbusch. Baltimore, MD: University Park Press, 97–122, $16.50.

This chapter focuses on a number of issues inherent to the team approach. Issues are first considered relative to professionals, such as the composition and philosophies of teams, and the roles of team members. The various components of the team assessment are described, including team leadership and aspects of the actual assessment, from screening to the parent conference and follow-up. Several issues are also considered relative to parents and other caregivers. These issues are presented in a question-answer format designed to help parents select a team (e.g., "What is the team philosophy?"). The final section presents a model for training in "interdisciplinariness." A philosophy is delineated, accompanied by a brief review of a training program developed by one clinic.

Holt, C. and Vanderheiden, G. 1976. Appendix B: 1974 Masterchart of communication aids. In *Non-vocal communication techniques and aids for the severely physically handicapped,* eds. G. Vanderheiden and K. Grilley. Baltimore, MD: University Park Press, 174–201, $12.50.

This appendix contains a variety of information on non-vocal communication aids including: (1) abbreviations and definitions (e.g., definitions for types of implementation, three basic approaches, and levels); (2) notes and footnotes explaining the information on the chart columns; (3) the Masterchart of Communication Aids—a table of information about existing communication aids including the name of aid and manufacturer, a general description, the type of input interface, output devices, etc.; and (4) a glossary of input interfaces including mechanical switches for the extremities, mechanical switches for a specific body part, pneumatic switches, touch switches, and so forth.

Hopper, C. and Helmick, R. 1977. Nonverbal communication and the severely handicapped: Some considerations. *Am. Assoc. Ed. Sever./Profound. Handicap. Rev.* 2: 47–52.

This paper covers three aspects in the development of non-vocal communication systems: (1) the maintenance of existing communication behaviors such as gestures, so that they may serve as the basis for more formal communication systems like American Sign Language; (2) instructional considerations in shaping these existing repertoires into more standardized systems; and (3) generalization of newly learned systems. The literature is discussed in each of these three areas and ideas are presented for further research on the use of manual communication with the severely handicapped.

Horstmeier, D.S. and MacDonald, J.D. 1978. *Ready, set, go: talk to me.* Columbus, OH: Charles E. Merrill Publishing Co., $5.95.

This book is intended for use by parents and professionals. It covers prelanguage and initial verbal communication skills. The content is based on a normal developmental sequence, with training being carried out continually in the child's environment. This book is a component of *The Environmental Language Intervention Program* (also authored by MacDonald), which was designed for and tested on developmentally delayed children.

The book includes a series of prescriptive packets intended to be adapted to the needs of each individual child. A diagnostic screening (test) is provided to assist in determining which prescriptive packet should be used. The authors also suggest how to adapt the program for classroom use. See Appendix B in this book for a review.

Horrocks, B.L. and Hollis, J.H. 1979. Nonspeech language training. In *Teaching the severely handicapped*, vol. IV, eds. R.L. York, and E. Edgar. Columbus, OH: Special Press, 219–37.

A brief review of Premack's chimpanzee research and of using plastic symbols to facilitate teaching language to nonverbal retardates is presented in this chapter. Terms such as cognitive mapping and linguistic mapping are defined and used to describe precommunication and communication behaviors. Several studies involving eight multihandicapped retarded institutionalized children are presented to illustrate specific teaching strategies. The studies suggest that even these severely handicapped individuals may be able to learn discriminations that can be used to develop a communication system.

Howard, G., ed. 1979. *Helping the handicapped: A guide to aids developed by the telephone pioneers of america*. Telephone Pioneers of America, 195 Broadway, New York, New York, 10017.

This handbook describes aids designed or produced by the Telephone Pioneers of America. It is not a catalog of equipment for sale, but rather a listing of devices and aids that may be constructed. "How to make it" information can be obtained from various Chapters of the Telephone Pioneers of America. These instructions typically include drawings, diagrams, and parts lists. Many of these devices can be built for under $100; Pioneer Chapters will often assist in the construction. The handbook is divided into six main areas according to the intended populations to be served: handicapped (general aids and devices); motion handicapped; retarded; hearing handicapped; speech handicapped; and visually handicapped. For each device listed, the following information is provided: name, purpose, description, background, cost, availability of plans, and contact group.

Hutchinson, B.B, Hanson, M.L. and Mecham, M.J. 1979. *Diagnostic handbook of speech pathology*. Baltimore, MD: Williams and Wilkins Company, 389 pp., $18.95.

This book covers in detail the many aspects of the diagnostic process. The need for developing interviewing skills such as taking case history information is stressed in establishing client-clinician communication. Specific chapters are devoted to the examination of specific disorders such as articulation, voice, and stuttering disorders. General testing procedures are discussed and a wide variety of published tests are described. Three appendices include resource information for evaluating tests and for locating test publishers.

Karnes, M.B. 1972. *GOAL: Language development*. Springfield, MA: Milton Bradley Company, 337 Model Lesson Plans.

GOAL stands for "Game Oriented Activities for Learning" specifically developed for use in day care centers, Headstart classrooms and regular pre-school and kinder-garten programs to enrich language learning. The language program also has been used with "children with learning disabilities in language and with somewhat older retarded children" (p. 1 of manual) as well as with children who are learning English as a second language. The program is based on the language processing model of the Illinois Test of Psycholinguistic Abilities (ITPA). Eleven checklists based on ITPA subtest areas (e.g., auditory reception, visual closure) are included to help place the student into the program. The kit (a large cardboard container) contains the program manual, 337 model lesson plans on separate file cards, and nine boxes of stimulus materials (e.g., pictures, cards, puzzle pieces, posters). Each lesson card provides: a specific objective, materials list, suggested procedures, and criterion activities to test for generalization of the task. The tasks are primarily designed for group administration, but the trainer can use them during sessions with individual children to establish specific skills.

Kent, L.R. 1974. *Language acquisition program for the retarded or multiply impaired.* Champaign, IL: Research Press, 185 pp., $7.95.

This program is primarily designed to elicit oral expressive language in severely handicapped individuals. Preverbal skills are taught, including attending and motor imitation. Verbal skills are developed in two sections: receptive and expressive. Assessment inventories and criterion for passing each objective are detailed. A chapter for modifying the program procedures for manual communication as a supplemental or alternative communication system is provided. See Appendix B in this book for a review.

Kipnis, C. 1974. *The mime book.* New York: Harper and Row Publishers, Inc., 226 pp., $8.95.

This book on mime techniques is divided into three sections. The first section covers the body, looking at both the body in isolation and the coordination of the whole body. The second section deals with illusion and covers movement, the mime as an object, and miming objects. The final section focuses on creating a world through pantomime and imagination. The outside borders on each page contain illustrations of mimes in various positions; when the pages are flipped rapidly, the illusion of the mime in action can be seen.

Kladde, A.G. 1974. Nonoral communication techniques: Project Summary #1, August 1967. In *Nonoral communication system project, 1964/1973,* ed. B. Vicker. Campus Stores, Publishers, 17 West College. The University of Iowa, Iowa City, IA, 52242, 59-104, $7.50.

This article presents information and ideas on communication board development and use. Factors for consideration in the use of nonoral communication systems include the following: (1) the selection of subjects (nine factors, such as the child's intellect and the extent of staff/parental interest and cooperation); and (2) selection of a technique (four factors such as the accuracy and range of the child's pointing ability). The development and use of frames and/or protective coverings are discussed. The type (e.g., pictures, words) and organization (e.g., through modification of the Fitzergald Key) of language materials on the communication board are discussed.

The author presents suggestions on helping the child to use the language he or she already has, in a functional way, through the use of a nonoral technique. Five general factors in planning therapy are presented and several case studies outlining the procedures are provided.

Kohl, F., Fundakowski, G., Menchetti, B., and Coleman, S. 1977. Manual communication training for severely handicapped students. In *The severely and profoundly handicapped child,* Illinois Office of Education, 105-21, free.

Following a very general discussion of the importance of communication (vocal and non-vocal) the authors present seven factors such as cost and communication potential, to be considered in selecting a non-vocal alternative or auxiliary communication system. The advantages and disadvantages of manual systems are discussed briefly. A task analysis is included, with a consideration of training items and a description of the phases of training. The training items used are listed; these consist of three sets of increasingly difficult items: situation-specific signs (e.g., "birthday"), common gestures (e.g., "come"), and home-based signs (e.g., "sister"). A data collection sheet is provided, with an explanation and example of its use. Instructional procedures are presented in the form of a figure showing training objectives and a sample flowchart.

Procedures for generalization are also suggsted. Two appendices complete the chapter. Appendix A covers the characteristics of the following manual sign systems: American Sign Language, Signed English, Seeing Exact English, and Manual English. Appendix B presents a glossary of selected training signs (those contained in the lexicon mentioned above). The sign name, a source of further information, a picture of the sign, the number of hands involved, hand and finger position, movement in space, and number of repeated movements is provided for each word.

Kopchick, G.A. and Lloyd, L.L. 1976. Total communication for the severely language impaired. A 24-hour approach. In *Communication assessment and intervention strategies*, ed. L.L. Lloyd, Baltimore, MD: University Park Press, 501–22, $16.50.

This chapter presents both rationale and methodology for a 24-hour communication program carried out in a residential setting. The term "total communication" refers here to a program "available throughout the client's total environment" (p. 503). A description of the 24-hour approach covered includes: considerations of such aspects as gaining administrative support; selecting clients, staff, a sign language system, and a teaching method; and staff training. A case study involving a schedule for one client is presented and a study involving 11 non-vocal adult clients is described.

Kotkin, R. and Simpson, S. 1976. A sign in the right direction: Language development for the non-verbal child. *Am. Assoc. Ed. Sever./Profound. Handicapp. Rev.* 1: 75–81.

The authors suggest several goals for the use of sign systems, ranging from the development of receptive vocabulary to the development of a major means of communication. Guidelines are then provided for the use of sign language with hearing children, based on these goals. For each goal, they consider the appropriate population(s), the behavioral characteristics noted, and a procedural summary. Prerequisites for using a sign system for the hearing child are discussed and advantages of sign systems are presented.

LeBlanc, J.M., Etzel, B.C., and Domash, M.A. 1978. A functional curriculum for early intervention. In *Early intervention—A team approach*, eds. K.E. Allen, V.A. Holm, and R.L. Schiefelbusch. Baltimore, MD: University Park Press, 331–81, $16.50.

This chapter addresses the development of a functional curriculum for a preschool classroom. Three major curriculum components are considered in some detail. First, a team approach to goal-setting is described. Relevant curriculum goals are identified for each child in terms of behaviors to be increased or decreased. Second, environmental arrangements for optimal learning are considered. Various ways in which teachers may provide optimal learning conditions are presented (e.g., instructions, imitation, reinforcement). Other environmental arrangements covered include peer involvement and use of materials (e.g., programming materials to reduce errors). Finally, on-going functional assessment of child behavior is described.

Lahey, M. and Bloom, L. 1977. Planning a first lexicon: which words to teach first. *J. Speech Hear. Dis.* 43: 340–50.

This article extends (and in some cases takes exception with) Holland's (1975) article. Three major considerations added are (1) the ease with which the concept can be demonstrated in the context, (2) the potential usefulness to the child of the words chosen as linguistic forms, and (3) organization of lexical items according to the ideas that they code. Both nonlinguistic and linguistic context are discussed, as well as the interaction of form and content in choosing words to teach. Reasons are given for excluding certain form/content interactions (.e.g, internal states, colors) in a first lexicon. An appendix is provided to aid in determining the interaction of form and content in choosing the first lexicon.

Lillie, D.L. and Trohanis, P.L., eds. 1976. *Teaching parents to teach*. New York: Walker and Company, 212 pp., $11.95.

This book presents a framework for planning and implementing parent involvement activities in preschool programs for handicapped children. The book is divided into four parts. Part 1 contains an introduction to parent programs, an overview of parent programs, which outlines the format of this book, and a discussion of parent-child and professional interaction. Part 2 considers four dimensions of the scope of parent programs: emotional support for parents; exchanging information; developing parent participation; and facilitating positive parent-child interactions. Each of these dimensions is considered in a separate chapter, with general and specific suggestions provided. Four perspectives on the operation of parent programs are covered in Part 3, including the following parent training models: center-based (University of Washington Child Development and Mental Retardation Center); home-center based (e.g., The Lunch Box Data System); home-based (Portage Project); and parent implemented (Regional Intervention Program, Nashville, Tennessee). One chapter is devoted to each of the four perspectives, covering descriptions of the programs listed above. The final part of this book contains an annotated bibliography.

Lloyd, L., ed. 1976. *Communication assessment and intervention strategies*. Baltimore, MD: University Park Press, 922 pp., $16.50.

This book contains 18 chapters and 7 appendices dealing with a wide range communication disorders in children. Six chapters deal primarily with the communication needs of the severely and profoundly retarded individual (see annotations for individual chapters for more information). Of particular value are the appendices for "Language Assessment Procedures" and "Language Intervention Systems: Programs Publishing in Kit Form." Each section provides author, title, publication information, a brief description, and comments about each assessment device or language program presented.

Lykos, C.M. 1971. *Cued Speech: Handbook for teachers*. Cued Speech Program, Gallaudet College, Kendall Green, Washington, D.C., 20002, 281 pp., $5.00.

This manual may be used by teachers of Cued Speech who are working directly with clients or with parent groups. A natural language approach is suggested for preschool children or older persons who have early language skills, while an analytical approach is recommended for clients who have more advanced language skills. Twelve lessons are presented to be used with the analytical approach, and numerous activities are provided for use with either approach. Exercises for hearing adults, such as teachers, clinicians, or parents, are include. Appendices contain supplementary materials such as transcription exercises.

Lyon, S., Baumgart, D., Stoll, A., and Brown, L. 1977. Curricular strategies for teaching basic functional object use skills to severely handicapped students. In *Madison's alternative for zero exclusion*, vol. VII, part 1, eds. L. Brown, P. Scheurman, and T. Crowner. Specialized Educational Services, Madison Metropolitan School District, 545 W. Dayton Street, Madison, WI, 53703, $9.00.

This task force covers training of functional object use skills. The three skill sequences comprising it are I — teaching person–object actions; II — teaching person–tool–object actions; and III — teaching person–tool-tool-object actions. The authors discuss a number of strategies for establishing curricular priorities and determining initial content. They also suggest ways to compensate if the client is severely impaired motorically.

Mallik, K.K. 1977. *Communication resources for the developmentally disabled: A guide for parents, paraprofessionals, and professionals.* The Job Development Laboratory, The George Washington University, Rehabilitation Medicine, 2300 Eye Street, N.W., Room 420, Washington, D.C., 20037, 255 pp., $6.00.

This is a collection of resources for persons working with the developmentally disabled. Chapter 1 covers screening instruments appropriate for use by the parent and paraprofessional and assessment tools for use by speech-language pathologists. In addition to identifying information, the following are included for each test: target; purpose/emphasis; format; users; cost; and subjective opinion. Chapter 2 reviews training materials, again separated according to those appropriate for parents and paraprofessionals and those intended for speech-language pathologists. The format for reviewing these training materials is the same as that for assessment tools. In Chapter 3, communication alternatives and devices are covered. This includes materials (e.g., books, articles) describing these alternatives and devices, plus descriptions of nearly 100 aids, including identifying information, type, portability, description and use, and cost of each aid. The final chapter provides a listing of source books, bibliographies, and major companies.

Mayberry, R. 1976. If a chimp can learn sign language, surely my nonverbal client can too. *ASHA* 18: 223-28.

The author asserts that "a decision to use sign language as a means of establishing communication in the normally hearing client for whom all else has failed, such as the autistic, severely retarded, and cerebral palsied, demands basic knowledge of the manual communication systems available" (p. 223). Therefore this paper briefly describes American Sign Language (ASL) and other recently developed systems, including Seeing Essential English (SEE1), Signing Exact English (SEE2), Signed English, and Linguistics of Visual English (LOVE). The author describes relationships between and among these systems, pointing out specific features of each, such as word order, and comparing them on the basis of availability and approximation to spoken English. She suggests some general guidelines for selecting a manual communication system (e.g., the availability of a teacher, the client's potential communication skills, etc.). Methods of teaching signs, including molding, shaping, and imitation, and structuring of sign language teaching (e.g., determining which signs to teach first) are also discussed.

McCormack, J.E. and Chalmers, A.J. 1978. *Early cognitive instruction for the moderately and severely handicapped.* Champaign, IL: Research Press Company, 165 pp. program guide, 333 pp. instructional program.

The program guide presents the rationale and details for implementing the entire instructional program. The program is designed for teachers, parents, or aides and has a training component (Volunteer Training Similation) to acquaint trainers with the program objectives and procedures. The skills targeted within the program are matching, sorting, constructing, recognizing, identifying, memory, and sequencing. The training steps are presented in a chart format with materials, instructions, expected responses, and correction procedures specified.

McDonald, E.T. 1976a. Conventional Symbols of English. In *Non-vocal communication techniques and aids for the severely physically handicapped,* eds. G. Vanderheiden and K. Grilley. Baltimore, MD: University Park Press, 77-84, $12.50.

This article presents a consideration of visual symbols and symbols in English grammar as a background for developing communication boards. Forms of visual symbols used include pictures, photographs, and letters of the alphabet. The levels of English grammar (e.g., words, sentences), and the development of language structure (e.g., through use of the Fitzgerald Key) are presented. The author discusses applying symbol systems to the communication board by giving general and specific examples and by using numerous figures.

McDonald, E.T. 1976b. Design and application of communication boards. In *Non-vocal communication techniques and aids for the severely physically handicapped,* eds. G. Vanderheiden and K. Grilley. Baltimore, MD: University Park Press, 105–19, $12.50

The author discusses entry skills necessary for using communication boards successfully, such as attention to visual stimuli and verbal symbols and a need or desire to communicate. The physical considerations (ambulation, vision, and posture) are also considered. Specific ways to assess and deal with these skills are presented. Methods of adapting the content and/or the board for an individual's physical problems are described, as well as general considerations in constructing communication boards. Finally, the author explains how to involve others in this process.

McDonald, E.T. 1980. Early identification and treatment of children at risk for speech development. In *Nonspeech language and communication: Analysis and intervention,* ed. R.L. Schiefelbusch. Baltimore, MD: University Park Press, 49–79, $24.95.

This chapter stresses the importance of developing communicative competence in severely handicapped clients, rather than focusing only on oral language. Types of information which might predict difficulty developing intelligible speech (history, developmental lags, examination findings) are briefly considered. Methods for training the clients to use a three-item communication board are presented. The author describes the content and organization of increasingly more complex communication boards. Numerous diagrams are included to clarify suggestions.

McDonald, E.T. and Schultz, A.R. 1973. Communication boards for cerebral-palsied children. *J. Speech Hear. Dis.* 38: 73–88.

Although the boards described in this article are intended for use with cerebral-palsied clients, many of the principles and suggestions would also be helpful for other populations, such as the severely mentally retarded. The authors stress the need to help parents understand and accept the use of communication boards. An evaluation of the child's physical capabilities and the construction and physical layout of the board for clients with different needs are included. Types and content of symbols, such as pictures, words or sentences, are discussed and a case study of the development and use of a communication board is provided.

McLean, J.E. and Snyder-McLean, L.K. 1978. *A transactional approach to early language training.* Columbus, OH: Charles E. Merrill Publishing Company, 280 pp., $9.95.

This book presents a transactional model of language acquisition which consists of three major components: cognitive, social, and linguistic. The authors suggest that the child's acquisition of language or of a linguistic code is shaped by the child's interactions with people in the environment. Two visual representations are presented as overviews of the model showing the relationships between the three major components. A detailed chapter on assessment presents skills to be tested, methods of assessing these skills, a list of procedures, and guidelines with references to relevant published instruments and assessment implications. Another chapter is devoted to treatment programs as viewed from the authors' transactional model. Suggestions for developing a treatment program and a review of some currently available programs are presented.

McLean, J., Yoder, D., and Schiefelbusch, R., eds. 1972. *Language intervention with the retarded: Developing strategies,* Baltimore, MD: University Park Press, $16.50.

This book contains twelve chapters by various authors, divided into two general sections: I-assessment and identification of goals, and II-treatment procedures, in which the strategies for language intervention are exemplified in several different programs. See chapter annotations for additional information.

McNaughton, S. 1976a. Bliss symbols — an alternative symbol system for the non-vocal pre-reading child. In *Non-vocal communication techniques and aids for the severely physically handicapped*, eds. G. Vanderheiden, and K. Grilley. Baltimore, MD: University Park Press, 85–104, $12.50.

The author presents background information on Blissymbolics and discusses the advantages of using the Bliss system for young non-vocal children, rather than teaching written symbols. A general introduction to Blissymbols and the construction of symbols (combining symbols or making up new ones) are provided. Other topics covered are techniques for expanding vocabulary, the role of the teacher, and the advantages and disadvantages of Blissymbols.

McNaughton, S. 1976b. Symbol communication programme at OCCC. In *Non-vocal communication techniques and aids for the severely physically handicapped*, eds. G. Vander-heiden and K. Grilley. Baltimore, MD: University Park Press, 132–43, $12.50.

This article presents specific and general information on using the Blissymbol program with children who have a range of physical problems, but who have near-normal or normal intelligence. The author discusses how children are introduced to the symbols, beginning with symbols of interest to the child and progressing to a 400 symbol display board. The features incorporated at each level are described. The author also considers the child's emotional development. Several examples of com-munication through Blissymbols are provided, including examples of symbols created by children.

McNaughton, S. and Kates, B. 1980. The application of Blissymbolics. In *Nonspeech Language and communication: Analysis and intervention*, ed. R.L. Schiefelbusch. Balti-more, MD: University Park Press, 303–21, $24.95.

The basic features of the Blissymbol system are presented, with numerous examples of symbols provided for clarity. Application of Blissymbols with severely handicapped persons is covered, with consideration of four issues basic to application (e.g., matching the system with the individual). General strategies are suggested for implementing a Blissymbolics instructional program. The discussion includes pre-requisite skills, advantages and disadvantages of the system, and results.

Melichar, J.F. 1977. *ISAARE*, vols. 1 to 7, Adaptive Systems Corporation, 1650 South Amphlett Boulevard, Suite 307, San Mateo, CA 94402, see prices below.

The Information System Adaptive Assistive Rehabilitation Equipment (ISAARE) pro-vides a means for aiding in the selection and location of equipment to meet the needs of the severely handicapped. It is composed of three parts: the six Index-Glossaries, encyclopedic-format descriptions of generic equipment (set, $30.00); the Locator Book, in which equipment items and manufacturers are cross-referenced ($18.00); and Mailing Labels and Check-In Log, to facilitate collection of equipment catalogue libraries ($20.00). A step-by-step "How-To" Book is also available ($5.00). An Institutional Use Set includes the above materials plus materials such as file folder labels for $69.50. The system can be accessed through the name of a desired item or the function the item must perform. A timeshared computer capability is also available. Six major categories of equipment are included, such as equipment for daily living skills. Sub-groupings for the communication category cover hearing, vision, touch, smell, taste, proprioception, internalization, and verbal and nonverbal expres-sion. Equipment descriptions consist of a diagram and a paragraph containing pertinent information such as parts of the equipment, other related equipment, and prerequisites for equipment use. The system is continually updated and the communication section is being expanded.

Melichar, J.F. 1978. ISAARE: A description. *Am. Assoc. Ed. Severe. Profound. Handicap. Rev.* 3:259–68.

This article presents an overview of the Information System on Adaptive, Assistive, and Rehabilitation Equipment (ISAARE). This system consists of a data base for storing and retrieving information about equipment for the severely handicapped. The author describes the system and its components, defines the terminology, demonstrates how to apply the system, and discusses its advantages over random flow information systems. A sample page showing entries in the system is provided.

Miller, J. 1977. On specifying what to teach: The movement from structure, to structure and meaning, to structure and meaning and knowing. In *Educational programming for the severely and profoundly handicapped*, ed. E. Sontag. Reston, VA: Council for Exceptional Children, 378–88, $14.95.

The author discusses the general trend in language teaching programs ranging from programs which bombard the child with verbal stimulation, to those which focus on structure and content, to those which emphasize the semantic aspect of language. The author briefly discusses a semantically based training program, and provides four operating principles (e.g., #4 - "first expansions of single-word utterances should be of relational functions previously expressed," p. 381). Miller notes "the inextricable relationship between semantics and cognition" (p. 381); he discusses methods for describing semantic development, taking the cognitive behavior of the child and the child's experiential history and present environmental situation into consideration.

Moores, D.F. 1980a. Alternative communication modes. In *Nonspeech language and communication: Analysis and intervention*, ed. R.L. Schiefelbusch. Baltimore, MD: University Park Press, 27–47, $24.95.

This chapter explores the use of alternative communication modes, both manual and symbolic, in moving toward "normalization" for the severely handicapped. A continuum of rationales are presented for selection and use of a non-vocal communication system. Three types of symbol systems are described: written, symbol, and visual-motor systems. The use of manual communication with severely handicapped, non-vocal children is considered.

Moores, D.F. 1980b. American Sign Language: Historical perspectives and current issues. In *Nonspeech language and communication: Analysis and intervention*, ed. R.L. Schiefelbusch. Baltimore, MD: University Park Press, 93–100, $24.95.

This chapter provides a brief summary of the roots of American Sign Language from the sixteenth century to the present. The cyclical controversy which has evolved around the acceptance of the use of sign language with the deaf is discussed. Recent issues regarding American Sign Language are described, including the development of pedagogical sign systems.

Moores, D.F. 1974. Non-vocal systems of verbal behavior. In *Language perspectives: Acquisition, retardation, and intervention*, ed. R. Schiefelbusch and L. Lloyd. Baltimore, MD: University Park Press, 377–418, $16.50.

This chapter provides a theoretical background for the consideration of manual linguistic systems. The author discusses the nature and use of sign languages and presents an overview of structural and functional characteristics of American Sign Language (ASL). Suggestions are made for the educational use of manual communication. The literature is reviewed relative to recent trends and results. The author attempts to dispel some common misconceptions regarding the use of sign systems.

Murdock, J. and Hartmann, B. 1975. *A language development program: Imitative gestures to basic syntactic structures*. Salt Lake City, UT: Word Making Productions, Inc., 60 West 400 South, 35 pp., $4.25.

This program is intended for "children whose language ability ranges from having no vocal verbalizations to those having syntactical (word order) and morphological (word form) skills below those of a normal 4-year-old child" (p.3). General information is provided regarding selection of words, reinforcers, testing procedures, setting and materials, procedures to eliminate inappropriate or nonattending behavior, teaching behavior, recording procedures, and generalization. Five learning categories are included in the program: I-preverbal motor and vocal imitation; II-phonological skills; III-semantic skills; IV-syntactical skills; and V-morphological skills. See Appendix B of this book for a review of the program.

Meyers, L.S., Grows, N.L., Coleman, C.L., and Cook, A.M. 1980. *An assessment battery for assistive device systems recommendations, part 1*. Assistive Device Center, California State University, 6000 J Street, Sacramento, CA 95819, 33 pp., currently free.

This report documents the assessment procedures used by the Assistive Device Center in working with physically and mentally disabled children and adults. The report is divided into five major sections: interview; sensory assessment; motor assessment; cognitive/language assessment; and device characteristics. Separate modules are described within each of these major sections. For each assessment task the following information is provided: purpose; materials (described in some detail); testing proceudre (described in fairly general terms, but with sufficient detail for replication); and applications. An initial evaluation form, available separately, provides space for recording results of many of the assessment tasks.

Nation, J.E. and Aram, D.M. 1977. *Diagnosis of speech and language disorders*. St. Louis, MO: C.V. Mosby Company, 453 pp., $21.95.

The authors view diagnosis as a professional skill which requires the speech-language pathologist to be aware of a vast amount of information. Normal language acquisition is presented as a base for judging disordered speech and language. A speech and language processing model is described and related to the identification of different disorders. Case management techniques, interpretation of assessment tools at a conference, and planning client follow-up are discussed. Six appendices include information such as administrative forms, and ways to improve report writing skills.

Nietupski, J. and Hamre-Nietupski, S. 1977. Nonverbal communication and severely handicapped students: A review of selected literature. In *Curricular strategies for teaching functional object use, nonverbal communication, problem solving, and mealtime skills to severely handicapped students*, vol. VII, part 1, eds. L. Brown, J. Nietupski, S. Lyon, S. Hamre-Nietupski, T. Crowner, and L. Gruenewald. Madison, WI: Department of Specialized Educational Services, 25 pp., $9.00.

This paper presents brief descriptions of various manual and symbolic systems appropriate for use with non-verbal, severely handicapped clients. Factors are discussed relative to deciding to initiate a non-vocal system and to selecting the most appropriate system. Advantages and disadvantages of each system are presented. Nine strategies for determining initial content are briefly described. A variety of instructional procedures such as imitation and hand shaping are described.

Nietupski, J., Stoll, A., Broome, D., and Brown, L. 1977. Curricular strategies for teaching selected problem solving skills to severely handicapped students. In *Curricular strategies for teaching functional object use, nonverbal communication, problem solving, and mealtime skills to severely handicapped students*, vol. VII, part 1, eds. L. Brown, J. Nietupski, S. Lyon, S. Hamre-Nietupski, T. Crowner, and L. Gruenewald.

Madison, WI: Department of Specialized Educational Services, Madison Metropolitan School District, 114 pp., $9.00.

This curriculum is centered around nine instructional components, such as methods, materials, and functional use of the problem solving skills taught. The content includes skills for successfully searching for and obtaining objects; these skills are related to the development of "object permanence" and "means-end relationship." The curriculum is divided into four skill sequences. For each skill sequence the following are provided: task analysis, example problems and solutions, and suggested curricular strategies. Procedures are suggested for "naturalized" assessment of problem solving skills, such as during feeding and playing.

Nugent, C.L. 1977. Rehabilitative speech and language pathology and nonoral communication. *Resources*, Los Angeles: Everett and Jennings, Inc., 1803 Pontius Avenue, Los Angeles, California, 90025, 8 pp., free.

This pamphlet describes the function of rehabilitative speech and language pathology with the patient having a speech and/or language deficit, generally resulting from neurological damage. The services provided to such patients in a rehabilitative facility are briefly discussed. Objectives and methods for evaluating the nonoral communicative candidate are presented, followed by brief consideration of the factors involved in selecting a nonoral communication system. Procedures are outlined for making the system applicable clinically, educationally, vocationally, and personally.

Oakander, S.M. 1980. *Language board instruction kit*, Exemplary/Incentive Dissemination Project, ESEA, Title IV-C, Non Oral Communication Center, Plavan School, 9675 Warner Avenue, Fountain Valley, CA 92708, 34 pp., $5.00.

This instruction kit is intended to serve as a step-by-step guide for determining goals, constructing a language board, and evaluating effectiveness of the board. Eight tasks are covered, with worksheets and suggestions for completing each. Examples of tasks are as follows: #1 — what are the goals; #4 — what are the motor skills; and #5 — which types of symbol systems can be used. Appendices include category suggestions for a customized vocabulary, suggested items for language boards, and sources for symbol systems.

O'Rourke, T.J. 1973. *A basic course in manual communication*. Silver Spring, MD: The National Association of the Deaf, 161 pp., $5.75.

This book contains 45 lessons, covering over 600 signs. For each lesson signs are presented through illustrations, with one or more possible English words that the sign can represent. Practice materials are provided in a separate section, with one practice sentence included for each of the possible meanings for each sign. Signs included in each lesson are not arranged in any functional grouping (such as items of clothing or verbs), nor is there any order of increasing difficulty across lessons. Rather, signs are grouped according to the type of handshape used. A final section of 72 signs includes the following: pronouns; affixes (e.g., -able, -ing); contractions; articles; the verb "to be;" and other function words. Appendices include a manual communication bibliography which lists prices and sources, and a selected annotated bibliography of books, films, and teaching media related to sign language.

Popovich, D. 1977. *A prescriptive behavioral checklist for the severely and profoundly retarded*. Baltimore: University Park Press, 431 pp., $14.95.

This book presents behavioral checklists for the following areas: motor development; eye-hand coordination; language development; and physical eating problems. The checklists, task analysis steps, and implementation suggestions for the language development area cover the following behavior: attending; physical imitation; auditory training; object discrimination; concept development; and sound imitation. Each implementation item describes the materials needed, prerequisite skills, and procedures to follow to meet the stated objective.

Reichle, J.E. and Yoder, D.E. 1979. Assessment and early stimulation communication in the severely and profoundly mentally retarded. In *Teaching the severely handicapped, vol. IV*, eds. R.L. York and E. Edgar. Columbus, OH: Special Press, 155–79.

The authors present a position that developmental and nondevelopmental approaches must be blended during assessment and curriculum planning to meet the needs of individual clients. A careful review of the literature pertaining to early communication behavior from a pragmatic viewpoint is presented. The need to consider awareness of a communication partner, communication turn-taking, establishing functions of symbols, and establishing individual meanings of symbols are discussed. An overview of precomprehension strategies from 8–24 months is summarized. The authors suggest ways to teach the following behavior: awareness, localization, tracking, line of regard, diverted gaze, imitation (stressing simultaneous motor and vocal imitation and mutual imitation), grasp and reach, functional use of objects, and pointing.

Rieke, J.A., Lynch, L.L, and Soltman, S.F. 1977. *Teaching strategies for language development*. New York: Grune and Stratton, 119 pp., $14.00.

The authors present issues and suggestions on how to assess a language disordered child's environment and how to establish vocal communication. Their approach is based on a developmental model which stresses the child's interactions with his environment. The authors refer to The Sequenced Inventory of Communication Development (Hedrick, Prather, and Tobin, 1975; see Appendix D in this book for more information) as a possible assessment tool to summarize a child's present abilities and to chart progress. Their discussion of "initiating behaviors," in which the trainer is required to "watch and listen for cues" (p. 31) from the child, receives particular emphasis. Eight case studies are provided as examples of implementing the language strategies.

Riekehof, L.L. 1978. *The joy of Signing*. Gospel Publishing House, Springfield, MO 65802, 336 pp., $12.95.

This manual "... is meant to provide the learner with knowledge of the basic traditional signs used by adult deaf persons today and with knowledge concerning the base on which new signs were developed" (p. 4). Signs are grouped into natural categories such as family relationships, location and direction, and nature. For each sign the following are provided: an illustration; potential English glosses of the sign; brief description of sign execution; origin, if known; and useage (e.g., sign embedded in a phrase or sentence). It is recommended that the phrases and sentences be used as practice materials.

Ruder, F. 1978. Planning and programming for language intervention. In *Bases of language intervention*, ed. R.L. Schiefelbusch. Baltimore, MD: University Park Press, 319–71, $14.50.

This chapter suggests "a strategy that incorporates a system for developing an individualized program for each language problem" (p. 321). The systematic approach includes both process components (e.g., initial evaluation, program development) and program components (e.g., target behaviors, branching steps). These components are described both theoretically and through the use of numerous examples, yielding development of a programmed approach for teaching a linguistic structure in the form of subject-verb-object. Each programming component is discussed "in terms of how to do it and how to specify and identify the overlap and interactions of the programming components with the process components" (p. 325).

Ruder, F. and Smith, M. 1974. Issues in language training. In *Language perspectives: Acquisition, retardation, and intervention,* eds. R. Schiefelbusch and L. Lloyd. Baltimore, MD: University Park Press, 565–605, $16.50.

Three basic issues are covered in this chapter. First, the authors consider the question of what (content) to train, with discussion centered around (a) syntactically based structural relationships, (b) semantically based structural relationships, or (c) a combination of a and b. Next, they discuss methodological issues, with primary emphasis on operant training, and the roles of imitation, comprehension, modeling, and expansion in language training. Finally, the authors review informal, formal and ongoing language assessments.

Schaeffer, B. 1980. Spontaneous language through signed speech. In *Nonspeech language and communication: Analysis and interventioin,* ed. R.L. Schiefelbusch. Baltimore, MD: University Park Press, 421–46, $24.95.

This chapter describes the use of signed speech, in which speech and sign are used simultaneously by both client and trainer. The author makes four propositions regarding the use of signed speech with autistic children, based on data from three clients. For example, it is asserted that "instruction in sign fosters spontaneous communication . . . " (p. 423). Each of these propositions is discussed, with numerous examples provided. Issues regarding communication mode and content, such as the role of imitation, are also presented.

Scheuerman, N., Baumgart, D., Sipmsa, K., and Brown, L. 1976. Toward the development of a curriculum for teaching non-verbal communication skills to severely handicapped students: Teaching basic tracking, scanning, and selection skills. In *Madison's alternative for zero exclusion,* vol. VI, part 3, eds. L. Brown, N. Scheuerman, and T. Crowner. Specialized Educational Services, Madison Metropolitan School Districts, 545 West Dayton Street, Madison, WI, 53703, $8.00.

The tracking skills section of this task force covers tracking people or objects through various paths (e.g., horizontal path) and barriers (e.g., transparent visual barrier). The second section covers the skills of attending, scanning, and selecting. Students are taught to scan and select items which are presented concurrently or consecutively. This is a naturalized curriculum, in which training takes place throughout the day in a variety of settings.

Schiefelbusch, R.L., ed. 1978a. *Bases of language intervention.* Baltimore, MD: University Park Press, 486 pp., $14.50.

This book includes information on the broad areas of language development, deficiency, and remediation, and is intended to serve specialists and students in those areas. Chapters cover such topics as pragmatics, assessment, and generalization. See chapter annotations for further information.

Schiefelbusch, R.L., ed. 1978b. *Language intervention strategies.* Baltimore, MD: University Park Press, 420 pp., $15.75.

This book describes a number of strategies that may be used with language-delayed and language-impaired individuals. The first chapter delineates a number of strategies that may be used by clinicians and researchers, the next six chapters present six program strategies, and the final chapter provides a perspective relating to all of the strategies. The six programs covered are (1) nonspeech language intervention, (2) a syntax-teaching program, (3) a functional program for nonverbal adolescents, (4) a milieu program for preschool children, (5) a parent-administered program for young children, and (6) a matrix-training system for language intervention. Individual chapters are annotated elsewhere in this bibliography.

Schiefelbusch, R.L., ed. 1980. *Nonspeech language and communication: Analysis and intervention*. Baltimore, MD: University Park Press, 529 pp., $24.95.

This book includes twenty chapters centering on the topic of nonspeech language and communication, perspectives on American Sign Language, assessment, strategies for the physically handicapped, autistic and severely retarded children, and interpretative issues. See individual chapter annotations for further information.

Schiefelbusch, R. and Lloyd, L.L., eds. 1974. *Language perspectives: Acquisition, retardation, and intervention*. Baltimore, MD: University Park Press, 680 pp., $16.50.

The intervention aspect of this book includes sections on non-vocal communication, early language intervention, and language intervention for the mentally retarded. See annotations of individual chapters for further information.

Schumaker, J.B. and Sherman, J.A. 1978. Parent as intervention agent: From birth onward. In *Language intervention strategies*, ed. R. Schiefelbusch. Baltimore, MD: University Park Press, 237–316, $15.75.

The authors provide an extensive review of research involving parents as initial language trainers for their normal developing children. Specific and contradictory evidence for the following parameters are detailed: models, prompts, and reinforcement in the natural environment; conditioning vocalizations in infants; the role of imitation; and the relationship between receptive and productive language. A section offering specific suggestions for parents to enhance the development of their child's language is presented. General guidelines for language enrichment include suggestions for increasing vocalizations, stimulating imitation, prompting spontaneous words, and increasing the child's utterances. Although the chapter focuses primarily on normal developmental data, much of the information can be applied to the language handicapped.

Schurman, J.A. 1974. Custom designing communication board frames: The role of the occupational therapist. In *Nonoral communication system project, 1964/1973*, ed. B. Vicker. Campus Stores, Publishers, 17 West College, The University of Iowa, Iowa City, 52242, 179–211, $7.50.

This paper is intended "to describe the procedures used by the occupational therapist to: (1) determine the child's physical skills, (2) identify the child's special needs in relation to the use of the communication board, and (3) show how this information is used to custom-design a communication board frame" (p. 179). Numerous figures and examples are provided to clarify the information presented, and a summary outline is available for duplication "to provide therapists with a convenient checklist when evaluating a patient for a nonoral communication system" (p. 208). A list of supply sources is also included.

Shane, H.C. 1980. Approaches to assessing the communication of non-oral persons. In *Nonspeech language and communication: Analysis and intervention*, ed. R.L. Schiefelbusch. Baltimore, MD: University Park Press, 197–224, $24.95.

This chapter covers assessment considerations which will assist in deciding whether to use a non-vocal system and, if so, which system to select. The author presents a model based on "Wepman's model;" it includes an integration component (forms of expression) and a transmission component (mode of expression). Components are described, such as vocal, nonlinguistic forms of expression (e.g., crying, grunting). Assessment approaches are suggested for each subcomponent of the model. Finally, seven guidelines are offered for finalizing clinical decisions with individual clients.

Shane, H.C. 1979. Approaches to communication training with the severely handicapped. In *Teaching the severely handicapped,* vol. IV, eds. R.L. York and E. Edgar.
Columbus, OH: Special Press, 155-79, $24.50.

In this chapter Shane introduces the concept of the communication spiral (figure 1, p.
159) as a framework for meeting two major communication objectives: (1) expressing
needs and wants, and (2) describing the here and now. Vocal and non-vocal communication are represented in the spiral concept with the emphasis that movement in
training can be horizontal (allowing vocal and non-vocal training to be done
simultaneously) as well as vertical (encouraging the client to move to higher levels of
representation or symbolic complexity). Regardless of the ultimate mode of communication chosen, Shane states that Level I—the physiological level and Level II—the
discrimination level, are prerequisites to vocal or non-vocal communication.

Shane offers useful guidelines to assist the trainer in the decision-making process
and provides suggestions for initial intervention procedures.

Siegel, G.M. and Spradlin, J.E. 1978. Programming for language and communication
therapy. In *Language intervention strategies,* ed. R. Schiefelbusch. Baltimore, MD:
University Park Press, 357-98, $15.75.

This chapter summarizes some of the issues presented throughout this edited book
regarding the general selection and implementation of language programs and communication therapy. The authors stress the need for clinicians "to remain sufficiently
knowledgeable and current in the literature to make informed evaluations concerning
the claims of various treatment methods" (p. 393). Implications for non-vocal
communication using alternative communication systems are discussed. The difficulties in differential diagnosis, the role of imitation in language training, and the
production before reception issue are reviewed.

Silverman, F.H. 1980. *Communication for the speechless.* Englewood Cliffs, NJ: Prentice-
Hall, Inc., 291 pp., $14.95.

Silverman presents a comprehensive review of nonspeech communication aids
classified according to response mode: gestural mode, gestural-assisted mode, and
neuro-assisted mode. Specific suggestions for selecting a nonspeech communication
mode are detailed. Many factors regarding intervention strategies such as gaining
acceptance, assessing the impact of the system, and maintaining the device are
discussed. Five appendices supplement the text with valuable information including a
comprehensive bibliography, sources of materials, sources of components for gestural
and neuro-assisted modes, construction details for inexpensive displays, and an
evaluation summary for selecting a nonspeech mode.

Silverman, H., McNaughton, S., and Kates, B. 1978. *Handbook of Blissymbolics for
instructors, Bliss symbol users, parents and administrators.* Toronto, Ontario: Blissymbolics
Communication Institute, 655 pp., $30.00

This handbook presents a general description of the Blissymbol System, including
devices for expanding the symbol vocabulary and a discussion of the syntax used with
the system. Instructions for drawing Blissymbols, with and without a template, are
provided. A second section deals with physical functioning considerations, including
positioning, handtraining, physical assessment and recommendations. Special information is presented for the cerebral-palsied Blissymbol user. The major portion of the
handbook covers the application of the system, including assessment (e.g., considerations in assessment and formal assessment devices available) and programming.
Programming is discussed in terms of the individual symbol user and an extension of
the system beyond the individual, including the class program, family involvement,
and community awareness. Programming for the individual includes general and
specific suggestions applicable to most symbol users (such as suggestions for

extending the program beyond the initial stage). In addition, special considerations are presented for the severely physically handicapped, mentally retarded, and preschool user. The socio-psychological implications of use of the Bliss system are also considered.

Simmons, V. and Williams, I. 1976. *STEPS UP to language for the learning impaired: Attending*, vol. 1. Tuscon, AZ: Communication Skill Builders, Inc., 37 pp., $10.00.

This program is designed for children up to the age of seven years but has been used successfully with older clients in special education programs. Systematic behavior management techniques are employed to establish the following attending behaviors: responses to auditory nonverbal cues; responses to name; eye contact for one second; attention for five seconds to continuous cueing; and attention with time lapse between cue and response. Each attention task is broken down into very small steps to allow the student to succeed. Each task serves as its own pre-test and post-test. A program data sheet is provided for record keeping.

Soltman, S.F. and Rieke, A., 1977. Communication management for the non-responsive child: A team approach. In *Educational programming for the severely and profoundly handicapped*, ed. E. Sontag. Division on Mental Retardation, Council for Exceptional Children, Reston, VA, 348–59, $14.95.

This chapter describes a comprehensive team approach to achieve a looking response in an unresponsive child functioning at a very low level. Six steps are included in the procedure and the person(s) responsible for each are identified. The steps are: assessment request, observations, systematic recording, sorting information, designing the intervention program, implementing the all-day program, and decisions for changes in the program. An example of the use of this approach is provided, including two sample communication behavior observation and recording forms, and an example of data sorting, a plan sheet, and the reminder board. The need for consistency and frequency of trials is noted.

Somerton, M.E. and Myers, D.G. 1976. Educational programming for the severely and profoundly mentally retarded. In *Teaching the severely handicapped*, vol. I, ed. N.G. Haring and L.J. Brown. New York: Grune and Stratton, 111–54, $24.50.

This chapter presents an overview of a program for the severely and profoundly retarded. The population to be served is carefully described, and general curriculum planning procedures are discussed. The curriculum presented here includes five broad developmental areas: sensory, motor, self-help, language, and perceptual cognitive. For each unit of instruction, the following is provided: competency checklist, instructional objective, readiness (prerequisites), procedures, task evaluation, materials and equipment. For some units, more than one cycle of instructional objective through task evaluation is presented. Selected readings and materials and equipment are suggested relative to the major curriculum areas.

Sontag, E., ed. 1977. *Educational programming for the severely and profoundly handicapped*. Reston, VA: Division on Mental Retardation, Council for Exceptional Children, 472 pp., $14.95.

This book includes five chapters on teaching strategies for communication and language, as well as numerous chapters in other areas related to communication. See the individual chapter annotations for more information.

Sternat, J., Messina, R., Nietupski, J., Lyon, S., and Brown, L. 1977. Occupational and physical therapy services for severely handicapped students: Toward a natural-ized public school service delivery model. In *Educational programming for the severely and profoundly handicapped*, ed. E. Sontag. Reston, VA: Division on Mental Retardation, Council for Exceptional Children, 263–78, $14.95.

Part III of this chapter covers "curricular suggestions for teaching severely handicapped students selected clusters of head control skills." An instructional sequence of nine skill clusters is presented, including head rotation, balancing, and righting. Task analyses are provided for selected head control skill clusters. Instructional strategies are suggested, including instructional considerations, assessment strategies, teaching procedures, and facilitatory/inhibitory events.

Stokoe, W.C. 1980. The study and use of sign language. In *Nonspeech language and communication: Analysis and intervention,* ed. R.L. Schiefelbusch. Baltimore, MD: University Park Press, 123–55, $24.95.

This chapter begins with a brief historical perspective on American Sign Language. The author describes the nature and elements of sign language, and argues for use of sign rather than speech-reading, as a more efficient use of visual input. Differences and similarities between American Sign Language and English are discussed. The social implications of sign language are considered in relation to the five levels of style. Bilingualism in American Sign Language and English is discussed in terms of both students and their teachers. Classroom research and application reported by the author supports use of a bilingual approach, in which the teacher carefully points out differences between the systems.

Stremel, K. and Waryas, C. 1974. A behavioral-psycholinguistic approach to language training. In *Developing systematic procedures for training children's language,* ed. L.V. McReynolds. ASHA Monographs 18: 96–132.

"This chapter presents a series of sequential language training programs and assessment procedures for the child who displays delayed or deficient language structures" (p. 96). The program steps are sequenced following a developmental model. Three sections of the program are outlined: (1) Early Language Training, (2) Early-Intermediate Training, and (3) Late-Intermediate Language Training. Behavior modification techniques are described to establish new behaviors. Entry level behaviors for the Early Language Training section include gross attention, comprehension of at least 10 functional nouns, and approximate imitation of a set of phonemes. Successful completion of Early Language Training section is required before moving to the other sections.

Stremel-Campbell, K., Cantrell, D., and Halle, J. 1977. Manual signing as a language system and as a speech initiator for the non-verbal severely handicapped student. In *Educational programming for the severely and profoundly handicapped,* ed. E. Sontag. Reston, VA: Division on Mental Retardation, Council for Exceptional Children, 335–47, $14.95.

This chapter presents a method for teaching sign language to non-vocal children. A rationale is advanced for the use and organization of such a system, based on a review of studies in children and animals (e.g., chimpanzees). The authors note several advantages of signing over other non-vocal systems and point out studies reporting the success of signing as a facilitator to vocal language and as an initiator of speech.

The authors discuss how to determine if a non-vocal approach is appropriate and, if so, which is best for the child. The determination of sign content (mostly American Sign Language and Signed English) and sequence (based on sign features and functional considerations) are considered. Training components included are assessment (general and sign imitation pretest) and training procedures (the use of time-delay with a handshaping-imitation-production sequence). The trainers always combine the English word (gloss) with the sign being taught or used. An example of the use of the training model with nine subjects is described, proceeding to the training of semantic relations expressed by two-sign combinations. The authors discuss the results of this training model with the subjects and present implications for future applications.

Striefel, S. 1974. *Managing behavior 7, Teaching a child how to imitate.* H and H Enterprises Inc., P.O. Box 3342, Lawrence, KS, 66044, 51 pp., $3.75.

This programmed manual is designed for use by professionals or lay people in teaching motor imitation skills to retarded children. Sections are included on the use of reinforcement, the analysis of entry behaviors, selecting and defining behaviors to be trained, procedures for training specific behaviors, how to overcome problems, and how to recognize when a child is ready for a more advanced program.

Struck, R. 1977. Santa Cruz Special Education Management Systems. *Behavioral characteristics progression* (BCP). Palo Also, CA: VORT Corporation, approx. 550 pp., $24.95.

Book three (Method Cards: Communication Skills 3) is divided into eleven strands (areas) dealing with communication skills. Each strand contains a series of method cards. Each method card provides a specific activity to meet a specified objective. Language comprehension, oral expression and manual communication can be taught with this system. Prerequisite abilities, type of setting, length of session and materials are included on each card. See Appendix B in this book for more information.

Swetlik, B. and Brown, L. 1977. Teaching severely handicapped students to express selected first, second, and third person singular pronoun responses in answer to "who-doing" questions. In *Teaching the severely handicapped*, vol. II, eds. N.G. Haring and L.J. Brown. New York: Grune and Stratton, 15–62, $19.50.

A ten-phase pronoun instructional program was designed for use with eight trainable retarded students in a public school system. Phase I required imitation of one-, two-, and three-word verbal responses (e.g., "I", "I am", "I am standing.") Phase X required the students to respond appropriately using first, second, and third person pronouns when asked "who is doing" (e.g., "he/she is running."). The intermediate phases included visually discriminating actions with verbal cues, visually discriminating people with name cues, and visually discriminating males and females using "he" and "she" (e.g., "touch a he."). A rationale for selecting the vocabulary is presented. Significant progress was noted when the client increased length of his/her response.

Tallal, P. 1980. Perceptual requisites for language. In *Nonspeech language and communication: Analysis and intervention*, ed. R.L. Schiefelbusch. Baltimore, MD: University Park Press, pp. 449–67, $24.95.

This chapter begins with a discussion of the concept of auditory perception, and a definition of the term. The Repetition Test, a test of auditory perception, is presented through a description of its eight subtests. Experimental results are discussed for using the test with four populations: children who have language disabilities; those who have developmental reading disabilities; normally developing children; and adult aphasics.

Tawney, J.W. 1977. Educating severely handicapped children and their parents through telecommunications. In *Teaching the severely handicapped*, vol. II, ed. N.G. Haring and L.J. Brown. New York: Grune and Stratton, 315–40, $19.50.

This chapter describes the present use of telecommunications to deliver educational services to homes of handicapped individuals from birth through school age who are unable to regularly attend specialized program centers. Five prototype programs are presented: The Utah Project, The Teaching Resources Center Project in New York, The New York State Department Project, The Purdue University Project in Indiana, and The University of Kentucky Project. Implications for the future use of television programming for lesson presentation and parental information are presented.

Thomas, M.A., ed. 1976. *Hey, don't forget about me.* Reston, VA: The Council for Exceptional Children, 1920 Association Drive, 208 pp., $7.50.

This book pools the knowledge of various contributors in the field of Special Education concerning the following topics: criterion of ultimate functioning, identification in infancy, the role of the parent, curriculum planning and deinstitutionalization. The issue of the over-use of one-to-one training in artificial, structured sessions at the expense of providing opportunities for growth in natural settings is presented. This softbound edition has an innovative format offering "key ideas" summarized in the side margins for quick reference.

Utley, B.L., Holvoet, J.F., and Barnes, K. 1977. Handling, positioning, and feeding the physically handicapped. In *Educational programming for the severely and profoundly handicapped*, ed. E. Sontag. Reston, VA: Division on Mental Retardation, Council for Exceptional Children, 279–99, $14.95.

This chapter considers skill development in physically handicapped children from a neurodevelopmental approach. Three major areas are addressed: assessment and measurement; proper positioning; and task analysis. The assessment portion covers reflexes and reactions, including oral reflexes. General positioning and handling techniques are described and technqiues for specific skills such as lifting and carrying, gross motor skills, fine motor skills, and feeding are presented. Sample programs are provided for each of those areas. These programs include positioning instructions, procedures, and data-keeping.

Vanderheiden, G.C., ed. 1978. *Non-vocal communication resource book.* Baltimore, MD: University Park Press, $12.50.

This book includes four documents which are published in a binder format, so they can be expanded and periodically updated. The current contents are as follows:
1. Illustrated digest of non-vocal communication and writing aids for severely physically handicapped individuals. The aids section is divided into four categories: communication aids; communication boards, charts, and laptrays; communication training aids; and assistive devices for communication. Each entry provides information on a number of factors such as type of aid, portability, description, options, and cost. An authors' packet is included so persons can send information on aids for inclusion in the directory.
2. 1977 master chart of communication aids which contains information about the type, approximate size, price range, and delivery of the aids; a list of sources for further information is also included.
3. Interface switch profile and annotated list of commercial switches. This document includes descriptions and illustrations of general categories of switches (e.g., push switches, pneumatic switches) and subcategoreis of each; a chart containing a review of commercial switches, their type, company, description and prices, is also presented.
4. 1977 bibliography on non-vocal communication techniques and aids, broken down into nine categories.
An update service is available for this book through the Trace Center. An entire new section, Accessories for Communication Aids, is planned.

Vanderheiden, G.C. 1976. Providing the child with a means to indicate. In *Non-vocal communication techniques and aids for the severely physically handicapped*, ed. G. Vanderheiden and K. Grilley. Baltimore, MD: University Park Press, 10–76, $12.50.

The three basic approaches for providing a means of indication — scanning, encoding, and directly selecting—are covered. Each is described briefly, followed by a more detailed look at specific techniques and a partial survey of the aids available for each mode of indicating. Numerous examples and figures are provided for all three modes.

The levels of implementation (unaided techniques, fundamental aids, simple electronic and mechanical aids, fully independent aids, and fully independent and portable aids), and the implications and advantages of each are discussed. Combinations of the three techniques are also described.

Vanderheiden, G.C. and Grilley, K., eds. 1976. *Non-vocal communication techniques and aids for the severely physically handicapped.* Baltimore, MD: University Park Press, 227 pp., $12.50.

This book is based on transcriptions of the 1975 Trace Center National Workshop Series on Nonvocal Communication Techniques and Aids. The major areas considered are the problem (e.g., identification of children at risk), the tools (e.g., Blissymbolics), and application and results (e.g., use of Bliss Symbols with the mentally retarded). Appendices include the following: (A) Additional information on Blissymbols and Blissymbol Programs, (B) 1974 Masterchart of Communication Aids, (C) Information and sample pages from *1976 Annotated Bibliography of Communication Aids,* and (D) Topical Bibliography. For more specific information, see descriptions of individual chapters.

Vanderheiden, G.C. and Harris-Vanderheiden, D. 1976. Communication techniques and aids for the nonvocal severely handicapped. In *Communication assessment and intervention strategies,* ed. L.L. Lloyd. Baltimore, MD: University Park Press, 607–52, $16.50.

The authors discuss "a simple model for expressive communication channel" (p. 611), relating this model to the nonvocal child. The process of selecting and developing a physical mechanism for indicating message elements is discussed in terms of the three basic approaches: scanning, encoding, and direct selection. The selection and development of a symbol system and vocabulary is covered, including general consideration and specific systems, such as picture vocabularies and Bliss Symbols. Applications of these non-vocal techniques (e.g., Blissymbolics) and aids (e.g., Auto-Com) are considered through discussion of specific studies. A suggested reading list is presented.

Vicker, B. 1974a. Advances in nonoral communication system programming: Project summary #2, August, 1973. In *Nonoral communication system project,* 1964/1973, ed. B. Vicker. Campus Stores, Publishers, 17 West College, The University of Iowa, Iowa City, 52243, 109–75, $7.50.

This paper focuses on several issues relating to the development and evolution of a nonoral communication project. The first topic considered is evaluation of the nonvocal child. General evaluation strategies and the use of formal and informal testing are discussed. Other general evaluation considerations, such as modifying tests to gain maximal information, are covered.

The topic of communication board display sheets and frames is discussed by considering three different wheelchair display trays: single sheet display, multiple display (sequential or simultaneous), and combination display.

Communication boards and supplementary notebooks or card sets are discussed in terms of selection of expressive vocabulary items, depiction of picture and word vocabulary entries, and content organization.

Vicker, B. 1974b. Communication board programming with a four-year-old child: A case report. In *Nonoral communication system project,* 1964/1973, ed. B. Vicker. Campus Stores, Publishers, 17 West College, The University of Iowa, Iowa City, 52242, 215–61, $7.50.

This paper "focuses on the expressive language training procedure developed for a very young cerebral palsied child who could not effectively use oral speech or manual language for communication purposes" (p. 215). In addition to providing a review of the client's needs and abilities, the author describes the program design rationale, program content, and program materials. Objectives, materials, procedures, and expected responses are listed for the three phases of the program: (1) presyntactical programming (e.g., location of vocabulary items, functional single-word utterances); (2) syntactical programming (e.g., phrase structure level-noun phrase + verb phrase, transformation level); and (3) index system programming (e.g., three category index opeations with people, color-number, and toy sections). An interim parent report is included, with examples of situations in which the family can help the child to successfully use the board.

Vicker, B., ed. 1974c. *Nonoral communication system project*, 1964/1973. Campus Stores, Publishers, 17 West College, The University of Iowa, Iowa City, Iowa, 52242, 261 pp., $7.50.

This monograph was prepared by speech-language pathologists and occupational therapists to describe an approach to nonoral programming: "the use of nonmechanical display materials that are designed to facilitate syntactic nonoral expression and are designed to accommodate the individual needs of children of varying ages and levels of educational skills" (p. 8-9). Appendices include sample communication display materials and communication board display frames. These appendices are contained in a separate packet and are useful as demonstration aids. See annotations of individual chapters for further information.

Vicker, B. 1974d. The communication process using a nonoral means. In *Nonoral communication system project*, 1964/1973, ed. B. Vicker, Campus Stores, Publishers, 17 West College, The University of Iowa, Iowa City, Iowa, 52242, pp. 17-56, $7.50.

This chapter covers three basic types of non-vocal communication systems: (1) idiosyncratic systems (e.g., self-devised gestures); (2) superimposed or second language systems (manual sign language, Blissymbols System); and (3) native language coding systems (handwritten communication, typing, fingerspelling, communication cards, and boards). Each of these sub-systems is described and discussed briefly; however, the major emphasis is on the communication board. The author discusses the variables of the non-vocal communication process as related to the message mode of the communication board or cards. Variables are considerd with regard to the sender (cognitive abilities, physical capabilities, educational skills, and motivat), the transmission system itself (accessibility/reliability of the system, flexibility, complexity of message transmission, message distortion, and ability to receive a non-vocal message, willingness to provide the speaker with his communication equipment, internal limitations on message comprehension, external limitations on message reception), and expectations for and recognition of communicative behavior. The author also discusses the use of picture + word cards for noncommunicative or quasi-communicative situations with non-vocal moderately to severely retarded children.

Waryas, C.L. and Stremel-Campbell, K. 1978. Grammatical training for the language-delayed child: A new perspective. In *Language intervention strategies*, ed. R. Schiefelbusch. Baltimore, MD: University Park Press, 145-92, $15.75.

The authors review current research regarding teaching grammatical structure in three types of training approaches: syntactic, semantic, and pragmatic. They emphasize that the speech-language pathologist should be familiar with all three and consider blending parts of each into an individualized program for each client. The authors present portions of a language program they have developed for clients "who possess some limited language ability" (p. 160). For more information on the program see the annotation for Stremel and Waryas (1974) in this bibliography.

Wetherby, B. and Striefel, S. 1978. Application of miniature linguistic system or matrix-training procedures. In *Language intervention strategies*, ed. R. Schiefelbusch. Baltimore, MD: University Park Press, 317–56, $15.75.

Experimental matrix training research conducted within both receptive and productive language modalities is reviewed in this chapter. The major emphasis in applying the miniature linguistic system to language disordered clients is on establishing generalized language skills. The need for training in language skills for use with other people and new situations is emphasized. Nine general categories of training principles are described (e.g., #3, use of concurrent training procedures).

Wilbur, R.B. 1980. Nonspeech symbol systems: Summary chapter. In *Nonspeech language and communication: analysis and intervention*, ed. R.L. Schiefelbusch. Baltimore, MD: University Park Press, 81–90, $24.95.

This summary chapter covers input and output requirements of various non-vocal systems. Two major issues are discussed in connection with non-vocal communication. The first issue deals with cautioning trainers to avoid overexpectations and to remain sensitive to the needs of clients. The second issue is the question of why non-vocal systems work, especially in facilitating speech. Several possible reasons for their success are suggested.

Wilber, R.B. 1976. The linguistics of manual language and manual systems. In *Communication assessment and intervention strategies*, ed. L. Lloyd. Baltimore, MD: University Park Press, 423–501, $16.50.

An in-depth discussion of manual language systems is presented. Nine manual systems are described and compared. Practical considerations regarding socialization, academic achievement, and emotional development are discussed. The author summarizes many research studies to illustrate specific issues of the oral-manual controversy in deaf education. Use of manual communication with populations other than the deaf is discussed. An extensive bibliography is included.

Wilson, P.S., Goodman, L., and Wood, R.K. 1975. *Manual language for the child without language: A behavioral approach for teaching the exceptional child.* Order from Eric Grossman, 14 Keefe Lane, Middletown, CT, 06457, 84 pp., $5.00 ($4.00 if prepaid).

This manual describes a method of teaching manual language to the client who has not acquired language normally (e.g., mentally retarded, autistic, aphasic), with emphasis on individualized programs. The first section is a behavioral language assessment, which considers what the child can do and how he or she learns. Areas covered are prerequisite independent skills (e.g., interaction skills), non-linguistic behaviors, language behaviors, and other significant information. Each of these is presented through explanations, examples, and questions. Chapter 2 is a preparation for teaching, with an evaluation of the concepts that the child is currently using and decisions regarding the language to be used during a "functional day." The final chapter describes the method of teaching signs for the words chosen in Chapter 2. The three phases of reception, reproduction, and expression are described in detail. See Appendix B in this book for a review of the program.

Woodcock, R. and Clark, C. 1969. *Peabody Rebus Reading Program teachers guide.* Circle Pines, MN: American Guidance Service, 71 pp., $4.25.

This reading program utilizes picture symbols to introduce reading to new or retarded readers. The student learns ". . . the reading process, rather than the complex abstract code of spelled words." The symbols used in this program could be used on communication boards or other devices for people who have difficulty with traditional orthography. The program is structured and is programmed in gradual self-reinforcing steps. The complete reading program has been developed in two levels: Readiness Level ($60.00) and Transition Level ($70.00). Each level has a kit which includes workbooks and numerous other materials (e.g., picture cards; sentence cards, answer strips).

Woolman, D.H. 1980. A presymbolic training program. In *Nonspeech language and communication: Analysis and intervention*, ed. R.L. Schiefelbusch. Baltimore, MD: University Park Press, 325–56, $24.95.

This chapter begins with a brief review of literature relative to language intervention strategies used with the mentally retarded, such as core vocabulary and total communication strategies. The author concludes that some nonverbal retarded persons are deficient in the prelinguistic skills necessary for entry into any of the five strategies reviewed. Woolman suggests that a visual-motor presymbolic program might be helpful with these clients. The visual attending/matching/memory program developed by Woolman is carefully described, and the appendix contains all program components for one of the program's 17 sub-objectives.

Worthley, W.J. 1978. *Sourcebook of language learning activities*. Boston, MA: Little, Brown and Company, 209 pp., $15.00.

This "sourcebook" offers the practicing speech-language pathologist learning activities "from an extremely low, non-verbal level up to orally produced sentences" (p. xi). The program is presented in "sets," which provide specific objectives, learning sequences and examples of trainer-client responses. A developmental model is used in sequencing the activities in order of difficulty. The appendices include record forms, "word finder" lists of the most frequently used words at certain ages, and a topic bibliography for further reference.

Wulz, S.V. and Hollis, J.H. 1980. Word identification and comprehension training for exceptional children. In *Nonspeech language and communication: Analysis and intervention*, ed. R.L. Schiefelbusch. Baltimore, MD: University Park Press, 357–87, $24.95.

This chapter focuses on the use of traditional orthography and the spoken word with non-vocal persons. A task analysis of word recognition is presented and six word recognition tasks are identified. Three experiments ". . . designed to study the acquisition of integrated single-word reading performance . . ." (p. 364) are described and the results are discussed. In general it is suggested that learning involved in non-vocal systems, such as Premack symbols, may not be different from the learning involved in reading.

York, R.L. and Edgar, E. 1979. *Teaching the severely handicapped*, vol. IV. Columbus, OH: Special Press, 424 pp., $24.50.

This book contains 18 chapters divided into three major sections: curriculum, communication, and delivery of services. The curriculum chapters cover programs designed for training the client in fine motor, self-care, recreational and prevocational skills. Assessment of oral-motor skills related to feeding problems is presented. Adaptive equipment, including a section on communication aids [see Barnes et al. (1979)], is described. The communication section consists of four chapters that are annotated individually [see Shane (1979), Reichle and Yoder (1979), Horrocks and Hollis (1979), and Harris et al. (1979)]. The delivery of services chapters discuss early intervention strategies as well as methods for developing individualized educational plans.

Yule, W. and Berger, M. 1976. Communication, language, and behavior modification. In *Behavior modification with the severely retarded*, eds. C.C. Kiernan and F.P. Woodford. Amsterdam, Holland: Associated Scientific Publishers, 33–65, $41.50.

The authors present some general findings regarding the use of technology in training language. They note that, although reinforcement and imitation have been found to be useful, "there is little evidence that functional speech generalizes beyond the immediate training setting" (p. 36). They suggest that operant training has been especially useful in teaching skills and enabling subjects to show linguistic skills that they were already capable of performing. The evidence for the primacy of cognitive development relative to language learning is discussed, and implications of this evidence are suggested. These authors suggest the use of a developmental model, and present a possible content, beginning at sounds and going to nouns, verbs, adjectives and questions; specifics are given for each category (e.g., sequence for questions should be what, where, when). The complexities of data collection are discussed, and a sample coding sheet is provided. The authors explore the possibility of teaching subjects to use single words in a variety of ways to convey different meaning.

Appendix B:
Review of Selected
Communication Programs

This Appendix covers a wide range of communication programs developed for the severely handicapped. These programs were selected because they meet one or more of the following criteria:

1. *available*—this includes programs that are easy to obtain and are relatively inexpensive;
2. *especially appropriate to a specific population*—these programs are directed toward specific client populations (e.g., deaf, mentally retarded) or trainer populations (e.g., parents, paraprofessionals);
3. *flexible*—these programs can be adapted for several handicapping conditions;
4. *comprehensive*—some programs are especially complete in the scope and/or the depth of their intervention programs.

Most programs contained in this Appendix meet more than one of these criteria. We have attempted to review samples of many different types of programs (child/adult, structured/unstructured), to give the reader a large selection. Clearly, this is not an exhaustive list of available programs. In addition, no one program will meet the needs of all severely handicapped clients. In fact, it is unlikely that a single program will meet the needs of even *one* client. Communication specialists should apply different programs at different points in the intervention process, combine more than one program, and devise original program components appropriate to the needs of individual clients. We hope that these programs can provide a starting point.

Each program is reviewed according to a standard set of factors:
A. Client
   1. Target population
   2. Prerequisites
   3. Entry level
   4. Exit level
B. Trainer
   1. Background
   2. Special training

C. Administration
  1. Equipment and materials
  2. Degree of structure
  3. Generalization

Each review begins with a general description of the program and ends with a list of special notes such as assessment tools included and problems regarding materials. Additional information about these and other programs is available in Appendix A. As in Appendix A, the entries in Appendix B are listed alphabetically by authors. Below is a topic index to assist the reader in locating a specific type of program.

Vocal Programs/Approaches

Bender and Valletutti (1976)
Bluma, Shearer, Frohman, and Hillard (1976)
Fredericks, Riggs, Furey, Grove, Moore, McDonnell, Jordan, Hanson, Baldwin, and Wadlow (1976)
Greenberger and Thum (1975)
Guess, Sailor, and Baer (1976)
Harris (1976)

Horstmeier and MacDonald (1978)
Kent (1974)
Murdock and Hartmann (1975)
St. Louis, Mattingly, Esposito, and Cone (1980)
St. Louis, Rejzer, and Cone (1980)
Struck (1977)
Tilton, Liska, and Bourland (1977)
Williams and Fox (1977).

Non-Vocal Gestural Programs/Approaches

*Guess, Sailor, and Baer (1976)
Lykos (1971)
Robbins (1978)
*St. Louis, Rejzer, and Cone (1980)
Skelly and Schinsky (1979)

*Snell (1974)
*Struck (1977)
*Williams and Fox (1977)
Wilson, Goodman, and Wood (1975).

Non-Vocal Symbolic Programs/Approaches

Carrier and Peak (1975)
Elder (1978)
*Guess, Sailor, and Baer (1976)
Hall, O'Grady, and Talkington (1978)
Hamre-Nietupski, Stoll, Holtz, Fullerton, Ryan-Flottum, and Brown (1977)

Montgomery (1980)
*St. Louis, Rejzer, and Cone (1980)
Silverman, McNaughton, and Kates (1978)
*Williams and Foxx (1977).

---

*These are vocal programs which have been adapted for non-vocal modes.

Bender, M., and Valletutti, P.J. 1976. *Teaching the moderately and severely handicapped, vol. II.* Baltimore, MD: University Park Press, 420 pp., $16.50.

General Description: This volume contains curriculum objectives, teaching strategies, and activities for training moderately and severely handicapped clients in the following skills:

1. Communication
2. Socialization
3. Safety
4. Leisure time

Only the communication section will be described below. The Communication Skills Curriculum is divided into two parts: Nonverbal and Verbal.

A. *Client*

1. *Target population*

This is intended for moderately and severely handicapped individuals including the severely physically impaired with normal intelligence and severely mentally retarded.

2. *Prerequisites*

None are specified for entrance into the program, but the tasks are developmentally sequenced so that later skills assume competency on earlier tasks.

3. *Entrance level*

a. The nonverbal curriculum begins with attention to the natural gesture of waving.

b. The verbal curriculum begins with eliciting nonspeech vocalizations (e.g., gurgling, laughing) and establishing an awareness to sound (e.g., student turns eyes and head in direction of noise).

4. *Exit level*

a. The nonverbal curriculum ends with the student using a combination of natural gestures and/or an alternate mode of communication (manual language or communication board) to adequately communicate needs, thoughts, and feelings.

b. Verbal — "The student speaks in the pattern of acceptable adult speech and does so with intelligible speech patterns" (p. 136).

B. *Trainer*

1. *Background*

The program is designed for teachers, paraprofessionals, speech-language pathologists, occupational and physical therapists as well as for parents or other primary caretakers.

2. *Special training*

No special training is required, although familiarity with behavior management techniques would be helpful.

C. *Administration*

1. *Equipment and materials*

a. Provided within the text are suggestions for a diagnostic checklist (that the teacher must generate from the sample provided). No specific forms for the assessment or program data collection are provided.

    b. All stimulus materials are provided by the trainer. A list of materials is provided at the end of each chapter.

  2. *Degree of structure*

    The program offers a general framework from which the teacher must individualize a program for each student. The authors give sample forms for the following information:

    a. Behavior Checklist

    b. Annual Performance Profile

    c. Weekly Planning Sheet

    Daily data recording procedures are left up to the discretion of the trainer.

  3. *Generalization*

    Throughout the activity suggestions, the trainer is encouraged to watch for situations in which the student may be reinforced for demonstrating maintenance of skills.

D. *Special notes*

  1. Suggestions for alternate modes of communication are presented.

  2. The program offers rather general objectives which the authors caution may need to be broken down into smaller steps.

  3. An extensive list of suggested readings is provided.

Bluma, S., Shearer, M., Frohman, A., and Hillard, J. 1976. *Portage guide to early education.* Cooperative Educational Services Agency 12, Box 564, Portage, WI, 53901. $32.00

General Description: This program provides an assessment device in the form of behavioral check lists which lead to specific program objectives and activities in the program card file. Five developmental areas are assessed and programmed: socialization, language, self-help, cognitive and motor. An infant stimulation section is included for use with infants and severely handicapped individuals.

A. *Client*

  1. *Target population*

    This is intended for children or adults who are functioning in the birth to six year range of abilities in the six developmental areas listed above.

  2. *Prerequisites*

    The program manual states that prerequisites for learning are attending, imitating, and compliance. Suggestions are presented for structuring situations to increase these skills throughout the client's daily activities as well as specifying program cards with activities related to increasing attention, imitation, and compliance on training tasks.

3. *Entrance level*

The discussion of each skill begins with items expected to be accomplished by a child between birth and one year. For example, in the language area, the client is expected to stop an activity when told "no" 75% of the time and to respond to a gesture with a gesture (e.g., wave "bye-bye").

4. *Exit level*

The exit level for the five major skills are tasks usually accomplished between the age of five and six years. In language, items such as tells address and answers questions like "what happens if. . . (you drop an egg)?" are presented.

B. *Trainer*

1. *Background*

The trainer's background is not specified. The program has been used successfully by parents and institutional aides as well as by professionals.

2. *Special training*

None is specified, but the user should be very familiar with the information contained in the manual, particularly with the behavioral objective section.

C. *Administration*

1. *Equipment and materials*

a. The following materials are included in the program:

(1) Manual–59 pages

(2) Checklist booklet for assessment–26 pages

(3) Card file–580 color coded activity cards

b. All stimulus items are provided by the trainer.

2. *Degree of structure*

This is a fairly low-structured curriculum. The program cards contain general information; the trainer is expected to specify the activity further to include progression criteria and to reduce the item into smaller teaching steps if necessary. Each card provides the following:

a. Age range for the task (e.g., 2–3)

b. Title or terminal objective (e.g., points to "big" and "little" upon request)

c. What to do: a list of three to five teaching suggestions. The authors caution that the trainer may need to modify the suggestions to meet individual needs of each client.

3. *Generalization*

Many of the teaching suggestions can be adapted for group activities and involve performing the tasks in different settings which would enhance generalization.

D. *Special notes*

1. The manual is concise and uses helpful examples in explaining behavioral terms and objectives.

2. The checklists and cards are color coded for easy reference.
3. The manual stresses the need for the trainer to constantly reassess the client's progress and to modify the procedures to meet individual needs.
4. The language area of the curriculum is oriented toward oral language. Alternate forms of communication are not discussed.

Carrier, J. and Peak, T. 1975. *Non-SLIP Kit: Non-speech language initiation program*. H and H Enterprises, Inc., P.O. Box 3342, Lawrence, KS, 66044, $238.00.

General Description: The advertised purpose of this program is "to give severely handicapped children (and some adults, including aphasics) some form of basic communication skill; it is essentially a language initiation program" (p. 1). Non-representational plastic forms are placed on a sentence tray to produce "utterances".

  A. *Client*

    1. *Target population*

    This program is intended primarily for persons for whom other methods have failed. It is used mainly with severely handicapped children, though it may be used with adults (such as aphasics) as well.

    2. *Prerequisites*

    The major behavioral/physical prerequisite is the ability to place forms on a board. Hollis and Carrier (1978) note that adaptations may be made for physically handicapped clients, such as mounting the symbols on blocks of wood, thus requiring even less precise hand movements.

    3. *Entrance level*

    The initial stages of the program require motor imitation of form placement on a tray and discrimination of form shapes.

    4. *Exit level*

    The client ends the program with an "utterance" type which is fairly complex, but stereotyped (e.g., "The horse is running on the sidewalk"). Since this is a language initiation program, the resulting language is not expected to be functional for the client. Speech may accompany symbol placement, but is not required.

  B. *Trainer*

    1. *Background*

    The trainer's background is open; however, a paraprofessional is the preferred trainer.

    2. *Special training*

    A course from a certified trainer is strongly recommended.

  C. *Administration*

    1. *Equipment and materials*

    All equipment needed is provided, except for individualized reinforcers. Materials included in the kit are the following:

    a. 59 symbols that represent words in the English language (e.g., "horse", "running", "sidewalk")

    b. A sentence tray

    c. Visual stimuli cards

    d. A manual covering rationale and procedures

    e. A set of step-by-step programs

  2. *Degree of structure*

  This is highly structured program, which is basically the same for all clients. Each of the programs (e.g., number matching program, labeling program) includes the following:

    a. Criterion

    b. Sequence

    c. Probes

    d. Pre- and post-test

    e. Data sheet

    f. Retention program

  3. *Generalization*

  No generalization procedures are provided within this program.

C. *Special notes*

  1. Complex response topographies such as speech, signing, or writing are not required.

  2. The program is based on Premack's (1970)[1] work with chimpanzees who also used plastic forms for communication.

  3. The program is intended to serve as a language initiator, not as a functional language system; thus, further programming will likely be needed after completion of the program to yield functional communication.

Elder, P.S. 1978. *Visual symbol communication instruction, part I: Receptive instruction.* DESEMO Project, University of Alabama in Birmingham, P.O. Box 313, University Station, Birmingham, AL, 35294, 74 pp., $7.50.

General Description: This program is intended to provide a methodology for teaching a visual symbol system, such as Blissymbolics, to individuals having receptive vocabulary skills. The 25 sequential steps comprise the following phases:

A. *Client*

  1. *Target population*

  This program is intended for non-vocal persons who exhibit receptive language which may be paired with visual symbols. In addition, candidates may be physically handicapped and/or mentally retarded, provided that they meet the entry requirements.

  2. *Prerequisites*

  Several specific, observable prerequisites are listed:

    a. Receptive language which may be paired with visual symbols

---

1. Premack, D. 1970. A functional analysis of language. *J. Exp. Anal. Beh.* 14: 107–25.

     b. Ability to attend to a task for approximately five minutes

     c. Eye contact for at least three seconds on command

     d. Interactive social behavior which would indicate a desire and a need to communicate

   3. *Entrance level*

   The client looks at a single symbol card.

   4. *Exit level*

   On command, the client looks at one of four symbol cards (one new and three previously learned).

B. *Trainer*

   1. *Background*

   The manual stresses that this program is appropriate for use by professionals or paraprofessionals.

   2. *Special training*

   No special training is required.

C. *Administration*

   1. *Equipment and materials*

     a. The manual, with instructions for constructing the Visual Communication Display, is provided.

     b. The trainer must provide the following:

       (1) Visual Communication Display — the list of materials and instructions for building one of two prototypes are included in the manual. Materials are estimated to cost approximately $25.00.

       (2) Symbol cards for the symbol system chosen (e.g., Blissymbolics, Rebus, pictures) must be provided, according to instructions listed in the manual.

   2. *Degree of structure*

   This is a highly structured program including 21 compulsory and 4 supplemental steps. Each step is presented in lesson plan form, with the following items carefully specified:

     a. Prerequisite skills

     b. Task objectives

     c. Necessary preparation and materials

     d. Criterion

     e. Basic procedures:

       (1) Teaching procedure

       (2) Reinforcement

       (3) Correction procedures

     f. Random schedules for symbol placement, verbal cueing, and card placement

     g. Data sheets.

   3. *Generalization*

   No generalization procedures or suggestions are provided.

D. *Special notes*

   1. It should be noted that this program is not designed to develop

linguistic concepts, but rather to teach visual symbols to represent already acquired vocabulary.

2. This protocol may be used with any type of visual symbol system, although field testing used Blissymbols.

3. A gestural response such as pointing or a visual response (eye gaze) may be used.

4. Eighteen program guidelines are provided to make the protocol easier to follow and to help the trainer avoid or solve potential problems. These guidelines deal with topics such as positioning, changing symbols, and reinforcement timing.

5. Retention is tested by rotating the previously learned symbols. In addition, suggestions are offered for periodic testing of all symbols learned.

Fredericks, H.D.B., Riggs, C., Furey, T., Grove, D., Moore, W., McDonnell, J. Jordan, E. Hanson, W., Baldwin, Y., and Wadlow, M. 1976. *The teaching research curriculum for moderately and severely handicapped*. Springfield, IL: Charles C. Thomas, 345 pp., $18.50

General Description: This curriculum guide provides detailed task analyses for the following skills: self-help, motor development, receptive oral language, writing, and cognitive. The information below relates to the receptive oral language and expressive oral language areas of the curriculum.

A. *Client*
1. *Target population*
The curriculum was designed for moderately and severely retarded, deaf and blind and multiply handicapped children who have performance age levels of 0–6 years, regardless of chronological age.

2. *Prerequisites*
The first four skills in the receptive oral language curriculum are to be presented in the following order and are prerequisites for entering the expressive oral language curriculum:
a. Responds to auditory cues
b. Responds to verbal sounds
c. Responds to name
d. Maintains eye contact

3. *Entrance level*
A placement test for language skills is included in the text.
a. The receptive oral language curriculum begins with attention to auditory cues.
b. The expressive oral language program begins with motor imitation, then motor and vocal imitation combined.

4. *Exit level*
a. The receptive oral language curriculum ends with comprehending commands which contain conditional clauses such as, "when I touch my nose, open the door," and demonstrating the

understanding of vocabulary such as identifying "first" and "last".

    b. The expressive oral language curriculum terminates when the client uses complete sentences to describe comparisons, relationships, and number and ownership of objects.

B. *Trainer*

  1. *Background*

The curriculum was designed for teachers who are familiar with behavior modification techniques. Paraprofessionals could use the program with careful supervision.

  2. *Special training*

None is specified, but knowledge of behavior management techniques is obviously needed.

C. *Administration*

  1. *Equipment and materials*

    a. The text provides specific program guidelines and objectives.

    b. The trainer must supply all the stimulus material.

  2. *Degree of structure*

Number and length of sessions are not specified. Each area (i.e., receptive and expressive language) is divided into the following framework:

    a. General behavior (e.g., identifies objects which have similar sounds.

    b. Terminal behavior (e.g., the child points to an object after receiving an auditory cue with two distractors.)

    c. Phases (e.g., Phase I — child points to object after receiving auditory cue. Phase II — child points to object after receiving auditory cue with one distractor.)

    d. Steps, which represent the suggested vocabulary to be presented for each phase (e.g., book, boot, boat).

  3. *Generalization*

Specific generalization activities are not provided; however, at the beginning of the text the authors mention that review is essential to ensure maintenance of previously learned skills. The teacher is encouraged to develop review activities during the course of the day to allow demonstration of acquired skills.

D. *Special features*

  1. Some modifications are suggested for students with physical impairments.

  2. The program follows a developmental model, but the authors suggest that higher level skills can be altered.

  3. No adaptations or implications for alternative forms of communication are mentioned.

Greenberger, S.M. and Thum, S.R. 1975. *STEP: Sequential testing and educational programming.* San Rafael, CA: Academic Therapy Publications, 235 pp., $22.50

General Description: "S.T.E.P., is a developmental framework of behavioral objectives which enables professionals who work with children to clearly describe the child's capacities, learning modalities, developmental levels, and the curriculum which will meet content needs." (p.11)

A. *Client*
1. *Target population*
   This is designed for children of preschool age though grade 5. Although the authors do not specify handicapping conditions, the materials appear to be designed for learning disabled children; however, limited portions of the program could be used with the severely or multi-handicapped population.
2. *Prerequisites*
   None are specified.
3. *Entrance level*
   Assessment and training begins at the sensory level (e.g., localizing auditory and visual stimuli).
4. *Exit level*
   The client communicates adequately with speech and writing.

B. *Training*
1. *Background*
   This program is designed for classroom teachers, but it is also considered a tool for other professionals—doctors, psychologists, reading specialists, and speech-language pathologists.
2. *Special training*
   No special training is required.

C. *Administration*
1. *Equipment and materials*
   a. The program manual contains the following:
      (1) The PAD - *p*lacement and *a*chievement *d*eterminer
      (2) Curriculum guide which specifies goals/objectives, assessment, learning/teaching activities, and suggested books and materials for each item in the program.
   b. The trainer provides all stimulus materials.
2. *Degree of structure*
   The placement and achievement determiner is a very structured framework for following the child's major progress; however, it would not be sensitive to the small changes that usually indicate progress for the severely handicapped. A system to collect daily data is not provided.
3. *Generalization*
   No generalization procedures are specified.

D. *Special notes*
1. The program is contained in a looseleaf notebook for easy reference and expansion.
2. The items are color coded according to learning processes for quick reference from the placement sheet into the program book.
3. No adaptation for alternate modes of communication is provided.
4. The teaching techniques are too general and in some cases inap-

propriate (e.g., for localization training—blindfold the child and have him play ping pong); therefore, the program should be used selectively.

Guess, D., Sailor, W., and Baer, D. 1976. *Functional speech and language training for the severely handicapped*, parts 1,2,3,4. H and H Enterprises, Inc., P.O. Box 3342, Lawrence, KS, 66044, $7.95 each.

General Description: This 60-step program consists of four parts:

Part 1 — Persons and Things (Steps 1–9)

Part 2 — Actions with Persons and Things (Steps 10–29)

Part 3 — Possession and Color (Steps 30–42)

Part 4 — Size and Relation and Location (Steps 43–60)

A. *Client*

1. *Target population*

This program is intended for people who lack language skills regardless of etiology (e.g., autistic, brain-damaged, profoundly retarded). It is appropriate for any age from preschool through adult.

2. *Prerequisites*

Prerequisites for Part 1 include the following:

a. Attending

b. Word imitation

In addition, Part 1 is a prerequisite for the other three parts of the program.

3. *Entrance level*

The client begins by imitating words.

4. *Exit level*

The program terminates with the client's production of 4–6 word sentences.

B. *Trainer*

1. *Background*

The trainer's background is open (e.g., teacher, paraprofessional, psychologist, speech-language pathologist).

2. *Special training*

No special training is required, although the authors strongly recommend a background in behavior management techniques.

C. *Administration*

1. *Equipment and materials*

a. The following are provided in the program:

(1) Manuals — $7.95 per part ($32.80 for all 4 parts)

(2) Answer sheet booklets (1 with each manual)

b. All stimulus items are provided by the trainer.

2. *Degree of structure*

This is a highly structured program; the authors suggest 30-minute sessions daily. Each program step specifies:

a. Training goal (objective)

b. Training items

     c. Procedures
       (1) Skill test
       (2) Computing percentage for skill test
       (3) Training instructions
     d. Criterion performance
       (1) At least 80% correct for one session (32 trials)
         OR
       (2) 12 correct responses in a row in one session
     e. Score forms
       (1) Skill test
       (2) Training step
       (3) Summary form
   3. *Generalization*

This program includes "programming for generalization steps directed toward parents, ward staff, and/or teachers."

D. *Special notes*
   1. Adaptations for communication boards and sign are being developed.
   2. Five language functions are taught:
     a. Reference — the idea that certain sounds (words) represent objects and events.
     b. Control — forms of requesting (to teach the power of language).
     c. Self-extended control — to teach clients to request more specific information.
     d. Integration — to teach clients to discriminate when to seek information through questions and when to respond with appropriate referents.
     e. Reception — teach concepts at the receptive level after they have been taught at the productive level.
   3. In this program, production is generally expected before reception is demonstrated.
   4. This program follows a remedial (as opposed to developmental) training model, based in part on data from subjects who have completed the program.

Hall, S.M., O'Grady, R.S., and Talkington, L.W. 1978. *Communication board training program for multihandicapped.* Zygo Industries, Inc., P.O. Box 1008, Portland, OR, 97207, 91 pp., $95.00.

General Description: This program is designed for use with the ZYGO Model 16 Communication Board. The following six levels are covered:
   1. Signal learning
   2. Stimulus-response learning
   3. Chaining learning
   4. Verbal association learning
   5. Multiple discrimination learning
   6. Concept formation learning

A. *Client*
   1. *Target population*

   This program is intended for persons who cannot use either verbal or manual communication systems. It is especially appropriate for clients with physical handicaps, from childhood through adulthood.

   2. *Prerequisites*

   The client must be able to operate a control mechanism to activate and to stop the scanner. The client must have some receptive language skills, since he or she must respond to verbal commands at each level before moving to a higher level (manual and verbal commands may be used).

   3. *Entrance level*

   The level of entry is determined on the basis of five placement tests. Failure on Test One indicates entry at Program One and so forth. The lowest entry point allows for direct eye contact through physical prompting.

   4. *Exit level*

   This program ends with the client indicating concepts of class, "yes/no," and "same/different" through production of one-symbol responses.

B. *Trainer*
   1. *Background*

   This program is designed so that ". . . any interested person with limited knowledge of communication" (p. 5) may serve as trainer. However, it is recommended that the program be coordinated by a Communication Therapist, if possible.

   2. *Special training*

   No special training is required.

C. *Administration*
   1. *Equipment and materials*
      a. The following materials are included in the kit:
         (1) Physical Abilities Checklist (PAC)
         (2) Training manual
         (3) Training flash cards, vocabulary displays, and masking panels
         (4) Score sheets (Daily Performance Report and Monthly Summary Report)
      b. The following must be purchased separately or must be provided by the trainer:
         (1) ZYGO Model 16 Communication Board
         (2) Suitable control mechanism (operating switch)
         (3) Stopwatch or watch with sweep second hand
   2. *Degree of structure*

   This is a highly structured program. Areas such as vocabulary may be adapted to the needs of the client. The following information is specified:

a. For each of five tests the manual describes the objective, the organization of the communication board, positions for trainer and client, and procedures.
b. For each of the six levels the following is provided:
    (1) Introduction: definition, examples, training goal, training materials, and instructions for positioning, arranging the communication board, and recording progress.
    (2) Training procedures: four training procedures are included for each level. For each procedure at each level, the manual specifies objectives, materials, positioning, and procedural steps (including antecedent, behavior, consequence, and procedures for recording).
3. *Generalization*

    No generalization steps are included within the training section. The authors provide one page of suggestions for further training, and note that, upon completion of this program "... actual *expressive* language work has only just begun" (p. 90).
D. *Special notes*
    1. This program is based on the seven-level learning hierarchy suggested by R.M. Gagne (*Conditions of Learning*, 1965). Thus, it is intended to simultaneously teach the client to use the Communication Board and to advance to levels needed for spontaneous communication.
    2. Within each training procedure of each learning level, four progressively dependent strategies are used: independent responding, verbal prompting, modeling, and "physical priming".
    3. The Physical Abilities Checklist, designed by "a person from the physical medicine field", may be used in initial and follow-up assessment. Areas such as sitting, head and arm control, vision, and hearing are assessed, and may help in selecting the optimum switch for a client.
    4. This program is intended to provide only a language learning strategy and initial functional use of the communication board. The client is not expected to develop multi-word utterances through this program.

Hamre-Nietupski, S., Stoll, A., Holtz, K., Fullerton, P., Ryan-Flottum, M., and Brown, L. 1977. Curricular strategies for teaching selected nonverbal communication skills to nonverbal and verbal severely handicapped students. In *Curricular strategies for teaching functional object use, nonverbal communication, problem solving, and mealtime skills to severely handicapped students*, vol. VII, part 1, eds. L. Brown, J. Nietupski, S. Lyon, S. Hamre-Nietupski, T. Crowner, and L. Gruenewald. Department of Specialized Educational Services, Madison Metropolitan School District, Madison, WI, 94-250, $9.00.

General Description: This curriculum focuses on three kinds of nonverbal communication mediators that may be used with severely handicapped individuals:

1. Communication boards and communication booklets
2. Generally understood gestures
3. Standardized signs

A. *Client*

   1. *Target population*

   This curriculum is appropriate for severely handicapped clients with various handicapping conditions, including physical disabilities.

   2. *Prerequisites*

   It is noted that the following skills should be taught prior to *or* concurrent with the skills in this curriculum: tracking, scanning, and selecting; using functional objects and problem solving; imitation, means-end, and object permanence skills.

   3. *Entrance level*

   Both curricular strategies (communication boards and gestures/ signs) start with teaching or verifying that the client attends to referents and performs appropriate actions with them in response to verbal and nonverbal cues.

   4. *Exit level*

     a. The final phase of the communication board program requires the ability to receive and to transmit a message of three or more symbols. Only a one-symbol response is required.

     b. The final phase of the gesture/sign program requires the ability to produce a sign, then perform an appropriate action using the correct referent.

B. *Trainer*

   1. *Background*

   The trainer's background is not specified. The curriculum uses a great deal of professional jargon; therefore, it is assumed that a teacher or speech-language pathologist would be the trainer.

   2. *Special training*

   No special training is required.

C. *Administration*

   1. *Equipment and materials*

     a. This curriculum is included in a book with several other curricula.

     b. Stimulus items must be provided by the trainer.

   2. *Degree of structure*

   This is a moderately structured curriculum. Each phase includes a very complex and lengthy objective, specifying features such as number of referents, number of representations, concurrent vs. consecutive presentations, presence or absence of cues, and distance of referents (within reach or not within reach). In addition, the following are provided:

     a. Suggested instructional procedures; these are general procedures (i.e., contextual cues to physical priming cues);

     b. A sample data sheet;

     c. A sample instructional protocol for one phase of the communication board curriculum;

     d. Example activities for teaching the skills; examples are presented for two phases for each curriculum area (e.g., comprehension of gestures/signs);

  3. *Generalization*

  Although no activities are specifically labeled for generalization, all example activities take place in the natural environment and deal with naturally occurring behaviors which enhances generalization.

D. *Special features*

  1. Production precedes comprehension for both the communication board and the gesture/sign curricula.

  2. The communication board curriculum includes alternative training sequences for concurrent or consecutive presentation of symbols.

  3. The authors suggest a concurrent instructional orientation, in which clients would be taught speech, and communication board use, as well as gestures and signs, if possible.

  4. Seven strategies are discussed for determining initial content, such as frequency of occurrence and student preference. Preference and frequency of occurrence checklists are included.

  5. A list of approximately 160 generally understood gestures are provided in Appendix A.

  6. Appendices B through C consist of lists of selected vocabulary for functional activities in several settings. The lists cover nouns, pronouns, verbs, adverbs, prepositions, and adjectives.

Harris, S.L. 1976. *Managing behavior 8, Behavior modification: Teaching speech to a nonverbal child.* Lawrence, KS: H and H Enterprises, Inc., 78 pp., $4.25.

General Description. This book was developed to provide parents of autistic children with information on how to help their child learn to talk. A four stage program is presented:

     Stage I: Teaching Attention

     Stage II: Teaching Nonverbal Skills

     Stage III: Teaching Verbal Imitation

     Stage IV: Teaching Functional Speech

A. *Client*

  1. *Target population*

  This program is designed primarily for autistic or schizophrenic children; however, it offers material that could be useful if modified for other populations (e.g., mentally retarded, selectively mute).

  2. *Prerequisites*

  None are specified, but the program assumes that the client has normal vision and hearing.

3. *Entrance level*

The program begins with establishing attention responses.

4. *Exit level*

The client is able to use three to five word phrases or sentences when asked specific questions, (e.g., Trainer: "Where is the key?" Client: "Next to box.").

B. *Trainer*

1. *Background*

This is specifically designed for parents. It might be advisable for the teacher or speech-language pathologists to introduce the program to the family and to follow their progress carefully.

2. *Special training*

None is specified although it may be helpful for the parent to discuss the behavior modification principles described in the book with a professional.

C. *Administration*

1. *Equipment and materials*

a. The program is completely described in the book. Samples of data sheets are included in the text.

b. All stimulus materials are provided by the trainer.

2. *Degree of Structure*

The program is described in detail with definitions of technical terms provided. Each stage of the program is divided into content steps. Each program step specifies:

a. pretest-materials needed, procedure, data collection, and criterion for baseline information;

b. training-materials needed, procedure, data collection, reward procedures, and criterion for moving to the next step.

3. *Generalization*

Although generalization is not presented as a specific section, suggestions and examples are provided throughout the book to encourage the child to use new skills at times other than during training sessions.

D. *Special notes*

1. This program is written with parents' emotional needs in mind.

2. It presents an overview of relevant historical information about autism in order to acquaint parents with research in that area.

3. Review questions are provided at the end of each chapter to help the parent focus on important information.

Horstmeier, D. and MacDonald, J. 1978. *Ready, set, go: Talk to me.* Columbus, OH: Charles E. Merrill Publishing Company, 134 pp., $5.95.

General Description: This developmental language program is intended for use by parents and professionals to aid in establishing prelanguage skills and initial verbal communication in children who do not have socially useful language. The following nine areas are covered through prescriptive packets:

(1) Preliminary skills

    (2) Functional play
    (3) Motor imitation
    (4) Receptive procedures - objects
    (5) Receptive procedures - actions
    (6) Following directions
    (7) Sound imitation
    (8) Single word production
    (9) Beginning social conversation

A. *Client*

  1. *Target population*

    This program was developed for "individuals who have yet to develop socially useful language." Thus, it is a noncategorical approach. The activities are geared for early childhood, but the approach has been successful with adults.

  2. *Prerequisites*

    No behavioral or physical prerequisites are listed for this program.

  3. *Entrance level*

    This program begins with attention.

  4. *Exit level*

    This program ends with "beginning social conversation," which consists of two- to four-word utterances

B. *Trainee*

  1. *Background*

    A parent or teacher would likely serve as the trainer, with a speech-language pathologist serving as a consultant.

  2. *Training*

    No specific training is required, and the manual is written with minimum professional jargon. It is assumed that the trainer will consult frequently with professionals.

C. *Administration*

  1. *Equipment and materials*

    a. The program consists of a manual and sample forms.
    b. Stimulus materials, such as toys and everyday materials, are provided by the trainer.

  2. *Degree of structure*

    This is not a highly structured program; it is assumed that "training" will be carried out continually in the child's environment, with 1-20 minute sessions of planned activities.

  3. *Generalization*

    Throughout the program generalization is stressed in suggestions for application of new skills to the environment. Suggestions are provided for mealtime activities and structured play activities.

D. *Special notes*

  1. A diagnostic screening test is included in the manual to assist in determining which prescriptive packets to use.
  2. The prescriptive packets included in this manual are intended to be adapted to the needs of each individual client.

3. A daily parent report form for describing success and giving examples is included with each packet.
4. One of the authors of this program is the parent of a retarded child.
5. Suggestions are given for adapting this program for classroom use.

Kent, L.R. 1974. *Language acquisition program for the retarded and multiply impaired.* Champaign, IL: Research Press, 185 pp., $6.95.

General Description: This book details a vocal language program that is divided into three sections: Pre-verbal, Verbal-Receptive, and Verbal-Expressive.

A. *Client*

1. *Target population*
   The program was primarily designed for severely retarded children, but has been successfully used with the visually handicapped, hearing handicapped, autistic, emotionally disturbed, and aphasic or brain damaged.

2. *Prerequisites*
   There are no specified prerequisites for entering this program. However, prerequisites of earlier trained skills are listed as the client progresses in the program.

3. *Entrance level*
   Even the most severely involved client can enter this program at the phase of preverbal attention or at the phase of eliminating interfering behaviors.

4. *Exit level*
   a. Verbal-Receptive exit level: the client comprehends four to six word commands containing a variety of vocabulary including nouns, verbs, adverbial "place-where" commands, and so forth.
   b. Verbal-Expressive exit level: the client produces three word phrases appropriately, such as "comb on table."

B. *Trainer*

1. *Background*
   The trainer's background is open (e.g., teacher, paraprofessional, psychologist, speech-language pathologist).

2. *Special training*
   None is required.

C. *Administration*

1. *Equipment and materials*
   a. The manual is provided.
   b. Any stimulus materials (common classroom and home objects) used in training are provided by the trainer.

2. *Degree of structure*
   This program is highly structured:
   a. Testing procedures are presented in the form of an initial inventory, final inventory, and retention check;
   b. Data recording is specified with criterion for movement to new

items indicated. The standard criterion is stated as "90% of the responses are correct on random sequence, including all items, two trials each. The trials on the same items are not necessarily successive" (p.10).

3. *Generalization*

No generalization procedures are specified.

D. *Special notes*

1. An adaptation of the program for manual communication is provided in Chapter 6 (see Snell, 1974, in this appendix).
2. The Pre-verbal section allows placement of the lowest functioning client in the program.
3. The client is moved through the program by section, phase, and part (which is the smallest training step in the program). When the client passes specific parts he or she moves on to the next phase.
4. A client may be trained at different phases in more than one section throughout the program; for example, during one training session the client may work on Receptive Expansion Phase II, Part 2—Placing objects in prepositional relationship to room parts; during another session he or she may work on Expressive Expansion Phase I, Part 2—Naming object in prepositional relationship to room part.

Lykos, C.M. 1971. *Cued speech: Handbook for teachers.* Cued Speech Program, Gallaudet College, Kendall Green, Washington, D.C., 20002, 281 pp., $5.00.

General Description: This manual is intended for teachers of Cued Speech who are working directly with clients and/or with parent groups. It is designed to be adapted to the needs of clients and/or parents.

A. *Client*

1. *Target population*

This manual is designed to be used with hearing-impaired clients, or with their parents. It could be adapted for use with other clients (e.g., selected aphasics, laryngectomees). It may be used with clients from preschool age through adults.

2. *Prerequisites*

Specific prerequisites are not listed in the manual. In some cases, Cued Speech may be introduced before the child has demonstrated the cognitive abilities necessary to decode it, just as we use vocal language with very young infants.

3. *Entrance level*

a. In the natural approach to Cued Speech, normal speech is cued, and the child is not required to respond.
b. In the analytical approach, used for more advanced clients, lessons are presented. The first lesson begins by demonstrating that homophenous words (e.g., aim, ape, cape) can be differentiated by adding cues.

4. *Exit level*

The program ends when the client is "able to read Cued Speech and understand it within the limits of his knowledge of spoken language" (p. 177). Clients should also develop expressive skills consistent with their knowledge of spoken language, through the exercises in the manual and general practice.

B. *Trainer*

1. *Background*

The trainer's background is not specified; however, it would likely be an educator of the deaf or a speech-language pathologist.

2. *Special training*

The trainer should be a fluent user of Cued Speech.

C. *Administration*

1. *Equipment and materials*

The manual provides a listing of activities and experiences, a set of lessons, practice exercises for hearing adults, and transcription exercises. Word lists for lessons and many materials for activities are included.

2. *Degree of structure*

This is a low-structured program designed to be adapted to individual clients or groups.

a. For activities, the following information is provided:
1. Name of activity;
2. List of materials, drawings or templates of materials;
3. Procedure, typically presented in a modified narrative format, giving steps for preparation, instructions, and suggestions for possible consequences; diagrams are frequently provided;
4. Variations, with several provided for each activity.

b. For lessons, the following information is provided:
1. General and specific procedures, presented in a modified narrative format, in a series of steps; diagrams and suggested materials (e.g., transparencies) are included;
2. Rules are presented within the procedures for each lesson (e.g., "RULE: Final consonants and consonants not followed by a vowel are cued at the side using the appropriate hand shape," p. 114);
3. Word lists and simple phrases are provided for practicing each rule.

3. *Generalization*

The Activities and Experiences section (pp. 11-89) provides numerous opportunities for generalization, through naturally occurring activities (e.g., Daily Procedures) and contrived activities (e.g., Story Telling and Dramatization).

D. *Special notes*

1. Exercises are provided for hearing adults, such as parents, teach-

ers, or clinicians learning Cued Speech. Listening, discrimination, and contrasting exercises are included (pp. 178–192).

2. Transcription exercises are presented, for use by two people practicing decoding and transmitting skills (pp. 223–275).

Montgomery, J., ed. 1980. *Non-oral communication, A training guide for the child without speech.* Title IV-C ESEA, Exemplary/Incentive Grant. Order from: Non-Oral Communication Center, Plavan School, 9675 Warner Avenue, Fountain Valley, CA, 92708, 200 pp., see below for prices.

General Description: This is a 200 page three-ring binder, guide-book for the assessment, training, and application of augmentative communication systems with non-speaking children. This curriculum was developed and field tested within a public school program with physically handicapped, non-oral children. The major areas are

1. assessing the non-oral child;
2. test modification;
3. vocabulary selection;
4. educational carryover;
5. monitoring the use of augmentative communication systems;
6. writing goals and objectives.

A. *Client*

1. *Target population*
   This guide is designed to be used with physically handicapped children who cannot speak.

2. *Prerequisites*
   The child must demonstrate
   a. communicative intent;
   b. visual attention span of 3–5 seconds.

3. *Entrance level*
   The child begins by following a visual cue which establishes a response method.

4. *Exit level*
   The child will be able to augment his or her limited oral speech with a consistent reliable output system.

B. *Trainer*

1. *Background*
   Suggested professionals to carry out the lessons would include speech language specialists, special education teachers, occupational and physical therapists. Aspects of the training can be conducted by supervised paraprofessionals.

2. *Special training*
   A Title IV-C, Non-Oral Communication Training Workshop is recommended.

C. *Administration*

1. *Equipment and materials*
   a. The following are provided in the program:

        (1) Guidebook ($10.00)

        (2) Sample lesson plans

        (3) Sample assessment forms

        (4) Language board instruction kit ($5.00)

    b. The following must be provided by the trainer:

        (1) Materials to construct necessary equipment

           (a) Tagboard

           (b) Sheets of plexiglass

           (c) Symbols (e.g., pictures, rub on letters, rebuses, or Blissymbols)

        (2) Stimulus items appropriate to each child

  2. *Degree of structure*

This is a moderately structured program. Specific instructions are given as examples, as well as sample lessons and evaluation guides. Discussions of test interpretation, interdisciplinary management, and evaluation criteria are equally important. The book serves as an overall guide to the beginning and intermediate steps of communication programming for the non-oral child. Lesson plans include:

a. Annual goal

b. Short term objective

c. Entry level skills

d. Materials

e. Dialogue

f. Criterion

g. Application to the classroom

  3. *Generalization*

The section on application to the classroom included in each lesson plan provides suggestions for generalization.

D. *Special notes*

  1. This curriculum includes lists of commercially available programs, tests and modification techniques, and an extensive bibliography.

  2. The role of advocacy is stressed in this guide.

  3. Sketches and diagrams of useful materials and step-by-step instruction for designing language/communication boards are included.

  4. A checklist of student characteristics is provided.

  5. This curriculum was field tested for three years with severely physically handicapped non-oral children, ages 3 to 16.

  6. This curriculum has been selected by the California State Department of Education as an exemplary program for statewide dissemination.

Murdock, J. and Hartmann, B. 1975. *A language development program: Imitative gestures to basic syntactic structures.* Salt Lake City, UT: Word Making Productions, Inc., 35 pp., $4.25.

General Description: This program consists of two placement tests (Expressive

Placement Test and Receptive Placement Test) and a series of language tasks divided into the following categories:

Receptive Tasks

Category I: Identifying Nouns-Discriminative Stimuli
Category II: Following Simple Directions
Category III: Identifying Prepositions
Category IV: Identifying Verbs
Category V: Identifying Adjectives
Category VI: Following More Difficult Directions

Expressive Tasks

Category I: Preverbal Motor and Vocal Imitation
Category II: Phonological Skills
Category III: Semantic Skills
Category IV: Syntactical and Morphological Skills

Client

1. *Target population*

"This program is written for children whose language ability ranges from having no vocal verbalizations to having syntactical (word order) and morphological (word form) skills below those of a normal 4-year-old child" (p. 3).

2. *Prerequisites*

Procedures are described for eliminating inappropriate or non-attending behaviors. Attention, defined as "sitting upright in a chair and looking at the instructor or other visual stimuli for 3 seconds or more" (p. 5), should be established before proceding into the program.

3. *Entrance level*

a. Receptive tasks begin with indicating the understanding of selected nouns (e.g., by touch or glance).
b. Expressive Tasks start with motor and vocal imitation presented simultaneously.

4. *Exit level*

a. Receptive Tasks end with the client being able to follow 2-3 part directions (e.g., "Go to the table and get the ball and give it to Sue").
b. Expressive tasks end with syntactical skills (early complete sentences having transformations), and morphological skills (such as pluralization of nouns).

B. *Trainer*

1. *Background*

The program was designed to be used by paraprofessionals under the direction of a classroom teacher or speech language pathologist. Understanding of behavior management techniques is required.

2. *Special training*

None is specified, but the trainer must be familiar with the program and behavior management techniques.

C. *Administration*
  1. *Equipment and materials*
     a. The manual provides samples of:
        (1) Placement Test Form
        (2) Data Recording Sheet
        (3) Generalization Training and Probing Cards
        (4) Suggested developmental tasks to be trained
     b. The trainer provides all stimulus materials.
  2. *Degree of structure*
     The program is designed for sessions up to 30 minutes in length with a minimum of 60 to 100 trials per session. The teaching procedures include the following information:
     a. What behaviors to reinforce
     b. When to reinforce
     c. Types of reinforcers
     d. Reinforcement schedule
     e. Criteria for movement—in most cases 10 consecutive correct responses or 80% correct responses for two consecutive sessions
  3. *Generalization*
     Specific suggestions are given to ensure generalization in the following situations:
     a. New physical settings
     b. With other people
     c. With different discriminative stimuli
     d. With similar tasks
D. *Special notes*
  1. A ten page appendix is provided which contains an ordered list of environmentally useful words with direct reference by item number to four commercially available stimulus programs.
  2. A five code recording system is described to record prompted as well as unprompted responses.
  3. The authors stress that vocabulary items should be functional and relevant.

Robbins, N. 1978. *Sign language curricula*. Perkins School for the Blind, Department for Deaf-Blind Children. Order from Howe Press, Perkins School for the Blind, Watertown, MA, 02172, $5.00.

General Description: The current curriculum includes three major areas:
  1. *Pre-linguistic manual communication*, covering receptive and expressive signals and gestures, and intended for use with all students following the curricula;
  2. *Sign language: conversational English*, including sub-areas such as one- and two-word grammar, use of inflections, and English questions; this is intended for students who demonstrate capacity for English language learning;

3. *Sign communication and everyday vocabulary*, covering receptive and expressive communication at the one- and two-word levels; this is intended for students with severe language learning disabilities, with cognitive level at the early pre-operational stage.

A. *Client*

1. *Target population*

These curricula are designed for deaf or severely handicapped students. As noted in the general description, there are several sub-groups, for which separate curricula are being or have been developed. The area on "Sign communication and everyday vocabulary" could be adapted to fit the needs of non-deaf populations such as mentally retarded or autistic clients.

2. *Prerequisites*

No prerequisites are listed for this program. However, it is apparent that attention skills would be required.

3. *Entrance level*

The pre-linguistic area begins with the client's appropriate non-verbal response to simple signals made in contact with his or her body (e.g., comes, when arm is pulled; opens mouth, when spoon is touched to it).

4. *Exit level*

The highest level area, "Sign language: conversational English", teaches everyday use of basic structures of English in conversations using signs plus fingerspelling. This area teaches conversational use of complex structures such as conjoined sentences, tag questions, and anaphonic pronouns.

B. *Trainer*

1. *Background*

The trainer's background is not specified. However, this curriculum does not appear to be appropriate for use by a paraprofessional, since training procedures are not specified.

2. *Special training*

The trainer would need to be fluent in sign language and fingerspelling, both receptively and expressively.

C. *Administration*

1. *Equipment and materials*

a. The manual provides the sequence of objectives and lists of vocabulary.

b. The trainer is expected to provide all other material. Since these curricula are designed to be carried out primarily during activities of daily living, most materials would be readily available.

2. *Degree of structure*

This is a moderately structured program. For each of the three curricula areas, the manual specifies the following:

a. Skills (e.g., asks by pointing and gesture for name of object, asks "why" questions including negative contractions).

b. Objectives: the conditions, the expected behavior, and the criterion. Numerous examples are provided.
These curricula do *not* suggest teaching procedures.
3. *Generalization*
This is intended to be an interactive, conversational-format program. Therefore, many criteria specify the client's use of skills in conversation. However, specific suggestions for generalization are not provided.
D. *Special notes*
1. A fourth track for this curriculum, *Ameslan*, is planned. It will cover structural features of American Sign Language. It is intended for students who show persistent use of Ameslan structures and have persistent difficulties in learning English structure.
2. These curricula focus on language in use rather than on language lessons involving drill and rote memory.

St. Louis, K.W., Mattingly, S., Esposito, A., and Cone, J.D. 1980. *West Virginia System: Receptive language curriculum for the moderately, severely, and profoundly handicapped.* The West Virginia System, Department of Psychology, Oglebay Hall, West Virginia University, Morgantown, WV, 26506, $71.00.

General Description: The Receptive Language Curriculum Binder contains the following information:
1. Discussion of language assessment
2. Procedures for developing individual educational plans
3. Detailed method cards divided into 25 sub-areas for teaching specific receptive language behaviors
4. A Scope, Sequence and Correspondence Chart as a cross-reference guide to selective commercially available tests and program
A. *Client*
1. *Target population*
The program was originally designed to meet the communication needs of the severely and profoundly retarded. However, it can be used with the mild and moderately retarded and adapted for use with non-vocal and multiply handicapped clients.
2. *Prerequisites*
None are stated for entrance into the program. However, each method card lists the general prerequisites needed for that particular objective (e.g., ambulation, vision, hearing and/or sign language). The objectives are sequenced so that earlier tasks may be prerequisites for later tasks.
3. *Entrance level*
The initial objectives require general awareness to auditory and/or gestural cues.
4. *Exit level*
The last two sub-areas require the ability to follow multi-concept directions and to understand stories.

B. *Trainer*

 1. *Background*

 This program is designed for classroom teachers and paraprofessionals who can consult a speech-language pathologist.

 2. *Special training*

 No special training is required, but knowledge of behavior management techniques would be helpful.

C. *Administration*

 1. *Equipment and materials*

 a. The curriculum binder includes

 1. detailed introduction to the West Virginia System and receptive language sub-areas;

 2. approximately 350 method cards sequenced in 25 subareas;

 3. recording information utilizing the "Universal Data Sheet;"

 4. the Scope, Sequence, and Correspondence Chart.

 b. The trainer provides all stimulus materials. Each method card states specifically what materials are needed for the training task.

 2. *Degree of Structure*

 Each method card follows a highly structured format to provide the following information:

 a. An objective written in behavioral terms (e.g., Given an object and the command, "Point to the (object)," the student must point to the object in three seconds.).

 b. Mastery criterion for movement onto the next objective (e.g., eight out of ten correct responses for two consecutive sessions).

 c. Suggested methods divided into steps for teaching the objective including correction procedures.

 3. *Generalization*

 One to three generalization method cards are included in each sub-area to encourage the trainer to check for maintenance of new skills in another setting or in a group activity.

D. *Special notes*

 1. The West Virginia System also has curricula available for training other adaptive skills (e.g., gross motor, feeding, recreation, toileting).

 2. This program can be used concurrently with The Expressive Language Curriculum (see St. Louis et al. 1980).

St. Louis, K.W., Rejzer, R., and Cone, J.D. 1980. *West Virginia system: Expressive language curriculum for the moderately, severely, and profoundly handicapped.* The West Virginia System, Department of Psychology, Oglebay Hall, West Virginia University, Morgantown, WV, 26506, $79.00.

General Description: The Expressive Language Curriculum Binder contains the following information:

 1. Discussion of language assessment

2. Procedures for developing individual educational plans
3. Detailed method cards divided into 25 sub-areas for teaching specific expressive language behaviors
4. A Scope, Sequence, and Correspondence Chart as a cross reference guide to selective commercially available tests and programs

A. *Client*

1. *Target population*

The program was originally designed to meet the communication needs of the severely and profoundly retarded. However, it can be used with the mild to moderately retarded and adapted for non-vocal and multiply handicapped clients of all ages.

2. *Prerequisites*

None are stated for entrance into the program. However, each method card lists the general prerequisites needed for that particular objective (e.g., use of hands, vision). The objectives are sequenced so that earlier tasks may be prerequisites for later tasks.

3. *Entrance level*

The initial objectives deal with making sounds and/or gestures in an attempt to determine if the client should be trained vocally and/or on a non-vocal system (e.g., communication board or manual communication).

4. *Exit level*

The client exits the program when he or she can relate experiences in complete sentences.

B. *Trainer*

1. *Background*

This program is designed for classroom teachers and paraprofessionals who can consult a speech-language pathologist.

2. *Special training*

No special training is required, but knowledge of behavior management techniques would be helpful.

C. *Administration*

1. *Equipment and materials*

a. The curriculum binder includes:
1. a detailed introduction to the West Virginia System and the expressive language sub-areas;
2. approximately 350 method cards sequenced into 25 sub-areas;
3. recording information utilizing the "Universal Data Sheet";
4. the Scope, Sequence, and Correspondence Chart.

b. The trainer provides all stimulus materials. Each method card states specifically the materials needed.

2. *Degree of structure*

Each method card follows a very structured format to provide the following information:

a. An objective written in behavioral terms (e.g., Given the direction, "Say (or sign) mama," the student must imitate the word (or sign) within three seconds).

b. Criteria for moving to the next objective (e.g., eight correct responses out of ten for two consecutive sessions).

c. Suggested methods for teaching including correction procedures.

3. *Generalization*

One to three generalization method cards are included in each sub-area to encourage the trainer to check for maintenance of new skills in other settings.

D. *Special notes*

1. The West Virginia System also has curricula available for teaching other adaptive skills (e.g., gross motor, dressing, vocational).

2. This program can be used concurrently with the Receptive Language Curriculum (see St. Louis et al. 1980, for more information).

3. This curriculum contains two sub-areas with specific suggestions and methods for adapting the vocal training program for use with non-vocal clients:

a. Sub-area 24—Adaptation of the Curriculum for Communication Boards

b. Sub-area 25—Adaptation of the curriculum for Manual Communication

Silverman, H., McNaughton, S., and Kates, B. 1978. *Handbook of Blissymbolics for instructors, users, parents and administrators.* Blissymbolics Communication Institute, 862 Eglinton Avenue East, Toronto, Ontario, Canada, M4G 2L1, 655 pp., $30.00.

General Description: This is not a program, but rather a reference guide for those who teach Blissymbolics. It covers a thorough description of the Blissymbol System, physical functional considerations (positioning, hand-training, physical assessment, interfacing), and application of the system.

A. *Client*

1. *Target population*

The Blissymbolics system was initially designed as a system of international communication by Bliss (1975). It has since been used with the communicatively handicapped, especially the non-vocal severely physically handicapped (such as cerebral-palsied persons) and the non-vocal mentally retarded.

2. *Prerequisites*

Although no prerequisites are listed directly, it is apparent that the client is expected to have reached the level of object permanence before this approach is initiated. The client would also need to have attention skills.

3. *Entry level*

This approach begins with positioning and handtraining for symbol usage. The program usually begins with visual matching and visual discrimination of symbols.

4. *Exit level*

Although there is no specific exit level for all users, the advanced stage includes advanced symbol strategies (e.g., symbol position), creative use of the system, complex sentence structure, story writing, and relating symbol-reading skills to word-reading.

B. *Trainer*

1. *Background*

As noted in the title, this handbook is intended for instructors, users, parents, and administrators. Instructors would typically be special educators or speech-language pathologists, although paraprofessionals could assist under supervision.

2. *Special training*

The authors stress that the *Handbook* ". . . is *not* intended as an independent, comprehensive instructional program in Blissymbolics. Workshop training is strongly recommended for instructors wishing to teach Blissymbolics" (Silverman, McNaughton, and Kates 1978, front inside cover). Training programs are offered through the Blissymbolics Communication Institute in Toronto, Canada.

C. *Administration*

1. *Equipment and materials*

a. In addition to a description of the system and its application, the manual includes the following:

1. Appendix 5—suggestions for materials to be used with preschool symbol users and with older children (27 suggestions, including illustrations or pictures);

2. Appendix 6—suggestions for toys and games (27 entries, including diagrams, illustrations, pictures, and specific instructions);

3. Appendix 7—aids to programming, including worksheet suggestions and examples;

4. Appendix 8—commercially available and teacher-made materials and other sources of information.

b. The trainer provides the communication board, symbols, worksheets, and so forth, many of which can be reproduced from suggestions in the *Handbook*. A master list of Blissymbolics is not included in this book, although instructions are provided for drawing Blissymbols with or without a template. A list of Blissymbols may be found in *Blissymbols for Use* (Hehner 1979).

2. *Degree of structure*

This is a very unstructured approach. The authors stress that ". . . much of the content of the *Handbook* is offered in the form of suggestions and alternative choices and not as outlines to be rigidly followed" (Silverman et al. 1978, p. 3). They do, however, request that instructors and users strictly adhere to the instructions for symbol construction and drawing, in order to maintain standard system forms.

3. *Generalization*

Numerous general suggestions for generalization are provided through use of games and worksheets, and through sections on "family involvement" and "extension into the community."

D. *Special notes*

1. Appendices of special interest but not listed above include:

a. Appendix 1—Syntax Supplement, describing the syntax recommended by C.K. Bliss;

b. Appendix 3—Display Types and Coding, covering various commercial or teacher-made display units and coding methods;

c. Appendix 4—Interfaces, describing a variety of interfacing equipment.

2. Three theoretical models for application of Blissymbolics are suggested:

a. Model One — Blissymbolics serves as a functional augmentative language for the client who has good receptive language.

b. Model Two — Blissymbolics serves as a communication medium for the young child during early stages of language development.

c. Model Three — Blissymbolics is used as a surface communication system for clients with lower intellectual levels.

3. A detailed, 207 page evaluation-study is presented.

Skelly, M. and Schinsky, L. 1979. *Amer-Ind gestural code based on universal american indian hand talk.* Elsevier North Holland, Inc., 52 Vanderbilt Avenue, New York, NY, 10017, 494 pp., $18.95

General Description: This is a text on Amer-Ind, based on the authors' extensive use of the code with a variety of severely handicapped clients. It includes three major parts:

Part 1   —Clinical Investigation (a review of the history of Amer-Ind and its use with the handicapped);

Part 2   —Clinical Application (a description of Amer-Ind, and a presentation of strategies for clinical testing and programming);

Part 3   —Clinical Signal Repertoire (a listing of 250 concept labels with illustrations).

A. *Client*

1. *Target population*

This program can be used with many populations (e.g., aphasics, oral-verbal apraxics, the mentally retarded); however, it is particularly suited to clients with symbolic deficiencies. Three major client groupings are recommended, with a separate treatment program for each:

Treatment Program A — Intact auditory comprehension of language (e.g., laryngectomees);

Treatment Program B — Impaired auditory reception of language (e.g., aphasics);

Treatment Program C — Developmentally impaired patients (e.g., the mentally retarded).

2. *Prerequisites*
   a. Eye contact
   b. Attention
   c. Physical imitation
   d. Pointing
   e. Shaping skills
3. *Entrance level*
   The lowest level program, Treatment Program C, begins with recognition and assisted imitation of signals modeled by the clinician. No linguistic input is used.
4. *Exit level*
   The highest level program, Treatment Program A, ends with use of signals at a level equivalent to propositional speech.

B. *Trainer*
1. *Background*
   It is assumed that the trainer will be a speech-language pathologist.
2. *Special training*
   The authors stress the importance of acquiring signal expertise before beginning to train clients. They recommend that potential trainers acquire Amer-Ind from an experienced, knowledgeable signaler. Workshops are also presented throughout the country, and a video program is available through the St. Louis Veterans Administration Hospital.

C. *Administration*
1. *Equipment and materials*
   a. This text includes description of three training programs and a list of 250 concept illustrations (signals).
   b. The trainer must provide materials such as color photographs and real objects which are typically readily available. The use of video equipment is highly recommended.
2. *Degree of structure*
   These are moderately structured programs. Each of the three programs specifies the following:
   a. Goal(s) and sub-goals
   b. Objectives
   c. Tasks
   d. Criteria
   For some tasks, exact procedures, including signal dialogue, are included in a script format.
3. *Generalization*
   These programs stress a reality approach, which should enhance generalization. In addition, numerous general suggestions for programming generalization are suggested.

D. *Special notes*
   1. Dr. Skelly is part American Indian, and was taught Hand Talk as a child by her Iroquois relatives.
   2. The first section of the text covers the results of numerous projects regarding the acquisition and the transmission of Amer-Ind.
   3. An *Amer-Ind* Scale of progress is presented and described. It is intended ". . . to record as briefly and meaningfully as possible the results of treatments by certain methods at certain levels of acquisition, execution, and transmission by the patient" (p. 97).
   4. Two other tests are included: *The Skelly Action Test of Auditory Reception of Language* (five forms with increasing levels of difficulty), and *The Skelly Comparative Apraxia Test: Oral and Manual.*
   5. A form is provided for analyzing patient strategies on the Leiter International Scale.

Snell, M. 1974. Sign language and total communication. In *Language acquisition for the retarded and multiply impaired*, ed. L.R. Kent. Champaign, IL: Research Press, pp. 147–85, $6.95.

General Description: This chapter is an adaptation of Kent's *Language Acquisition Program*. It is designed to establish signing responses in clients with very low or no expressive language skills.
   A. *Client*
      1. *Target population*
      This adaptation could be used with non-verbal hearing impaired, severely retarded, emotionally disturbed, and brain-damaged clients.
      2. *Prerequisites*
      None are specified, but the client must be visually alert and have at least moderate control over both hands to produce the signs presented.
      3. *Entrance level*
      Training begins with establishing attention using signs such as "sit", "look", and "quiet."
      4. *Exit level*
      Three-sign responses, such as "hat on table."
   B. *Trainer*
      1. *Background*
      The trainer's background is not specified, but it is stressed that the trainer must be thoroughly familiar with the signs being taught. A classroom teacher, paraprofessional, or speech-language pathologist who knows sign could administer the program.
      2. *Special training*
      The trainer should know the signs to be taught before training is begun, so that the signs are presented consistently in a smooth manner. This would require training all the staff and family

members involved with the client so that they may encourage the client to communicate.

C. *Administration*
    1. *Equipment and materials*
        a. The program is presented in book form. A limited signing vocabulary is presented for initial phases of the program.
        b. All stimulus materials are provided by the trainer. A source list is given for reference in expanding the signed vocabulary.
    2. *Degree of structure*
    This program is structured similarly to Kent's *Language Acquisition Program* using the section, phase, and part strategy. The criterion for progression through the program is the same (see Kent 1974 in Appendix A and B).
    3. *Generalization*
    Although generalization activities are not specified, the signs must be used consistently throughout the client's daily activities to develop this communication system.

D. *Special notes*
    1. The signs presented are generally part of American Sign Language (Ameslan).
    2. A total communication approach is stressed in which signs and speech are presented simultaneously throughout the program.
    3. A signed vocal imitation phase is included to encourage vocalizations from the client, utilizing the motor imitation repertoire taught earlier.

Struck, R. 1977. Santa Cruz Special Education Management System. *Behavioral characteristics progression* (BCP). Palo Alto, CA: VORT Corporation, $99.95.

General Description: This curriculum consists of an observation booklet and five books of method cards. Fifty-nine strands comprise the curriculum (e.g., health, toileting, attention span), with method cards provided for 49 of the strands. The method cards are arranged into five books:
    1. Self-Help Skills (9 strands)
    2. Motor Skills (12 strands)
    3. Communication Skills (11 strands)
    4. Social Skills (12 strands)
    5. Learning Skills (6 strands)

A. *Client*
    1. *Target population*
    This curriculum is intended for use with severely handicapped individuals from preschool to adult age groups. Nine strands have been developed to make it appropriate for use with clients having severe sensory and/or physical impairments (e.g., sign language, speechreading, orientation, wheelchair use).
    2. *Prerequisites*
    Although no general behavioral or physical abilities are listed for

the entire program, each Method Card lists pupil abilities required for that activity.

3. *Entrance level*

The entrance level varies considerably according to strand.

4. *Exit level*

Since this is not a correlated program, skills are cumulative only within strands. Thus, exit levels also vary according to strand.

B. *Trainer*

1. *Background*

The trainer's background is open. It is likely that the trainer for the Communication section would be a special education teacher or a speech-language pathologist, though an aide or parent could serve as trainer.

2. *Special training*

No special training is required for most strands. However, the sign language trainer should, of course, have a good knowledge of the sign system used.

C. *Administration*

1. *Equipment and materials*

a. Materials provided with the program include an observation booklet and five pages of method cards.

b. The trainer provides everyday items, game materials, and reinforcers.

2. *Degree of structure*

This is a moderately structured program with regard to scope and sequence of objectives, and procedures for activities. Follow-up, such as daily data-keeping, error correction, and generalization, is very loosely structured or omitted. Some objectives have more than one method card, while others have no method cards. Method cards include the following information:

a. Title of the activity

b. Identifying information (strand, objective)

c. Pupil abilities required (e.g., vision, sign language)

d. Interest level (preschool to adult)

e. Pupil grouping (independent to large group)

f. Activity length

g. Number of adults required

h. Materials and equipment

i. Instructions presented in a modified narrative format

3. *Generalization*

This curriculum is very school and activity centered; it makes no specific provisions for generalization across persons, places, materials, or cues. Since many of the training activities are contrived, game-type events, repeated practice is unlikely and generalization should not be expected without special training.

D. *Special notes*

1. Method cards for this curriculum were developed by 250

California professionals. Each participant wrote up 10–15 of his or her most successful, creative, or fun teaching techniques, then matched them to an objective. Therefore, some objectives have more than one method card (all of them unrelated), while others have no method cards.

2. Some objectives related to communication may be found in volumes other than the Communication volume (e.g., in the social and learning skills books).

3. Computerization of this system is currently in progress; this could aid in determining objectives and methods most appropriate for specific clients.

4. The Communication section includes the following strands: Auditory Perception, Pre-articulation, Articulation, Language Comprehension, Language Expression, Listening, Sign Language, Fingerspelling, Speech Reading, Articulation I, Articulation II.

5. The Sign Language and Fingerspelling strands would be appropriate for use with non-vocal clients, whether hearing or deaf.

Williams, W. and Fox, T., eds. 1977. Communication. In *Minimum objectives system for pupils with severe handicaps: Working draft number one*, vol. 1. Center for Special Education, University of Vermont, Burlington, VT, 142 pp., $10.00.

General Description: This developmentally-based program consists of four major programming areas:

(1) Communication
(2) Motor
(3) Self-care
(4) Social

A. *Client*

1. *Target population*

The minimum objectives were developed for use with severely handicapped students in the public schools. They are appropriate for clients from birth through adulthood.

2. *Prerequisites*

No behavioral or physical prerequisites are listed for this program.

3. *Entrance level*

The communication area begins with "activation," which includes objectives such as decreasing behaviors that interfere with instruction and learning, and responding to sound.

4. *Exit level*

Several fairly complex linguistic structures (e.g., "before," verb tenses, plurals) are taught; the program ends with fairly simple overall utterances and a short mean length of utterance.

B. *Trainer*

1. *Background*

The trainer's background is open; however, a teacher or speech-language pathologist would likely administer the program in the public schools.

2. *Special training*

No special training is required, but it is suggested that the trainer solicit the assistance of a communication specialist to help assess and design communication programs.

C. *Administration*

1. *Equipment and materials*

a. A complete manual ($10.00) is provided.

b. The trainer must provide everyday materials such as cups, cookies, and so forth.

2. *Degree of structure*

This is a structured program, although it is recommended that it be tailored to fit the needs of the individual. Each minimum objective is first discussed in narrative form, including information such as description and rationale. Each minimum objective specifies

a. behavioral objective, including:

(1) Condition

(2) Behavior

(3) Acquisition criterion.

b. potential strategies, activities, or training sequences.

c. performance levels, a scoring system ranging from six points for independence to one point for full assistance and zero points for no response.

Data sheets and assessment forms are also provided.

3. *Generalization*

An excellent strategy for generalization is provided in the mastery assessment. Mastery is assessed across time, people, cues to respond, materials, and settings. A mastery score sheet is provided. This strategy could be used with any program.

D. *Special notes*

1. This is a coordinated program; the four areas (communication, motor, self-care, social) are taught concurrently.

2. Functional alternatives are utilized to make client behaviors as normative as possible and to allow for independence. Potential sequences are suggested for adapting the program for signing (pp. 61–65) or for communication board use (pp. 58–61).

3. Updatings are planned annually or biannually; a new edition is currently in press.

4. A number of bibliographies relating directly to communication (e.g., general, signing, communication boards, pronouns) and to general graining procedures (e.g., task analysis, behavior management, decreasing behaviors) are provided.

5. The program includes a section on how to develop an Individualized Educational Program (IEP) Plan (pp. 34–40).

Wilson, P.S., Goodman, L., and Wood, R.K. 1975. *Manual language for the child without language: A behavioral approach for teaching the exceptional child.* Order from Eric Grossman, 14 Keefe Lane, Middletown, CT, 06457, 84 pp., $5.00 ($4.00 if prepaid).

General Description: Manual Language is defined by the authors as ". . . the simultaneous pairing of a sign and a spoken word" (introduction). A "Behavioral Language Assessment" is presented followed by a three phase training program:

        Phase I — Reception

        Phase II — Reproduction

        Phase III — Expression

  A. *Client*

    1. *Target population*

    This program is intended for individuals who have little or no understanding of speech and/or limited or no intelligible expressive oral language. It has been used with hearing impaired, autistic, profoundly mentally retarded and aphasic children. It could be adapted for adults.

    2. *Prerequisites*

    The following are required:

    a. Attending skills

    b. Imitates signs or gestures naturally

    c. Client is non-vocal, but visually alert

    3. *Entrance level*

    The client demonstrates understanding (reception) of a sign.

    4. *Exit level*

    The client spontaneously uses the sign in an appropriate situation.

  B. *Trainer*

    1. *Background*

    The trainer's background is not specified. From the book it appears directive enough to be used by classroom teachers, or by aides with supervision from the teacher.

    2. *Special training*

    No special training is specified.

  C. *Administration*

    1. *Equipment and materials*

    a. An 84-page manual is provided.

    b. Any stimulus items (common classroom and home objects) used in training are to be provided by the trainer.

    2. *Degree of structure*

    a. The authors suggest a very structured daily classroom schedule designed as a "Functional Day" to fully assess the client's independent skills (e.g., grooming, dressing, etc.) and to aid in selecting the vocabulary to be taught.

    b. The three phase teaching strategy contains levels and steps within each phase to ensure successful learning.

    c. Sample forms are illustrated in the manual with permission for copying provided.

    d. Criteria for moving to new items is not specified.

  3. *Generalization*

The terminal goal of each phase is for the client to spontaneously use the sign correctly in a variety of different situations. However, the authors caution that "True spontaneous language cannot be taught" (p. 79).

D. *Special notes*

  1. The client must demonstrate reception of the sign even if he/she already shows reception of the spoken word.

  2. Prompting procedures are detailed to ensure initial success and to allow systematic fading of the prompts to establish independent responses.

Appendix C:
Organizations, Agencies, and Publications

This appendix covers selected sources of further information on the severely handicapped. It includes organizations such as the Association for Retarded Citizens, governmental agencies such as the Bureau of Education for the Handicapped, and publications such as *Communication Outlook*. For each entry information is included regarding the services provided, particularly in relation to the severely communication-impaired.

The following index is an alphabetical listing of all the entries in this appendix.

Adaptive Systems Corporation
1650 S. Amphlett Blvd.
Suite 307
San Mateo, CA 94402
(415) 573-6114

This corporation distributes *ISAARE,* Information System Adaptive Assistive Rehabilitation Equipment. In brief, ISAARE consists of an alphabetic file of equipment catalogues, a six-volume Index-Glossary set, and a Locator Book. It is intended to aid in selecting and locating equipment to meet the needs of the severely and profoundly handicapped. Further information on this system is presented in Appendix B (see Melichar 1977).

Alexander Graham Bell
Association for the Deaf
3417 Volta Place, N.W.
Washington, D.C. 20007
(202) 337-5220

This organization includes professionals and parents concerned with providing services to the deaf. The group conducts information collection and dissemination, including personalized information to parents, access to the Volta Bureau Library, and numerous pamphlets and reprints. Publications include a journal, *The Volta Review;* a newsletter, *Newsounds;* and an annual *Monograph.* Several books are published each year by the organization, and they distribute other books. Several special interest sections have been organized, such as the International Parents Organization. Public education is attempted through dissemination of information and the mass media. The association also serves as a leading advocate of oral education of the hearing impaired and engages in advocacy activities through its Children's Rights Program. A regular active membership including all benefits is $30.00 per year.

American Annals of the Deaf
5034 Washington Avenue, N.W.
Washington, D.C. 20016
(202) 363-1327

The *American Annals of the Deaf* is an educational journal published six times a year. The April issue each year is a reference issue, including information such as teacher training data and a comprehensive listing of services for the deaf. The other five issues are literary issues containing articles and research reports on deafness. The subscription rate for one year is $17.50. A large variety of books and pamphlets on deafness are available through this organization; many of these are free or can be obtained for a nominal reprinting charge.

American Foundation for the Blind (AFB)
15 West 16th Street
New York, NY 10011
(212) 620-2000

This organization has two national and four regional offices serving the needs of persons with vision problems. There are national consultants in a number of areas such as Children and Youth, Rehabilitation, and Special Population Groups. The AFB publishes numerous books, periodicals, and newsletters intended for rehabilitation professionals and others concerned with vision problems. The *Journal of Visual Impairment,* published ten times per year, is available at a cost of $11.00 for one year. It covers a wide range of topics such as legislation, technology, employment, and social issues. The AFB also distributes a number of products for the blind and visually impaired. A library also has information regarding visual impairment; anyone may borrow materials at no charge, either in person or by mail.

American Radio Relay League (ARRL)
225 Main Street
Newington, CT 05111

This organization is concerned with providing services to Amateur Radio Operators. The Club and Training Department provides assistance in areas such as licensing for use of amateur radio equipment. One aspect of this aid involves learning Morse Code. Several publications, including *Tune in the World with Ham Radio* and *ARRL Code Kit*, aid in learning code. The organization also provides names of licensed instructors of Morse Code.

American Speech-Language-Hearing Association (ASHA)
10801 Rockville Pike
Rockville, MD 20852
(301) 897-5700 or
(800) 638-6868 (toll free)

ASHA is the national professional organization for speech-language pathologists and audiologists. It is an accrediting agent for programs in speech-language pathology and a certifying agency for speech-language pathologists. ASHA publishes three quarterly and one monthly journal, plus frequent monographs and reports. Numerous pamphlets are also available through this organization. ASHA members serve a wide range of communication-handicapped clients in addition to the severely handicapped.

Assistive Device Center
California State University, Sacramento
6000 J Street
Sacramento, CA 95819
(916) 454-6422

This organization provides direct services to clients with severe communication handicaps, research activities, and dissemination of information. It publishes technical reports on various facets of the program, such as an assessment battery developed at the center for making recommendations on assistive device systems (see Appendix A, Meyers et al. 1980, for a review of that report).

The Association for the Severely Handicapped (TASH)
1600 West Armory Way
Garden View Suite
Seattle, WA 98119
(206) 283-5055

This organization is a coalition of teachers, parents, therapists, and other concerned people working for quality education for the severely handicapped. TASH serves as an advocate for that population in areas such as developing specialized teacher training personnel. They provide an information department which answers specific questions regarding education and services for the severely handicapped. Membership in TASH entitles members to a monthly newsletter covering information on programs, conferences, and new resources, and a quarterly journal which stresses practical application of instructional procedures with the severely handicapped. The organization also publishes a variety of materials, including an annual volume, *Teaching the Severely Handicapped*.

Blissymbolics Communication Institute (BCI)
862 Eglinton Avenue, E.
Toronto, Ontario
Canada M4G 2L1
(416) 425-7835

General membership costs $25.00 per year. Members receive the following publications three times per year: *BCI Bulletin*, which includes news about Blissymbolics and BCI; BCI *Newsletter*, which contains articles submitted by parents, instructors, users, and others. A variety of products are available from BCI, including books, Blissymbol stamps, various teaching aids, and professional materials. A wide variety of training programs is offered, ranging from orientation presentations through special interest training sessions and internships. A loan library of videotapes, slides and books is provided.

Bureau of Education for the Handicapped (BEH)
U.S. Office of Education
Washington, D.C. 20202

BEH works with exceptional children who are mentally retarded, hard of hearing, deaf, speech impaired, visually impaired, seriously emotionally disturbed, orthopedically impaired or otherwise health impaired; or who have specific learning disabilities; or who are gifted and talented. BEH is divided into five service divisions: (1) Division of Assistance to States; (2) Division of Innovation and Development; (3) Division of Personnel Preparation; (4) Division of Media Services; (5) Office of Gifted and Talented. Inquiries about grant applications and other information should be directed to the appropriate division.

Closer Look
Box 1492
Washington, D.C. 20013

Closer Look is a national resource center for parents of children with handicaps. All publications and information packets provided by this center are free of charge. The packets provide suggestions for parents in coping with daily problems and finding services from preschool through young adulthood. Although most information is geared to parents, professionals are encouraged to use the materials in their coordinated work with parents.

Communication Outlook
Artificial Language Laboratory
Computer Sciences Department
Michigan State University
East Lansing, MI 48824

This quarterly newsletter is the principal publication of the International Action Group for Communication Enhancement. It covers areas of international interest such as review of current literature, new aids, conference notices, funding, reader viewpoints, and general articles and features regarding non-vocal communication. A question and answer exchange by readers is also included. Subscription is $12.00 per year for four issues.

The Council for Exceptional Children
1920 Association Drive
Reston, VA 22091
(703) 620-3660
Information Hot Line: (800) 336-3728

This is an umbrella organization for professionals serving handicapped or gifted children. Twelve divisions exist within the organization, including Division for Children with Communication Disorders, Division on Physically Handicapped, Division on Mental Retardation. Each division publishes a journal and/or a newsletter. CEC also publishes several periodicals (*Exceptional Children, Teaching Exceptional Children,* and *Exceptional Child Education Resources*) and a variety of books, bibliographies, and nonprint media (e.g., films). An information Hot Line is available for information regarding access to services such as computer search reprints. Membership is $25.00 in most states, with an additional fee for division membership.

Dissem/Action
3705 S. George Mason Drive
Suite C-4 South
Falls Church, VA 22041
(703) 931-4420/4421

This project is sponsored by the Division of Personnel Preparation, Bureau of Education for the Handicapped. The organization operates a clearinghouse on personnel preparation in special education. They provide names of individuals who are excellent resources for specific kinds of information. They also publish a newspaper, *Counterpoint,* twice yearly. This newspaper covers issues and presents information regarding special education personnel preparation projects throughout the United States.

ERIC Clearinghouse on Handicapped and Gifted Children
The Council for Exceptional Children
1920 Association Drive
Reston, VA 22091

ERIC, The Educational Resources Information Center, consists of a network of 16 clearinghouses that gather literature in specialized fields. This clearinghouse provides the following services: acquires abstracts and indexes literature for inclusion in ERIC reference publications; publishes a variety of materials, such as bibliographies, monographs and newsletters; conducts individualized computer searches of the ERIC database; and distributes information such as spot bibliographies and fact sheets.

Everest and Jennings "Resources"
1803 Pontius Avenue
Los Angeles, CA 90025
(213) 478-1057

This is a commercial company which produces Zygo Communication Sysems and other products for the handicapped. This company publishes *Resources,* a newsletter distributed four times a year at no charge. Articles are contributed by professionals such as occupational therapists or speech-language pathologists. In addition, articles are occasionally reprinted from other journals. A number of these articles are on the topic of non-vocal communication.

The Exceptional Parent
P.O. Box 4944
Manchester, NH 03108

This organization publishes *The Exceptional Parent,* a journal appropriate for parents and professionals dealing with handicapped children. There are six issues per year, at a cost of $10.00 for the first year. The Exceptional Parent Bookstore distributes two types of books, most at discount prices. Special books are books of interest to readers concerned with the life of children with disabilities. General books are those which provide practical guidance about children in general.

The Foundation Center
888 7th Avenue
New York, NY 10009

This organization publishes "A Bibliography of State Foundation Directories." This publication provides an update of state and regional directories of funding sources. They will furnish information on directories serving any locality in the United States. This organization also published the *National Data Book*, a two volume set which profiles all of the more than 21,000 nonprofit organizations in the United States which are currently active in issuing grants.

Gallaudet College
Kendall Green
7th and Florida Avenue, N.E.
Washington, D.C. 20002

Gallaudet serves deaf individuals in a number of ways, in addition to providing higher education for the deaf. Information concerning Cued Speech can be obtained from the Office of Cued Speech Programs. A newsletter, *Cued Speech News*, is issued several times per year. Information concerning Signed English is also available from Gallaudet. The Gallaudet College Press publishes in a variety of areas, such as the Signed English Series. In addition, the Bookstore distributes materials published by several commercial companies, including numerous sign language texts.

Mime Workshops

American Movement Institute
Webster College
470 East Lockwood, N.E.
St. Louis, MO

Bond Street Theatre Coalition
2 Bond Street
New York, NY 10012
(212) 244-4270

Celebration Mime Theatre
R.D. 1, Box 44
South Paris, ME 04281
Attention: Tony Montanaro

Colorado Mountain College
Box 2208
Breckenridge, CO 80424
(303) 453-6757
Attention: Tom Hart

Performing Arts Center
Grand Valley State Colleges
Allendale, MI 49401

School for Movement Theatre
Davis and Elkins College
Elkins, WV 26241
(304) 636-1900, ext. 274
Attention: Julie Pedretti

These addresses represent several groups throughout the country who offer training in mime and related art forms. Most of the organizations listed provide workshops or summer courses. For example, the School for Movement Theatre offers two, four, and six week sessions for both novices and professional performers. Master classes with well-known instructors are available in areas such as illusions of pantomime, rhythms of mime, fundamental principles of mime, corporeal mime, and acrobatic mime and juggling. Offerings differ from session to session.

National Association for Retarded Citizens (ARC)
2709 Avenue E East
Arlington, TX 76011

ARC is a "grassroots" organization which focuses on services and advocacy at the local level. The national organization offers a wide variety of publications, including books, pamphlets, and periodicals. *Mental Retardation News*, a newspaper, and *The ARC*, the official publication of the ARC, are published bimonthly, at a cost of $3.50 each. Pamphlets providing general information about retardation are provided at no charge.

National Association of the Deaf (NAD)
814 Thayer Avenue
Silver Spring, MD 20910

Individual membership of $15.00 per year entitles the member to a subscription to the monthly publication, *The Deaf American*. Publications about all facets of deafness and rehabilitation of the deaf are available through NAD; some of these are published by other companies or organizations.

National Association of the Physically Handicapped
76 Elm Street
London, OH 43140
(614) 852-1664

This association attempts to advance the social, economic, and physical welfare of physically handicapped adults. The organization focuses on encouraging legislation to benefit the physically handicapped and increasing public awareness. They sponsor an education and research committee and publish a newsletter concerning their activities.

The National Center, Educational Media, and Materials for
    the Handicapped (NCEMMH)
The Ohio State University
College of Education
356 Arps Hall
Columbus, OH 43210

This organization offers training and other inservice support sessions designed and conducted to facilitate use of their products. Products include a variety of books and programs related to intervention with exceptional individuals. A quarterly magazine, *The Directive Teacher*, intended for teaching personnel is available without charge in the United States. Each issue focuses on a major theme, such as language instruction.

National Center for Law and the Handicapped, Inc. (NCLH)
P.O. Box 477
University of Notre Dame
Notre Dame, IN 46556
Attention: Information Specialist

The NCLH is a national legal advocacy organization for the handicapped, staffed by attorneys and public information professionals. Their major activities include advocacy through input to federal agencies, legislators, and professional and consumer organizations; developing public awareness through workshops and conferences; and providing numerous publications on law and the handicapped. A bimonthly journal, *Amicus*, reports on news, legislation, and litigation affecting the handicapped.

Other publications include a national directory of attorney and advocacy organizations which assist the handicapped and monographs on a variety of topics (e.g., *Right to Habilitation*, $3.00; *Community Living: Zoning Obstacles and Legal Remedies*, $3.00).

The National Easter Seal Society (NESS)
2023 West Ogden Avenue
Chicago, IL 60612

This organization provides direct services to persons with a variety of disabilities through its approximately 2,000 facilities and programs. NESS offers a variety of pamphlets, reprints, and other publications on topics such as cerebral palsy, speech, language, hearing, and use of volunteers. Serial publications distributed by NESS include *Easter Seal Communicator*, which is printed four times per year and covers events and personalities regarding NESS (free); *Rehabilitation Literature*, an interdisciplinary journal published six times per year for professional personnel and students ($15.00).

National Library Service for the Blind and Physically Handicapped
Library of Congress
Washington, D.C. 20542

This is a free national library service providing recorded and braille materials to blind and physically handicapped persons. Playback equipment is loaned for use with books and magazines that are recorded. Two catalogs are available that list by state *Volunteers Who Produce Books* and *Library Resources for the Blind and Physically Disabled*. An information sheet entitled *Facts* is also available from this address.

National Society for Autistic Children (NSAC)
1234 Massachusetts Avenue, N.W.
Suite 1017
Washington, D.C. 20005
(202) 783-0125

This is a national advocacy center serving people with autism and their families. The organization provides information and referral on topics such as education and treatment programs and techniques; taxes, guardianship, and estate planning; and organizing for better community services. The $15.00 yearly membership fee includes subscription to *Advocate*, the NSAC newsletter. The NSAC Bookstore offers numerous publications on the subject of autism.

Non-Oral Communication Center
Plavan School
9675 Warner Avenue
Fountain Valley, CA 92708
(714) 964-2014

This organization disseminates information on non-oral communication. Examples of materials provided are a newsletter covering special projects and breakthroughs in the field as well as stories about and by students at the Center; a film, *To Say I Am*, accompanied by a 19-page viewers guide with resource material; and an appendix of manufacturers of non-oral communication devices. This is a very "applied" organization which offers numerous suggestions on basic problems such as funding and measuring communication aid effectiveness.

Northeast Communication Group
c/o Judith A. Hoyt
Association for Human Services
42 Arnold Street
Westfield, MA 01085

This regional organization addresses a number of areas with regard to communication for the handicapped. Goals in the area of education include influencing preservice training programs relative to the needs of non-vocal people, organizing films and exhibits to increase public awareness, and providing seminars. Advocacy services include development of an information and referral service and an augmentative resource guide for New England. A newsletter is currently being planned.

Office for Handicapped Individuals
Office of Health and Welfare
Department of Health and Human Services
Washington, D.C.

The primary objectives of this agency are "to serve as the focal point within the Department of Health, Education, and Welfare for advocacy, review, coordination, information and planning related to Department-side policies, programs, procedures and activities relevant to the physically and mentally handicapped; and to operate for the Department a national information resource program known as the clearinghouse on the handicapped" (from the Catalog of Federal Domestic Assistance, 1979, p. 360).

Pacific Northwest Nonvocal Communication Group (PNWNVCG)
Communication Disorders Division
Children's Orthopedic Hospital and Medical Center
Box C-5371
Seattle, WA 98105

This group is currently concerned with four primary areas: education (of those working with the non-vocal and the public); dissemmination of information and materials; advocacy for non-vocal people; and membership. The education program involves yearly all-day workshops and evening seminars. The organization publishes the *PNWNVCG Newsletter*, which is issued quarterly. It focuses on local news and features as well as updating information such as "publications of interest."

Regional Centers for Services to Deaf-Blind Children
c/o New England Regional Center for
Services to Deaf-Blind Children
Perkins School
175 North Beacon Street
Waterton, MA 02172

There are eight multistate and eight single state centers for services to deaf-blind children. Although these centers differ in their approaches, they typically provide services such as resource lending libraries and representation and advocacy for the deaf-blind at the federal, state, and local levels. Addresses for these centers may be obtained from the New England Center.

Registry of Interpreters for the Deaf, Inc.
814 Thayer Avenue
Silver Spring, MD 20910

This organization registers individuals to serve as interpreters for the deaf. The requirements for becoming an interpreter are very comprehensive. The interpreter must master skills such as interpreting from spoken English to American Sign Language and vice versa, and transliterating spoken English to Manually Coded/pidgin sign and vice versa. A list of registered interpreters in your area may be obtained from the Registry. A newsletter, *Views*, is published by this organization.

Southern California Communication Group
834 22nd Street
Santa Monica, CA 90403

This organization is intended "to encourage the development of community resources for non-vocal severely physically handicapped individuals." A bimonthly newsletter, *Speakeasy*, is available for $3.00 per year. It covers activities of the group, announcements (e.g., conferences), suggestions, and human interest stories.

Superintendent of Documents
Government Printing Office
Washington, D.C. 20402

This office offers more than 24,000 different publications, periodicals, and subscription services for sale. There are 270 subject bibliographies which list publications on a single subject or field of interest. These subject bibliographies are free of charge. Subject bibliographies of particular interest to those concerned with services to the communication handicapped are Children and Youth, Hearing and Hearing Disabled, the Handicapped.

The Swedish Institute for the Handicapped
The Library
Box 303
S-161 26 Bromma, SWEDEN

This organization is building up a system for computerized literature retrieval in several rehabilitation fields, including technical aids for the communication impaired. This file, labeled TALDOC, currently contains about 700 references to books, reports, journal articles, and data sheets. The system is under constant updating. The material is made accessible through a list including complete bibliographic information and alphabetical indexes on authors, institutions, and descriptors. A thesaurus (list of descriptors with cross-references) is also provided.

Telephone Pioneers of America
195 Broadway
New York, NY 10017
(212) 393-3252

This is a volunteer organization of telephone people throughout the United States and Canada. It comprises 94 chapters which develop their own programs. Many chapters have developed special devices to aid the blind, hearing, speech, motion and retarded handicapped. A manual entitled "Helping the Handicapped — A Guide to Aids Developed by the Telephone Pioneers of America" is available at this address. See Appendix A for more information. The address of the chapter serving a region can be obtained by writing the address provided here.

Trace Research and Development Center
314 Waisman Center
1500 Highland Avenue
Madison, WI 53706
(608) 262-6966

This organization is a research, development, and resource center in the area of augmentative communication systems for severely handicapped clients. The group has five major programs, with various projects and plans under each of these programs. The five programs and examples of projects are communication processes program (e.g., testing use of wearable biofeedback aids); research, development, and availability (e.g., development of Blissymbol Printing Communication Aid); information and resource program (e.g., Trace publication series and reprint series); training and inservice program (e.g., "Where to Begin" workshop series); and client services program (e.g., consultative service delivery program).

United Cerebral Palsy Associations, Inc. (UCPA)
66 East 34th Street
New York, NY 10016

This organization offers a variety of informational pamphlets on cerebral palsy, including one entitled "Helping the Patient With Cerebral Palsy to Communicate." A wide variety of publications, audio-visuals, and reprints are offered, many free of charge for a single copy. In addition, UCPA publishes two periodicals at no charge: *UC People*, a bimonthly newsletter, and *Word from Washington*. The various departments of UCPA (e.g., Professional Services, Public Relations, Volunteer Development Committee) also have additional listings regarding books, and audio-visual materials, and so forth.

Appendix D:
Assessment Procedures
and Tools

This appendix presents a listing of primary areas of assessment for severely communication impaired clients. For each area, the goal(s) of assessment are described, indicating how the information obtained relates to programming. Sample procedures, references, or assessment tools are suggested for each area. References and tools are listed alphabetically at the end of this appendix, with bibliographic information provided for each.

This appendix is not intended to be an exhaustive listing of information on assessment, but merely an overview of the process. Throughout this book we have provided numerous ideas for assessment strategies, such as using frequency of occurrence checklists to aid in selecting initial content. Some of these strategies emphasize the importance of assessing factors such as the client's environment as well as directly assessing the client. Additional resources relating to assessment are annotated in Appendix A of this book. The reader's attention is especially directed to three texts which review a number of assessment devices: Darley (1979); Hutchinson, Hanson, and Mecham (1979); and Nation and Aram (1977).

Table D-1
Pre-linguistic Communication Assessment

Area	Goal(s) of Assessment	Procedures/Resources/Tools*
Attention Physical Attention	To determine: ability to sit for training, to attend to the trainer, to maintain on-task behavior	Chart client's length of sitting, attention to caregiver, and attention to interesting stimuli (e.g., television). Take baseline during initial training attempts. *Environmental Prelanguage Battery* *The West Virginia Assessment and Tracking System*
Visual Attention	ability to (1) fixate on an object; (2) visually track a moving object; and (3) scan an array of objects for a specific item	Present an object that is visually stimulating (e.g., a bright, moving toy or mirror). Once client fixates on it, move it horizontally, vertically, or circularly, noting range of tracking. For scanning, present tsks which require locating a missing item within a group of tems. "Sensorimotor functions and cognitive development"
Sensory Activity Auditory Discrimination	ability to receive and discriminate spoken language	Perform hearing screening and refer to audiologist if necessary.
Visual Acuity & Discrimination	ability to receive and discriminate visual stimuli	Perform vision screening and refer to ophthalmologist if necessary.
Oral-motor functioning	ability to inhibit abnormal oral reflexes	"Handling, positioning, and feeding the physically handicapped" "Feeding reflexes and neural control"
Cognitive Skills	level of sensorimotor development	*Albert Einstein Scales of Sensorimotor Development* *Assessment in Infancy: Ordinal Scales of Psychological Development*
	general intellectual abilities	*Arthur Adaptation of the Leiter International Performance Scale* (1952) ages: 2–18 years *Callier-Azusa Scale* (designed for deaf-blind and multiply handicapped) ages: birth to 9 years *Infant Cognitive Development Scale*, ages: 4–20 months
Functional Object Use	variety of action patterns used by the clients	Present a variety of objects and note whether client acts differently on different objects (e.g., does he or she put all objects in mouth?).
	appropriate use of objects	Present a variety of objects and note whether client acts on each according to its intended function (e.g., pushes truck, feeds self). "Training prerequisites"

*Items in this column include commercially available tools or assessment devices (italicized) and procedures that are described in chapters of books (in quotation marks). These materials are listed alphabetically at the end of this appendix.

Table D-2
Vocal Communication Assessment

Area	Goal(s) of Assessment	Procedures/Resources/Tools*
Speech Production Examination of the Oral Mechanism	To determine: structure and function of the oral mechanism	*Oral Speech Mechanism Screening Examination* Also see table D-1: Oral-Motor Functioning
Vocalization	spontaneous vocalizations	Observe during periods of high vocalization (e.g., bath time); chart types and frequency of vocalization. "Training prerequisites"
	vocal imitation	Imitate sounds the client makes and new sounds; chart imitation. "Training prerequisites" *Oliver: Parent-Administered Communication Inventory* *Environmental Prelanguage Battery*
Articulation	production of speech sounds in words, sentences, and conversational speech	Conduct conversational speech sampling, using procedures as in "Conversational speech behaviors." *Arizona Articulation Proficiency Scale* *Goldman-Fristoe Test of Articulation* *Templin-Darley Tests of Articulation*
Receptive Language Vocabulary	Identification of objects and actions	*Environmental Prelanguage Battery*
	identification of pictures	*Assessment of Children's Language Comprehension,* part A *Peabody Picture Vocabulary Test* *Vocabulary Comprehension Scale*
	understanding of basic concepts	*Boehm Test of Basic Concepts* *The Basic Concept Inventory*
Syntax	comprehension of syntactical forms	*Test for Auditory Comprehension of Language*
Directions	ability to follow directions with and without contextual support	*Environmental Prelanguage Battery* *Skelly Action Test of Auditory Reception of Language*
General Abilities, including the ones above	overall receptive language level	*Communication Assessment for the Non-verbal Pupil* *Sequenced Inventory of Communication Development*

Table D-2, continued

Area	Goal(s) of Assessment	Procedures/Resources/Tools*
Expressive Language Vocabulary	ability to label objects, actions, and pictures	*Preschool Language Scale* *Houston Test of Language Development*
Syntax and Semantic Relations	ability to use grammatical structures appropriately in two or more word utterances under imitative conditions	*Carrow Elicited Language Inventory* *Oral Language Sentence Imitation Diagnostic Inventory*
	ability to use grammatical structures appropriately in two or more word utterances under spontaneous or elicited conditions	*Clinical Oral Language Sampling* *Developmental Sentence Analysis*
Functional Use of Language	ability to integrate content, form, and use in structured or naturally-occurring situations	*Language Development and Language Disorders* (Chapters XI and XII)

*Items in this column include commercially available tools or assessment devices (italicized) and procedures that are described in chapters of books (in quotation marks). These materials are listed alphabetically at the end of this appendix.

Table D-3
Gestural Communication Assessment

Area	Goal(s) of Assessment	Procedures/Resources/Tools*
Motoric Control		
Hands	To determine: fine motor control voluntary control speed of hand movement motor imitation	Observe client in activities of daily living, such as buttoning, eating; see *Manual Language for the Child Without Language* *Oseretsky Tests of Motor Proficiency* *Teaching Research Motor-Development Scale for Moderately and Severely Retarded Children*
Arms	voluntary control and range of motion	Place an imaginary cup at person's midline 10″ from his body and instruct him to: lift 6″; extend by reaching; rotate as if to pour; pull back; cross midline; reposition if necessary (from *Assessment Battery for Assistive Device System Recommendations*, part 1
Facial Musculature	ability to portray emotions through facial expression	Observe on natural occasions (sad, happy, angry); ask client to pretend
Comprehension of Gestures		
Vocabulary	identification of gestures for objects, actions, and so forth	Observe client's responses to various signals, signs, or gestures, natural and formal *Sign Language Curricula (Level 1, Unit 1)* *Action Test for Amer-Ind Signal Comprehension*
Pre-Expression Skills		
Hand Preference	dominant hand, to be used for one-handed signs	Observe which hand the client uses in reaching for objects or supporting self
Functional Use of Objects	ability to demonstrate functional use of objects	Items from curricula may be used (e.g., "Curricular Strategies for Teaching Basic Functional Object Use to Severely Handicapped Students"
	ability to pantomime functional use of objects	Show client an object or picture and have him or her pantomime its use. Manual Expression Subtest, *Illinois Test of Psycholinguistic Abilities*
Motor Imitation	generalized and specific imitative skills	Items from curricula may be used (e.g., *West Virginia System Expressive Language Curriculum*)
Sign/Signal Imitation	ability to imitate specific signs or signals	Devise an imitation pre-test, consisting of 10–20 items; note the levels of prompting needed by the client.

Table D-3, continued

Area	Goal(s) of Assessment	Procedures/Resources/Tools*
Espression of Gestures		
Natural Gestures	ability to produce natural gestures which code meaning	Observe how client alerts others to needs and deires using gestures; obtain parental and teacher reports; structure situations in which client must use gestures to communicate.
Signs and Signals	ability to produce signs or signals which code meaning	Check for spontaneous use of signs or signals to which client has been exposed.
Visual Discrimination	ability to discriminate between different visual configurations (e.g., handshapes)	If client comprehends same/different concept, present pairs of gestures and have him or her judge whether they are the same or different.
Receptive Language	(see table D-2)	see table D-2

*Items in this column include commercially available tools or assessment devices (italicized) and procedures that are described in chapters of books (in quotation marks). These materials are listed alphabetically at the end of this appendix.

Table D-4

Symbolic Communication Assessment

Area	Goal(s) of Assessment	Procedures/Resources/Tools*
Motoric Skills Upper Extremities Face and neck Trunk and Lower Extremities	To determine: range of motion, speed, accuracy, and reliability of response for selecting input switch(es) and means of indicating	Procedures for evaluating accuracy, speed, force (etc.) are described in *Muscle Testing*; they are summarized in *Communication for the Speechless* *Assessment Battery for Assistive Device Systems Recommendations, part 1*
Visual Perceptual Skills	levels of development in skills such as figure-ground discrimination, position in space, perception of symbols in varying sizes	Experiment with symbols varying along the following dimensions: type (e.g., pictures, Bliss), size, location, boldness; see *West Virginia System: Expressive Language Curriculum* *Frostig Development Test of Visual Perception Assessment Battery*
Tracking and Scanning	(see table D-1, Visual Attention)	see table D-1, Visual Attention
Receptive Language	(see table D-2, Receptive Language)	see table D-2, receptive language
Visual Matching	ability to match object to object, object to object, object to symbol, symbol to symbol	Present objects and their symbolic representation (pictures, words) for client to match.
Reception of Symbols	ability to comprehend that symbols represent objects, actions, emotions, and so forth	Present array of symbols and have client indicate the one named or demonstrated (i.e., through pantomime); for orthographic symbols (e.g., words), this may be extended to include reading vocabulary through a sentence completion test (see *Assessment Battery for Assertive Device Systems Recommendations, part 1*)
Expression through symbols	ability to communicate desires, information, and so forth through symbols, as well as to demonstrate skills of sequencing, encoding, etc.	Make symbol system accessible to client and observe whether he or she uses it responsively or spontaneously. *Assessment Battery for Assistive Device Systems Recommendations, part 1, Cognitive/Language Level Module.*
Selection of Communication Aid	preferences and needs of teacher, therapist, parent and client regarding various device options	*Assessment Battery for Assistive Device Systems Recommendations, part 1, Device Characteristics Module.*

*Items in this column include commercially available tools or assessment devices (italicized) and procedures that are described in chapters of books (in quotation marks). These materials are listed alphabetically at the end of this appendix.

Listing of References and
Assessment Devices Cited in Appendix D

Action Test of Amer-Ind Signal Comprehension (1979), Skelly, M.; In Skelly, M. and Schinsky, L., *Amer-Ind Gestural Code Based on Universal American Indian Hand Talk*; Elsevier North Holland, Inc., 52 Vanderbilt Avenue, New York, NY 10017.

Albert Einstein Scales of Sensorimotor Development (1969), Corman, H.H. and Escolona, S.K.; Albert Einstein College of Medicine, Child Development Project, 1165 Morris Park Avenue, Bronx, NY 10461.

An Assessment Battery for Assistive Device System Recommendations. part I (1980), Meyers, L.S., Grows, N.L., Coleman, C.L., and Cook, A.M.; Assistive Device Center, California State University, Sacramento, Sacramento, CA 95819.

Arizona Articulation Proficiency Scale (1974), Fudala, J.B.; Western Psychological Services, 12031 Wilshire Boulevard, Los Angeles, CA 90025.

Arthur Adaptation of the Leiter International Performance Scale (1952), Arthur, G.; The Psychological Service Center Press, Washington, D.C.

Assessment in Infancy: Ordinal Scales of Psychological Development (1975), Uzgiris, I.C. and Hunt, J.; University of Illinois Press, Urbana, IL 61801.

Assessment of Children's Language Comprehension (1969, 1973), Foster, R., Giddan, J., and Stark, J.; Consulting Psychologists Press, Inc., 577 College Avenue, Palo Alto, CA 94306.

The Basic Concept Inventory (1967), Engelmann, S.E.; Follett Educational Corporation, P.O. Box 5705 (Dept. DM), 1010 West Washington Blvd., Chicago, IL 60607.

Boehm Test of Basic Concepts (1969, 1971), Boehm, A.; Psychological Corporation, 304 East 45th Street, New York, NY 10017.

Callier-Azusa Scale (1975), Stillman, R.; Callier Centre for Communication Disorders, University of Texas, 1966 Inwood Road, Dallas, TX 75235.

Carrow Elicited Language Inventory (1974), Carrow, E.; Learning Concepts, 2501 North Lamar, Austin, TX 78705.

Clinical Oral Language Sampling, (1978) Barrie-Blackley, S., Musselwhite, C.R., and Rogister, S.H.; Interstate Printers and Publishers, 19-27 North Jackson Street, Danville, IL 61832.

Communication Assessment for the Non-Verbal Pupil, Soltman, S., In *Educational Methods for Deaf-Blind and Severely Handicapped Student, vol. 1*; Texas Education Agency, Special Education Developmental Services Center for Deaf-Blind, 201 East Eleventh Street, Austin, TX 78701.

Communication for the Speechless, Chapter 7 (1980), Silverman, F.; Prentice-Hall, Inc., Englewood Cliffs, NJ 07632.

"Conversational speech behaviors" (1979), Faircloth, M.A. and Blasdell, R.C.; In Lass, N.J., ed. *Speech and Language: Advances in Basic Research and Practice*, vol. 2; Academic Press, 111 Fifth Avenue, New York, NY 10003.

"Curricular strategies for teaching basic functional object use to severely handicapped students" (1977), Lyon, S., Baumgart, D., Stoll, A., and Brown, L.; In L. Brown, J. Nietupski, S. Lyon, S. Hamre-Nietupski, T. Crowner, and L. Gruenewald, eds. *Curricular Strategies for Teaching Non-verbal Communication, Functional Object Use, and Problem Solving Skills to Severely Handicapped Students*, vol. VIII, part 1; Department of Specialized Educational Services, Madison, WI.

Developmental Sentence Analysis (1974), Lee, L.L.; Northwestern University Press, 1735 Benson Avenue, Evanston, IL 60201.

Diagnosis of Speech and Language Disorders (1977), Nation, J.F. and Aram, A.M.; The C.V. Mosby Company, St. Louis, MO.

Diagnostic Handbook of Speech Pathology (1979), Hutchinson, B.B., Hanson, M.L., and Mecham, M.J.; Williams and Wilkins Company, Baltimore, MD.

Environmental Prelanguage Battery (1978), Horstmeier, D.S. and MacDonald, J.D.; Charles E. Merrill Publishing Co., 1300 Alum Creek Drive, Columbus, OH 43216.

Evaluation of Appraisal Techniques in Speech and Language Pathology (1979), F.L. Darley, ed.; Addison-Wesley Publishing Company, Reading, MA.

"Feeding reflexes and neural control." (1978), Radtka, S.; In J. Wilson, ed. *Oral-Motor Function and Dysfunction in Children*; Division of Physical Therapy, Chapel Hill, NC 27514.

Frostig Developmental Test of Visual Perception, rev. ed. (1966), Frostig, M.; Consulting Psychologists Press, Inc., 577 College Avenue, Palo Alto, CA 94306.

Goldman-Fristoe Test of Articulation (1972), Goldman, R. and Fristoe, M.; American Guidance Service, Inc., Publishers Building, Circle Pines, MN 55014.

"Handling, positioning, and feeding the physically handicapped" (1977), Utley, B.L., Holvoet, J.F., and Barnes, K.; In E. Sontag, ed. *Educational Programming for the Severely and Profoundly Handicapped*; Division on Mental Retardation, Council for Exceptional Children, 1920 Association Drive, Reston, VA 22091.

The Houston Test of Language Development (1958, 1963), Crabtree, M.; Houston Test Company, P.O. Box 35152, Houston, TX 77035.

Illinois Test of Psycholinguistic Abilities (1961, 1968), Kirk, S.A., McCarthy, J.J., and Kirk, W.D.; University of Illinois Press, Urbana, IL 61801.

Infant Cognitive Development Scale (1971), Mehrabian, A. and Williams, M.; In *Journal of Psycholinguistic Research* 1: 113–26.

Language Development and Language Disorders (1978), Bloom, L. and Lahey, M.; John Wiley and Sons, New York, NY.

Manual Language for the Child Without Language (1975), Wilson, P.S., Goodman, L., and Wood, R.K.; Eric Grossman, 14 Keefe Lane, Middletown, CT 06457.

Muscle Testing: Techniques of Manual Examination, 3rd ed. (1972), Daniels, L. and Worthingham, C.; W.B. Saunders, Philadelphia, PA.

Oliver: Parent-Administered Communication Inventory (1978), MacDonald, J.D.; Charles E. Merrill Publishing Co., 1300 Alum Creek Road, Columbus, OH 43216.

Oral Language Sentence Imitation Diagnostic Inventory (1977), Zachman, L., Huisingh, R., Jorgenson, C., and Barrett, M.; LinguiSystems, Suite 806, 1630 Fifth Avenue, Moline, IL 61265.

Oral Speech Mechanism Screening Examination (1981), St. Louis, K.O. and Ruscello, D.M.; University Park Press, Baltimore, MD.

Oseretsky Tests of Motor Proficiency (1964), Doll, E.A. ed.; American Guidance Service, Inc., Publishers Building, Circle Pines, MN 55014.

Peabody Picture Vocabulary Test (1959, 1965), Dunn, L.M.; American Guidance Service, Inc., Publishers Building, MN 55014.

Preschool Language Scale (1969), Zimmerman, I.L., Steiner, V.G., and Evatt, R.I.; Charles E. Merrill Publishing Co., 1300 Alum Creek Drive, Columbus, OH 43216.

"Sensorimotor functions and cognitive development" (1978), Robinson, C.C. and Robinson, J.H.; In M.E. Snell, ed. *Systematic Instruction of the Moderately and Severely Handicapped*, pp. 102–53; Charles E. Merrill Publishing, 1300 Alum Creek Drive, Columbus, OH 43216.

Sequenced Inventory of Communication Development (1975), Hedrick, D.L., Procther, E.M., and Tobin, A.R.; University of Washington Press, Seattle, WA.

Sign Language Curricula (1978), Robbins, N.; New England Regional Center for Services to Deaf-Blind Children, Perkins School for the Blind, Watertown, MA.

Skelly Comparative Apraxia Text: Oral and Manual (1979), Skelly, M.; In Skelly, M. and Schinsky, L., *Amer-Ind Gestural Code Based on Universal American Indian Hand Talk*; Elsevier North Holland, 52 Vanderbilt Avenue, New York, NY 10017.

Skelly Action Test of Auditory Reception of Language (SATAR) (1979), Skelly, M.; In Skelly, M. and Schinsky, L., *Amer-Ind Gestural Code Based on Universal American Indian Hand Talk*; Elsevier North Holland, Inc., 52 Vanderbilt Avenue, New York, NY 10017.

"Speech performance, dysphagia and oral reflexes in cerebral palsy" (1980), Love, R.J., Hagerman, E.L., and Taimi, E.G.; In *J. Speech Hear. Dis.* 45: 59–75.

Teaching Research Motor-Development Scale for Moderately and Severely Retarded Children (1972), Charles C Thomas; Springfield, IL 62717.

The Templin-Darley Tests of Articulation, 2d ed. (1969), Templin, M.C. and Darley, F.L.; University of Iowa Bureau of Educational Research and Service, Extension Division, C-20 East Hall, Iowa City, IA 52242.

Test for Auditory Comprehension of Language (1970), Carrow, E.; Learning Concepts, 2501 North Lamar, Austin, TX 78705.

"Training prerequisites to verbal behavior" (1978), Bricker, D. and Dennison, L.; In M.E. Snell, ed. *Systematic Instruction of the Moderately and Severely Handicapped*; Charles E. Merrill Publishing Company, 1300 Alum Creek Drive, Columbus, OH 43216.

Vocabulary Comprehension Scale (1976), Bangs, T.E.; Learning Concepts, 2501 North Lamar, Austin, TX 78705.

West Virginia System Expressive Language Curriculum (1980), St. Louis, K., Rejzer, R., and Cone, J.D.; Department of Psychology, Oglebay Hall, West Virginia University, Morgantown, WV 26506.

The West Virginia Assessment and Tracking System (WVAATS) (1978), Cone, J.D.; (Unpublished manuscript, available from author) Department of Psychology, Oglebay Hall, West Virginia University, Morgantown, WV 26506.

References

Abkarian, G.G., Dworkin, J.P., and Brown, S.R. 1978. An adventitiously non-verbal child: Signed English as a transitional step in Reye's Syndrome. A paper presented at the American Speech-Language-Hearing Association Convention, San Francisco, CA.

Allen, J. 1977. *The other side of the elephant: Theatre activities for classroom learning.* Buffalo, NY: DOK Publishers, Inc.

Allen, K., Holm, V., and Schiefelbusch, R. 1978. *Early intervention—A team approach.* Baltimore, MD: University Park Press.

Alpert, C. 1980. Procedures for determining the optimal nonspeech mode with the autistic child. In *Nonspeech language and communication: Analysis and intervention,* ed. R.L. Schiefelbush. Baltimore, MD: University Park Press, 389–420.

American Indian Sign 1974. A video-cassette distributed by the Learning Resources Center, Veterans Administration Hospital, St. Louis, MO.

Amerind video dictionary 1974. A series of four videocassettes distributed by the Learning Resources Center, Veterans Administration Hospital, St. Louis, MO.

Anderson. J.D. 1980. Spatial arrangement of stimuli and the construction of communication boards for the physically handicapped. *Ment. Retard.* 18: 41–42.

Anthony, D. 1966. Seeing Essential English. Unpublished manuscript, Ypsilanti, MI.

Anthony, D. 1971. *Seeing essential english,* vols. 1 and 2. Anaheim, CA: Educational Services Division, Anaheim Union School District.

Apffel, J.A., Kelleher, J., Lilly, M.S., and Richardson, R. 1975. Developmental reading for moderately retarded children. *Ed. Train. Ment. Retard.* 10: 229–36.

Arnold, L.E. ed. 1978. *Helping parents help their children.* New York: Brunner/Mazel Publishers.

ARRL code kit. Newington, CT: The American-Radio Relay League (no date).

ASHA Task Force, 1980. *A report on third-party reimbursement of speech-language pathology and audiology services.* Rockville, MD: American Speech-Language-Hearing Association.

Ashcroft, S.C. and Henderson, F. 1963. *Programmed instruction in Braille.* Pittsburgh, PA: Stanwik House, Inc.

Ashton-Warner, S. 1971. *Teacher.* New York: Bantam.

Auenback, A. 1968. *Parents learn through group discussion: Principles and protection of parent group education.* New York: John Wiley.

(Anon.) 1979. Autocuer feasibility study. *Cued Speech News.* Washington, D.C.: Office of Cued Speech Programs, Gallaudet College.

Azrin, N.H., Kaplan, S.J., and Foxx, R.M. 1973. Autism reversal: Eliminating stereotyped self-stimulation of retarded individuals. *Am. J. Ment. Deficiency* 78: 241–48.

Babbini, B.E. 1974a. *Manual communication: Fingerspelling and the language of signs. A course of study outlines for instructors.* Urbana, IL: University of Illinois Press.

Babbini, B.E. 1974b. *Manual communication: Fingerspelling and the language of signs. A course of study for students.* Urbana, IL: University of Illinois Press.

Baer, D.M. 1978. The behavioral analysis of trouble. In *Early intervention—A team approach,* eds. K.E. Allen, V.A. Holm, and R.L. Schiefelbusch. Baltimore, MD: University Park Press, 57–93.

Baer, D.M., Peterson, R., and Sherman, J. 1967. The development of imitation by reinforcing behavioral similarity to a model. *J. Exper. Anal. Beh.* 10:405–16.

Baker, B.L. 1976. Parent involvement in programming for the developmentally disabled. In *Communication assessment and intervention strategies,* ed. L.L. Lloyd. Baltimore, MD: University Park Press, 691–733.

Baker, C. and Padden, C.A. 1978a. *American Sign Language: A look at its history, structure and community.* Silver Spring, MD: T. J. Publishers, Inc.

Baker, C. and Padden, C.A. 1978b. Focusing on nonmanual components of American Sign Language. In *Understanding language through sign language research,* ed. P. Siple. New York: Academic Press, 27–57.

Balick, S., Spiegel, A. and Greene, G. 1976. Mime in language therapy and clinician training. *Arch. Phys. Med. and Rehab.* 57:35–38.

Bannatyne, A.D. 1968. *Psycholinguistic color system: A reading, writing, spelling and language program.* Urbana, IL: Learning Systems Press.

Barrie-Blackley, S., Musselwhite, C., and Rogister, S. 1978. *Clinical oral language sampling.* Danville, IL: The Interstate Printers and Publishers.

Bassin, J. and Kreeb, D.D. 1978. *Reaching out to parents of newly diagnosed retarded children.* St. Louis, MO: St. Louis Association for Retarded Children.

Bates, E. 1976. *Language and context: The aquisition of pragmatics.* New York: Academic Press.

Beadles, R.L. and Brown, J.N. 1979. A feasibility study for the development of a speech autocuer. Final report (NASA Contract No. NAS5-25541), Research Triangle Park, NC.

Beck, R. 1977. Interdisciplinary model: Planning distribution and ancillary input to classrooms for the severely/profoundly handicapped. In *Educational programming for the severely and profoundly handicapped,* ed. E. Sontag. Reston, VA: Division on Mental Retardation, Council for Exceptional Children, 397–404.

Bender, M. and Valletutti, P.J. 1976a. *Teaching the moderately and severely handicapped: Behavior, self-care and motor skills,* vol. I. Baltimore, MD: University Park Press.

Bender, M. and Valletutti, P.J. 1976b. *Teaching the moderately and severely handicapped,* vol. II. Baltimore, MD: University Park Press.

Bender, M., Valletutti, P.J., and Bender, R. 1976. *Teaching the moderately and severely handicapped:* vol. III. Baltimore, MD: University Park Press.

Beukelman, D.R. and Yorkston, K. 1977. A communication system for the severely dysarthric speaker with an intact language system. *J. Speech Hear. Dis.* 42: 265–70.

Beukelman, D.R. and Yorkston, K.M. 1980. Nonvocal communication: Performance Evaluation. *Arch. Phys. Med. Rehab.* 61: 272–75.

Bigge, J.L. 1977. Severe communication problems. In *Teaching individuals with physical and multiple disabilities,* eds. J.L. Bigge and P.A. O'Donnell. Columbus, OH: Charles E. Merrill, 104–36.

Bliss, C.K. 1965. *Semantography—Blissymbolics.* Sydney, Australia: Semantography Publications.

Bliss, C.K. and McNaughton, S. 1975. *The book to the film: "Mr. Symbol Man."* Sydney, Australia: Semantography Publications.

Bloom, L. and Lahey, M. 1978. *Language development and language disorders.* New York: John Wiley and Sons.

Bluma, S., Shearer, M., Frohman, A., and Hillard, J. 1976. *Portage guide to early education.* Portage, WI: Cooperative Educational Services.

Bonvillian, J.D. and Nelson, K.E. 1976. Sign language acquisition in a mute autistic boy. *J. Speech Hear. Dis.* 41:339–47.

Bonvillian, J.D. and Nelson, K.E. 1978. Development of sign language in autistic children and other language handicapped individuals. In *Understanding language through sign language research,* ed. P. Siple. New York: Academic Press.

Bornstein, H. 1973. A description of some current sign systems designed to represent English. *Am. Ann. Deaf* 118: 454–63.

Bornstein, H. 1974. Signed English: A manual approach to English language. *J. Speech Hear. Dis.* 39: 330–43.

Bornstein, H. 1979. Systems of sign. In *Hearing and hearing impairment*, eds. L.J. Bradford and W.G. Hardy. New York: Grune and Stratton Inc.

Bornstein, H., Hamilton, L.B., Saulnier, K.L. and Roy, H.L., eds. 1975. *The signed english dictionary for preschool and elementary levels*. Washington, D.C.: Gallaudet College Press.

Bornstein, H., Saulnier, K., and Hamilton, L. 1979. Signed English: A first evaluation. *Am. Ann. Deaf* 125:467–81.

Borrild, K. 1972. Cued Speech and the mouth-hand system. In *International symposium on speech communication ability and profound deafness*, ed. G. Fant. Washington, D. C.: A. G. Bell Association for the Deaf.

Bove, L. 1980. *Sesame street sign language fun*. New York: Random House.

Bosma, J.F. 1975. Anatomic and physiologic development of the speech apparatus. In *The nervous system: Human communication and its disorders*, vol. 3, ed. D.B. Tower. New York: Raven Press

(Anon.) 1978. *Braille instruction and writing equipment*. Washington, D. C.: National Library Service for the Blind and Physically Handicapped.

Bricker, W. and Bricker, D. 1974. An early language training strategy. In *Language perspectives—Acquisition, retardation and intervention*, eds. R. Schiefelbusch and L. Lloyd. Baltimore, MD: University Park Press, 431–68.

Bricker, D.D. and Dennison, L. 1978. Training prerequisites to verbal behavior. In *Systematic instruction of the moderately and severely handicapped*, ed. M.E. Snell. Columbus, OH: Charles E. Merrill Company, 157–78.

Bricker, D.D., Dennison, L., and Bricker, W.A. 1975. Constructive interaction—adaptation approach to language training. *MCCD Monograph Series No. 1*. Mailman Center for Child Development, Miami, Florida: University of Miami.

Bricker, D.D., Dennison, L., Watson, L., and Vincent-Smith, L. 1973. *Language training program for developmentally delayed children*. Nashville, TN: Institute on Mental Retardation and Intellectual Development Publications.

Bricker, D.D., Ruder, K.F., Vincent, L. 1976. An intervention strategy for language-deficient children. In *Teaching special children* eds. N.G. Haring and F.L. Phillips. New York: McGraw-Hill.

Brown, H.E.D. 1979. Developing reliable physical responses in non-vocal children for use with communication devices. A paper presented at the American Speech-Language-Hearing Association Convention, Atlanta, GA.

Brown, L., Nietupski, J., and Hamre-Nietupski, S. 1976. Criterion of ultimate functioning. In *Hey, don't forget about me*, ed. M.A. Thomas. Reston, VA: The Council for Exceptional Children, 2–15.

Brown, R. 1973. *A first language*. Cambridge, MA: Harvard University Press.

Cansler, D., Martin, G. and Valand, M. 1975. *Working with families*. Winston-Salem, NC: Kaplan Press.

Carlson, F. and James, C.A. *Picsyms Dictionary* (in progress).

Carlson, F. and James, C.A. 1980. Picsyms system and symbol system, unpublished paper.

Carr, E.G., Binkoff, J.A., Kologinsky, E., and Eddy, M. 1978. Acquisition of sign language by autistic children: Expressive labelling. *J. Appl. Beh. Anal.* 11: 489–510.

Carrier, J.K. Jr. 1974. Application of functional analysis and a nonspeech response mode to teaching language. In *Developing systematic procedures for training children's language*, ed. L.V. McReynolds. ASHA Monograph 18.

Carrier, J.K., Jr. 1976. Application of a nonspeech language system with the severely language handicapped. In *Communication assessment and intervention strategies*, ed. L.L. Lloyd. Baltimore, MD: University Park Press, 523–47.

Carrier, J.K. Jr. and Peak, T. 1975. *Non-speech language initiation program (Non-Slip)*, Lawrence, KS: H. and H. Enterprises.

(Anon.) 1979. *Catalog of federal domestic assistance*. Washington, D. C.: Superintendent of Documents, United States Government Printing Office.

Chapman, R.S. 1974. Discussion summary: Developmental relationship between receptive and expressive language. In *Language perspectives—Acquisition, retardation, and intervention*, eds. R.L. Schiefelbusch and L.L. Lloyd. Baltimore, MD: University Park Press, 335–44.

Chapman, R.S. and Miller, J.F. 1975. Early two and three word utterances: Does production preceded comprehension. *J. Speech Hear. Res.* 18: 355–71.

Chapman, R.S. and Miller, J.F. 1980. Analyzing language and communication in the child. In *Nonspeech language and communication: Analysis and intervention*, ed. R.L. Schiefelbusch. Baltimore, MD: University Park Press, 159–96.

Chappell, G.E. and Johnson, G.A. 1976. Evaluation of cognitive behavior in the young child. *Lang. speech, hear. serv. schools* 7 : 17–27.

Chen, L.Y. 1971. Manual communication by combined alphabet and gestures. *Arch. Phys. Med. Rehab.* 52: 381–84.

Chen, L.Y. 1968. "Talking Hands" for aphasic patients. *Geriatrics* 23: 145–48.

Christopher, D.A. 1976. *Manual communication*. Baltimore, MD: University Park Press.

Clark, C.R. 1977. Research Report # 107: A comparative study of young children's ease of learning words represented in the graphic systems of Rebus, Bliss, Carrier-Peak and traditional orthography. Unpublished paper, Minneapolis, MN: Research, Development and Demonstration Center in Education of Handicapped Children.

Clark, C.R., Davies, C.O., and Woodcock, R.W. 1974. *Standard rebus glossary*. Circle Pines, MN: American Guidance Service.

Clark, C.R. and Greco, J.A. 1973. *MELDS glossary of rebuses and signs*. Minneapolis, MN: Research, Development and Demonstration Center in Education of Handicapped Children.

Clark, C.R., Moores, D.F., and Woodcock, R.W. 1975. *The minnesota early language development sequence*. Minneapolis, MN: Research, Development and Demonstration Center in Education of Handicapped Children.

Clark, C.R. and Woodcock, R.W. 1976. Graphic systems of communication. In *Communication assessment and intervention strategies*, ed. L.L. Lloyd. Baltimore, MD: University Park Press, 549–605.

Clark, W.P. 1885. *Indian sign languages*. Philadelphia, PA: L. R. Hammersley and Company.

Clarke, B.R. and Ling, D. 1976. The effects of using Cued Speech: A follow-up study. *Volta Rev.* 78: 23–34.

Cohen, C., Montgomery, J., and Yoder, D. 1979. *Phonic Mirror HandiVoice seminar manual*. Mill Valley, CA: H. C. Electronics, Inc.

Cohen, M., Gross, P., and Haring, N.G. 1976. Developmental pinpoints. In *Teaching the severely handicapped*, vol. 1, eds. N.G. Haring and L. Brown. New York: Grune and Stratton, 35–110.

Committee on Supportive Personnel 1979. *American Speech and Hearing Association, Guidelines for the employment and utlization of supportive personnel in audiology and speech-language pathology. Asha* 21: 980–84.

Copeland, K., ed. 1974. *Aids for the severely handicapped*. New York: Grune and Stratton.

Cornett, R.O. 1967. Cued Speech. *Am. ann. Deaf* 112: 3–13.

Cornett, R.O. 1974. The learning of English by the deaf. *Teaching english to the deaf*. Washington, D. C.: Gallaudet Colelge English Department.

Cornett, R.O. 1975. Cued Speech and oralism: An analysis. *Audiol. Hear. Ed.* 1: 26–33.

Cornett, R.O. 1978. If you have a deaf child. Washington, D. C.: Gallaudet College, Office of Cued Speech Programs.

Cornett, R.O. 1979. What? When? How? Some answers to parents questions about kids' speech. *Cued Speech News* 12: 4–5.

Craig, E. 1976. A supplement to the spoken word—The Paget-Gorman sign system. In *Methods of communication currently used in the education of deaf children*, ed. Royal National Institute for the Deaf. Letchworth, England: The Garden City Press.

Creech, R. 1979. Utilizing the Phonic Mirror Handi-Voice in communication programming. A workshop. Atlanta, GA.

Crickmay, M. 1966. *Speech therapy and the Bobath approach to cerebral palsy*. Springfield, IL: Charles C. Thomas.

(Anon.) 1979. *Cued Speech News*, no. 5. Washington, D.C.: Office of Cued Speech Programs, Gallaudet College.

Dalgaard, J., Newhoff, M., and Barnes, G. 1979. "Show Me...": Enhancing receptive and expressive language through pantomime. A paper presented at the American Speech-Language-Hearing Association Convention, Atlanta, GA.

De Haven, D. 1978. The nonoral evaluation. *Communicat. Outlook* 1: 8.

Deich, R.F. and Hodges, P.M. 1978. *Language without speech*. New York: Brunner/Mazel.

De Pape, D. 1980. Communication aids and systems clinic. Unpublished paper, Communication Aids and Systems Clinic, University of Wisconsin Hospital and Clinics, Center for Health Sciences, Madison, WI.

Dolan, E.T. and Burton, L.F. 1976. *The Severely and profoundly handicapped: A practical approach to teaching*. New York: Grune & Stratton.

Duffy, L. 1977. An innovative approach to the development of communication skills for severely speech handicapped cerebral palsied children. Master's Thesis, University of Nevada, Las Vegas, NV.

Dunn, L.M. 1959. *Peabody picture vocabulary test*. Circle Pines, MN: American Guidance Services, Inc.

Dunn, L.M. and Smith, J.E. 1969. *Peabody language development kits: Level P, I, II, III*. Circle Pines, MN: American Guidance Service.

Dunn, M.L. 1979. An analysis of the motor component of imitative sign production. A miniseminar presented at the American Speech-Language-Hearing Association Convention, Atlanta, GA.

Ebert, R.S. 1979. A training program for community residence staff. *Ment. Retard.* 17: 257-59.

Eichler, J. 1975. ETRAN Eye Signalling System, Preliminary annotated bibliography of communication aids no. 22. In *Participants resource book on non-vocal communication techniques and aids*. Madison, WI: Cerebral Palsy Communication Group, University of Wisconsin.

Elder, P. 1978. *Visual symbol communication instruction: Part I, receptive instruction*. Birmingham, AL: DESEMO Project.

Elder, P. and Bergman, J. 1978. Visual symbol communication instruction with non-verbal, multiply-handicapped individuals. *Ment. Retard.* 16: 107-12.

Enderby, P. and Hamilton, G. 1979. 'SPLINK'—A new communication aid for the speech handicapped and deaf. A paper presented to the National Rehabilitation Association of America Conference, Chicago, IL.

Englemann, S. and Osborn, J. 1976. *Distar language I*. Chicago, IL: Science Research Associates, Inc.

Fant, L.J. 1977. *Sign language*. Joyce Motion Picture Company.

Fantz, R.L. and Nevis, S. 1967. The predictive value of changes in visual preferences in early infancy. In *Exceptional infant: The normal infant*, ed. J. Hellmuth. New York: Bruner/Mazel.

Fitzgerald, E. 1949. *Straight language for the deaf*. Washington, D.C.: The Volta Bureau.

Flavell, J.E., Flavell, J.E., and McGimsey, J.F. 1978. Relative effectiveness and efficiency of group vs. individual training of severely retarded persons. *Am. J. Ment. Deficiency* 83: 104-9.

Fothergill, J., Luster-Carpenter, M.J., Vanderheiden, G.C., and Holt, C.S. 1978. Illustrated digest of non-vocal communication and writing aid for severely, physically handicapped individuals. In *Non-vocal communication resource book*, ed. G.C. Vanderheiden. Baltimore, MD: University Park Press.

Foxx, R.M. and Azrin, N.H. 1973a. The elimination of self-stimulatory behavior by overcorrection. *J. Appl. Beh. Anal.* 6: 1–14.

Foxx, R.M. and Azrin, N.H. 1973b. *Toilet training the retarded.* Champaign, IL: Research Press.

Fredericks, H.D.B., Riggs, C., Furey, T., Grove, D., Moore, W., McDonnell, J., Jordon, E., Hanson, W., Baldwin, Y., and Wadlow, M. 1976. *The teaching research Motor Development Scale for moderately and severely Retarded.* Springfield, IL: Charles C. Thomas.

Frishberg, N. 1979. Historical change: From iconic to arbitary. In *The signs of language*, eds. E.S. Klima and U. Bellugi. Cambridge, MA: Harvard University Press, 67–83.

Fristoe, M. 1975. *Language intervention systems for the retarded: A catalog of original structured language programs in use in the U. S.* Montgomery, AL: State of Alabama, Department of Education.

Fristoe, M. and Lloyd, L.L. 1977. Manual communication for the retarded and others with severe communication impairment: A resource list. *Ment. Retard.* 15: 18–21.

Fristoe, M. and Lloyd, L.L. 1978. A survey of the use of non-speech communication systems with the severely communication impaired. *Ment. Retard.* 16: 99–103.

Fristoe, M. and Lloyd, L.L. 1979. Signs used in manual communication training with persons having severe communication impairments. *AAESPH Rev.* 4: 364–73.

Fristoe, M. and Lloyd, L.L. 1980. Planning an initial expressive sign lexicon for persons having severe communication impairment. *J. Speech Hear. Dis.* 45: 170–90.

Fristoe, M., Lloyd, L., and Wilbur, R. 1977. Non-speech communication systems and symbols. A short course presented at the American Speech-Language-Hearing Association Convention, Chicago, IL.

Fry, E. B. 1964. A diacritical marking system to aid beginning reading instruction. *Elemen. Engineering* 41: 526–29.

Fulwiler, R. and Fouts, R. 1976. Acquisition of sign language by a non-communicating, autistic child. *J. Aut. Child. Schiz.* 6: 43–51.

Gagne, R.M. 1965. *Conditions of learning.* New York: Holt, Rinehart, and Winston.

Garcia, E. and De Haven, E. 1974. Use of operant techniques in the establishment and generalization of language. : A review and analysis. *Am. J. Ment. Deficiency* 79: 169–78.

Gardner, H., Zurif, E., Berry, T., and Baker, E. 1975. Visual communication in aphasia. Unpublished manuscript, Aphasia Research Center, Boston, University School of Medicine and Psychology Service, Boston Veterans Administration Center, Boston, MA.

Gaylord-Ross, J. 1977. The development of treatment technqiues for the remedication of self-injurious behavior in the classroom and home. Annual Reports, N. Y. Bureau of Education for the handicapped, Washington, D. C.

Gershon, M. and Biller, H.B. 1977. *The other helpers: Professionals and non-professionals in mental health.* Lexington, MA: D. C. Heath.

Giddings, W., Norton, J., Nelson, P., McNaughton, S., and Reich, P. 1979. Development of a Blissymbol Terminal: An interactive TV display to enhance communication for the physically handicapped. A paper presented at the 6th Man-Computer Communications Conference, Ottawa, Canada.

Ginsburg, H. and Opper, S. 1969. *Piaget's theory of intellectual development: An introduction.* Englewood Cliffs, NJ: Prentice-Hall, Inc.

Goddard, C. 1977. Application of symbols with deaf children. *Blissymbolics, Communication Institute Newsletter*, no. 3.

Golbin, A. 1977. Breathing and Speech. In *Cerebral palsy and communication: What parents can do*, ed. A. Golbin. Washington, D. C.: George Washington University, 63–76.

Goodenough-Trepagnier, C. 1978. Language development of children without articulate speech. In *Recent advances in the psychology of language: Part A, language and mother-child interaction*, ed. R.N. Campbell and P. Smith. New York: Plenum Press, 421–26.

Goodenough-Trepagnier, C. and Deser, T. 1980. Rate of output with a SPEEC non-vocal communication board. A paper presented at the International Conference on Rehabilitation Engineering, Toronto, Canada.

Goodenough-Trepagnier, C. and Prather, P. In press. Communication systems for the non-vocal, based on frequent phoneme sequences. *J. Speech and Hear. Dis.* (in press).

Goodenough-Trepagnier, C. and Prather, P. 1979. *Manual for teachers of SPEEC.* Boston, MA: Biomedical Engineering Center, Tufts-New England Medical Center.

Goodman, L., Wilson, P.S., and Bornstein, H. 1978. Results of a national survey of sign language programs in special education. *Ment. Retard.* 16: 104-6.

Goodrich, E. 1979. Modern voice generation techniques. *Communicat. Outlook* 2: 6.

Gray, B. and Ryan, B. 1973. *A language program for the non-language child.* Champaign, IL: Research Press.

Greenberger, S.M. and Thum, S.R. 1975. *S.T.E.P.: Sequential testing and educational programming.* San Rafael, CA: Academic Therapy Publications.

Grinnell, M.F., Detamore, K.L., and Lipke, B.A. 1976. Sign it successful—Manual English encourages expressive communication. *Teach. Except. Child.* 8: 123-24.

Guess, D., Keogh, W., and Sailor, W. 1978. Generalization of speech and language behavior. In *Bases of language intervention*, eds. R. Schiefelbusch and L. Lloyd. Baltimore, MD: University Park Press.

Guess, D. Sailor, W., and Baer, D. 1974. To teach language to retarded children. In *Language perspectives—Acquisition, retardation and intervention*, eds. R. Schiefelbusch and L. Lloyd. Baltimore, MD: University Park Press, 529-63.

Guess, D., Sailor, W., and Baer, D. 1976. *Functional speech and language training for the severely handicapped.* Lawrence, KS: H. and H. Enterprises.

Guess, D., Sailor, W., and Baer, D. 1977. A behavioral-remedial approach to language training for the severely handicapped. In *Educational programming for the severely and profoundly handicapped*, ed. E. Sontag. Reston, VA: Division on Mental Retardation, Council for Exceptional Children, 360-77.

Guess, D., Sailor, W., and Baer, D. 1978. Children with limited language. In *Language intervention strategies*, ed. R.L. Schiefelbusch. Baltimore, MD: University Park Press. 101-43.

Guess, D., Sailor, W., Rutherford, G., and Baer, D. 1968. An experimental analysis of linguistic development: The productive use of the plural morpheme. *J. of Appl. Beh. Anal.* 1:225-35.

Gustason, G., Pfetzing, D., and Zawolkow, E. 1980. *Signing exact english.* Silver Spring, MD: Modern Signs Press.

Hall, S.M., O'Grady, R.S., and Talkington, L.W. 1978. *Communication board training program for multihandicapped.* Portland, OR: Zygo Industries, Inc.

Halliday, M.A.K. 1973. *Explorations in the functions of language.* London: Edward Arnold.

Hamblin, K. 1978. *Mime: A playbook of silent fantasy.* Garden City, NY: Dolphin Books.

Hamre-Nietupski, S., Stoll, A., Holtz, K., Fullerton, P., Ryan-Flottum, M., and Brown, L. 1977. Curricular strategies for teaching selected nonverbal communication skills to nonverbal and verbal severely handicapped students. In *Curricular strategies for teaching functional object use, nonverbal communication, problem solving and mealtime skills to severely handicapped students*, vol. VII, part 1, eds. L. Brown, J. Nietupski, S. Lyon, S. Hamre-Nietupski, T. Crowner, and L. Grunewald. Madison, WI: Department of Specialized Educational Services, Madison Metropolitan School District, 94-250.

Harris, D. 1978. Descriptive analysis of communication interaction processes involving non-vocal, severely physically handicapped children. Ph. D. Dissertation, University of Wisconsin, Madison, WI.

Harris, D. and Vanderheiden, G. 1980. Enhancing the development of communicative interaction. In *Nonspeech language and communication: Analysis and intervention*, ed. R. Schiefelbusch. Baltimore, MD: University Park Press, 227-57.

Harris, S.L. 1976. *Managing behavior 8, Behavior modification: Teaching speech to a nonverbal child.* Lawrence, KS: H. and H. Enterprises.

Harris, S.L. 1975. Teaching language to nonverbal children—with emphasis on problems of generalization. *Psych. Bulle.* 82: 565-80.

Harris-Vandeheiden, D. 1976. Blissymbols and the mentally retarded. In *Non-vocal communication techniques and aids for the severely physically handicapped*, ed. G.C. Vanderheiden, and K. Grilley. Baltimore, MD: University Park Press, 120–31.

Harris-Vanderheiden, D., McNaughton, S., and McDonald, E. 1976. Some remarks on assessment. In *Non-vocal communication techniques and aids for the severely physically handicapped*, eds. G.C. Vanderheiden and K. Grilley. Baltimore, MD: University Park Press, 152–68.

Harris-Vanderheiden, D. and Vanderheiden, G.C. 1977. Basic Considerations in Development of Communicative and Interactive Skills for Non-Vocal Severely Handicapped Children. In *Educational Programming for Severely and Profoundly Handicapped*, ed. E. Sontag. Reston, VA: Division on Mentally Retarded, Council for Exceptional Children, 323–34.

Hart, B. and Rogers-Warren, A. 1978. A milieu approach to teaching language. In *Language intervention strategies*, ed. R.L. Schiefelbusch. Baltimore, MD: University Park Press, 193–235.

Hart, V. 1977. The use of many disciplines with the severely and profoundly handicapped. In *Educational programming for the severely and profoundly handicapped*, ed. E. Sontag. Reston, VA: Division on Mental Retardation, Council for Exceptional Children, 391–96.

Hatten, J., Goman, T., and Lent, C. 1976. *Emerging language 2*. Tucson, AZ: Communication Skill Builders, Inc.

Hayden, A.H. and McGinness, G.D. 1977. Bases for early intervention. In *Educational programming for the severely and profoundly handicapped*, ed. E. Sontag. Reston, VA: Division on Mental Retardation, the Council for Exceptional Children, 153–65.

Haynes, U. 1976. *Staff development handbook*. New York: United Cerebral Palsy Associations, Inc.

Hehner, J. 1979. *Blissymbols for use*. Toronto, Canada: Blissymbolics Communication Institute.

Henegar, M.G. and Cornett, R.O. 1971. *Cued speech handbook for parents*. Washington, D. C.: Cued Speech Program, Gallaudet College.

Herst, J., Wolfe, S., Jergensen, G. and Pallen, S. 1976. *Developmental profiles: Sewell Early Education Developmental Program*. Denver, CO: Sewell Rehabilitation Center.

Higgins, J. and Mills, J. 1978. Techniques for developing communication systems with non-oral individuals. A workshop presented at Los Gatos Rehabilitation Center, Los Gatos, CA.

High, E.C. 1977. Positioning for Speech. In *Cerebral palsy and communication: What parents can do*, ed. A. Golbin. Washington, D. C.: George Wahington University, 11–26.

Hobson, P.A. and Duncan, P.D. 1979. Sign learning and profoundly retarded people. *Ment. Retard.* 17: 33–37.

Hogg, J. 1975. Normative development and educational program planning for severely educationally sub-normal children. In *Behavior modification with the severely retarded*, eds. C.C. Kiernan, and F.P. Woodford. Amsterdam, Holland: Associated Scientific Publishers.

Holland, A. 1975. Language therapy for children: Some thoughts on context and content. *J. Speech Hear. Dis.* 40: 514–23.

Hollis, J.H. and Carrier, J.K., Jr. 1978. Intervention strategies for non-spech children. In *Language-internvention strategies*, ed. R.L. Schiefelbusch. Baltimore, MD: University Park Press, 57–100.

Holm, V.A. and McCartin, R.E. 1978. Interdisciplinary child development team: Team issues and training in interdisciplinariness. In *Early intervention—A team approach*, eds. E. Allen, V.A. Holm and R.L. Schiefelbusch. Baltimore, MD: University Park Press, 97–122.

Holt, C.S. Buelow, D., and Vanderheiden, G.C. 1978. Interface switch profile and annotated list of commercial switches. In *Non-vocal communication resource book*, ed. G.C. Vanderheiden. Baltimore, MD: University Park Press.

Horstmeier, D.S. and MacDonald, J.D. 1978a. *Environmental prelanguage battery*. Columbus, OH: Charles E. Merrill Publishing Co.

Horstmeier, D.S. and MacDonald, J. 1978b. *Ready, set, go; talk to me*. Columbus, OH: Charles E. Merrill Publishing Company.
Howard, G., ed. 1979. *Helping the handicapped: A guide to aids developed by the Telephone Pioneers of America*. New York: Telephone Pioneers of America.
Huttenlocher, J. 1974. The origins of language comprehension. In *Theories in cognitive psychology*, ed. R. Solso. New York: Halsted Press.
Jaffe, M., Blackstone, S., and Hanna, R. 1980. Total Communication: Intervention strategies. A short course presented at the Three Rivers Conference, Pittsburgh, PA.
Jarrow, J.E. and Northrup, B.K. 1979. Non-verbal options in communication. . . .Who, What, Where, When, Why, How!?! A miniseminar presented at the American Speech-Language-Hearing Association Convention, Atlanta, GA.
Jensema, C.K. 1979. Communication methods used with deaf-blind children: making the decision. *Am. Anns. Deaf* 124: 7–8.
Jernberg, A.M. 1979. *Theraplay*. San Francisco: Jossey-Bass, Inc.
Kahn, J.V. 1978. Acceleration of object permanence with severely and profoundly retarded children. *AAESPH Rev.* 3: 16–22.
Kapisovsky, M.M. 1978. The use of sign language with nonverbal hearing children: A review of the literature. Unpublished Master's Thesis, Boston University, Boston, MA.
Karnes, M.B. 1972. *GOAL: language development*. Springfield, MA: Milton Bradley Company.
Kates, B. and McNaughton, S. 1975. *The first application of blissymbolics as a communication medium for non-speaking children: history and development, 1971–1974*. Toronto, Canada: Blissymbolics Communication Institute.
Keenan, J.S. and Brassel, E.G. 1975. *Aphasia language performance scale*. Murfreesboro, TN: Veterans Administration Hospital.
Keeney, T. and Wolfe, J. 1972. The acquisition of agreement in English. *J. Verb. Learn. Verb. Beh.* 11: 698–705.
Kent, L.R. 1974. *Language acquisition program for the retarded and multiply impaired*. Champaign, IL: Research Press.
Kimble, S.L. 1975. Signed English: A language teaching technique with totally nonverbal, severely mentally retarded adolescents. A paper presented at the American Speech-Language-Hearing Association Convention, Washington, D. C.
Kipnis, C. 1976. *The mime book*. New York: Harper & Row.
Kirk, S.A., McCarthy, J.J. 1968. and Kirk, W.D. *The Illinois test of psycholinguistic abilities*. rev. ed. Urbana, IL: University of Illinois Press.
Kladde, A.G. 1974. Non-oral communication techniques: Project Summary No. 1, August, 1967. In *Non-oral communication system project 1964/1973*, ed. B. Vicker. Iowa City, IA: Campus Stores, Publishers, The Univerity of Iowa, 57–104.
Klima, E.S. and Bellugi, U. 1979. *The signs of language*. Cambridge, MA: Harvard University Press.
Koegel, R.L. and Covert, A. 1972. The relationship of self-stimulation to learning in autistic children. *J. Appl. Beh. Anal.* 5: 143–57.
Koepp-Baker, H. 1971. The cleft palate team. In *Cleft lip and palate*. eds. W.C. Grabb, S.W. Rosenstein, and K.R. Bzoch. Boston, MA: Little, Brown and Company.
Kohl, F., Fundakowski, G., Menchetti, B., and Coleman, S. 1977. Manual communication training for severely handicapped students. In *The severely and profoundly handicapped child*, Illinois Office of Education, 105–21.
Konstantareas, M.M. and Leibovitz, S.F. 1978. Auditory-visual versus visual communication with autistic and autistic-like children. A paper presented at the American Speech-Hearing-Language-Hearing Association Convention, Chicago, IL.
Konstantareas, M.M., Oxman, J., and Webster, C.D. 1978. Iconicity: Effects on the acquisition of sign language by autistic and other dysfunctional children. In *Understanding language through sign language research*, ed. P. Siple. New York: Academic Press 213–37.

Kopchick, G.A. and Lloyd, L.L. 1976. Total Communication for the severely language impaired: A 24-hour approach. In *Communication assessment and intervention strategies,* ed. L.L. Lloyd. Baltimore, MD: University Park Press, 501–22.

Koselka, M.J., Hannah, E.P., Gardner, J.O., and Reagan, W. 1975. Total communication therapy for a non-deaf child and his family. A paper presented at the American Speech and Hearing Association Convention, Washington, D. C.

Krogman, W.M. 1979. The cleft palate team in action. In *Cleft palate and cleft lip: A team approach,* H.K. Cooper, R.L. Harding, W.M. Krogman, M. Mazaheri, and R.T. Millard. Philadelphia: W.B. Saunders Company.

Kuhn, D. 1973. Imitation Theory and Research from a Cognitive Perspective. *Hum. Devel.* 16: 157–80.

Lahey, M. 1974. Use of prosody and syntactic markers in children's comprehension of spoken sentences. *J. Speech Hear. Res.* 17: 656–68.

Lahey, M. and Bloom, L. 1977. Planning a first lexicon: which words to teach first. *J. Speech Hear. Dis.* 42: 340–50.

Lane, H. 1977. Notes for a psychohistory of American Sign Language. *Deaf Am.* 30: 3–7.

Leathers, D.G. 1976. *Nonverbal communication systems.* Boston, MA: Allyn and Bacon, Inc.

Leonard, L. 1975. Modeling as a clinical procedure in language training: *Lang. Speech Hear. Serv. Schools* 6: 72–85.

Levett, L.M. 1969. A method of communication for nonspeaking severely sub-normal children. *Brit. J. Dis. Communic.* 4: 64–6.

Levett, L.M. 1971. A method of communication for nonspeaking, severely subnormal children—trial results. *Brit. J. Dis. Communic.* 6: 125–28.

Liddell, S.K. 1978. Nonmanual signals and relative clauses in American Sign Language. In *Understanding language through sign language research,* ed. P. Siple. New York: Academic Press, 59–90.

Liebergott, J.W. 1980. Facilitating communication and linguistic abilities in preschool language impaired children. A short course at the Three Rivers Conference on Communicative Disorders, Pittsburgh, PA.

Liebman, R. 1977. Feeding therapy and speech: Some problems of oral motor control. In *Cerebral palsy and communication: What parents can do,* ed. A. Golbin. Washington, D. C.: George Washington Univerity, 27–44.

Lovaas, O.I., Berberich, J.P., Perloff, B.F., and Schaeffer, B. 1966. Acqusition of imitative speech by schizophrenic children. *Science* 151: 705–7.

Love, R.J., Hagerman, E.L., and Taimi, E.G. 1980. Speech performance, dysphagia and oral reflexes in cerebral palsy. *J. Speech Hear. Dis.* 45: 59–75.

Lykos, C.M. 1971. *Cued speech handbook for teachers.* Washington, D. C.: Cued Speech Program, Gallaudet College.

Lyon, S., Baumgart, D., Stoll, A., and Brown, L. 1977. Curricular strategies for teaching basic functional object use skills to severely handicapped students. In *Curricular strategies for teaching nonverbal communication, functional object use and problem-solving skills to severely handicapped students, vol. VIII, part 1,* eds. L. Brown, J. Nietupski, S. Lyon, S. Hamre-Nietupski, T. Crowner and L. Grunewald. Madison, WI: Department of Specialized Educational Service.

MacDonald, J.D. 1978. *Environmental language inventory.* Columbus, OH: Charles E. Merrill Publishing Co.

MacDonald, J.D. and Blott, J. 1974. Environmental language intervention: The rationale for a diagnostic and training strategy through rules, context and generalization. *J. Speech Hear. Dis.* 39: 244–56.

McCormack, J.E. and Audette, R.H. 1977. Developing twenty-four hour service plans for severely handicapped learners. *AAESPH Rev.* 2: 209–16.

McCormack, J.E. and Chalmers, A.J. 1978. *Early cognitive instruction for the moderately and severely handicapped.* Champaign, IL: Research Press Company.

McDonald, E.T. 1976. Conventional symbols of English. In *Non-vocal communication technique and aids for the severely physically handicapped,* eds. G.C. Vanderheiden and K. Grilley. Baltimore, MD: University Park Press, 77–84.

McDonald, E.T. 1980. Early identification and treatment of children at risk for speech development. In *Nonspeech language and communication: analysis and intervention*, ed. R.L. Schiefelbusch. Baltimore, MD: University Park Press, 49–79.

McDonald, E.T. and Crane, B. 1964. *Cerebral palsy*. Englewood Cliffs, NJ: Prentice-Hall, Inc.

McDonald, E.T. and Schultz, A. 1973. Communication boards for cerebral palsied children. *J. Speech Hear. Dis.* 38: 73–88.

McLean, J.E. and Snyder-McLean, L.K. 1978. *Transactional approach to early language training*. Columbus, OH: Charles E. Merrill Publishing Company.

McLean, L. and McLean, J. 1974. A language training program for nonverbal autistic children. *J. Speech Hear. Res.* 35: 186–93.

McNaughton, S. 1978. Blissymbolics. A paper presented at the Council for Exceptional Children Congress, Winnipeg, Manitoba.

McNaughton, S. and Kates, S. 1980. The application of Blissymbolics. In *Nonspeech language and communication: Analysis and intervention*, ed. R.L. Schiefelbusch. Baltimore, MD: University Park Press, 303–21.

Mallery, G. 1881. Sign language among North American Indians compared with that among other peoples and deaf mutes. In *First annual report of the Bureau of Ethnology to the Secretary of the Smithsonian Institution* 1879–1880, Washington, D. C.: Government Printing Office, 263–552.

Mallik, K. 1977. *Communication resources for the developmentally disabled: A guide for parents paraprofessionals, and professionals*. Washington, D. C.: The George Washington University Job Development Laboratory.

Markowicz, H. 1977. *American Sign Language: Fact and fancy*. Washington, D. C.: Gallaudet College.

Mayberry, R.I. 1976. If a chimp can learn sign language, surely my nonverbal client can too. *Asha* 18: 223–28.

Mayberry, R.I. 1978. Manual communication. In *Hearing and deafness*, 4th ed., eds. H. Davis and S.R. Silverman. New York: Holt, Rinehart, and Winston.

Melichar, J.F. 1977. *ISAARE*, volumes 1 to 7. San Mateo, CA: Adaptive Systems Corporation.

Melichar, J.F. 1978. ISAARE: A description. *Am. Assoc. Ed. Severe. Profound. Handicapp. Rev.* 3: 259–68.

Miller, A. 1968. *Symbol and accentuation—A new approach to reading*. Santa Ana, CA: Doubleday Multimedia.

Miller, J. 1977. On specifying what to teach: The movement from structure, to structure and meaning, to structure and meaning and knowing. In *Educational programming for the severely and profoundly handicapped*, ed. E. Sontag. Reston, VA: Division on Mental Retardation, Council for Exceptional Children.

Miller, J.F., Chapman, R.S., Branston, M.B., Reichle, J. 1980. Language comprehension in sensorimotor stages V and VI. *J. Speech Hear. Res.* 23: 284–311.

Miller, J.F., Reichle, J. and Rettie, M. 1977. Sensorimotor, stage 5—children's responses to requests and demands in a free play task. Unpublished manuscript.

Miller, J.F. and Yoder, D.E. 1972. A syntax teaching program. In *Language intervention with the retarded: Developing strategies*, eds. J.E. McLeary, D.E. Yoder and R.L. Schiefelbusch. Baltimore, MD: University Park Press.

Miller, J.F. and Yoder, D. 1974. An ontogenetic language teaching strategy for retarded children. In *Language perspectives—acquisition, retardation and intervention*, eds. R.L. Schiefelbusch and L.L. Lloyd. Baltimore, MD: University Park Press, 505–28.

Miller, M.A., Cuvo, A.J. and Borakove, L.S. 1977. Teaching naming of coin values—comprehension before production versus production alone. *J. Appl. Beh. Anal.* 10: 735–36.

Mills, V. 1972. Board of Education of the District of Columbia. 348 F. Supp. 866, D.C.D.C.

(Anon.) 1977. *Mime directory: Human resources, vol. 1*. New York: International Mimes and Pantomimists.

(Anon.) 1978. *Mime directory: Bibliography, vol. 2.* New York: International Mimes and Pantomimists.

Montgomery, J. 1980a. Measuring communication aid effectiveness. *Non-oral Communicat. Center Newsletter* 3: 1–3.

Montgomery, J., ed. 1980b. *Non-oral communication: A training guide for the child without speech.* Title IV-C ESEA, Exemplary/Incentive Grant.

Montgomery, J. 1979. Potential funding sources for the purchase of non-oral communication systems. In *Phonic Mirror HandiVoice seminar manual*, eds. C. Cohen, J. Montgomery and D. Yoder. Mill Valley, CA: H. C. Electronics, Inc., 166–67.

Moores, D.F. 1969. Cued speech: Some practical and theoretical considerations. *Am. Ann. Deaf* 114: 23–27.

Moores, D.F. 1980. American Sign Language: Historical perspectives and current issues. In *Nonspeech language and communication: Analysis and intervention*, ed. R.L. Schiefelbusch. Baltimore, MD: University Park Press, 93–100.

(Anon.) n.d. *Morse Code for the radio amateur.* London, England: Radio Society of Great Britain.

Mueller, H. 1975a. Feeding. In *Handling the young cerebral palsied child at home*, ed. N.R. Finnie. New York: E. P. Dutton & Co., Inc., 113–32.

Mueller, H. 1975b. Speech. In *Handling the young cerebral palsied child at home*, ed. N.R. Finnie. New York: E. P. Dutton & Co., Inc., 133–40.

Murdock, J. and Hartmann, B. 1975. *A language development program: Imitative gestures to basic syntactic structures.* Salt Lake City, UT: Word Making Productions, Inc.

Musselwhite, C.R. and Thompson, E.R. 1979. Functional fine motor skills curriculum. Unpublished manuscript.

Myers, L.S., Grows, N.L., Coleman, C.L. and Cook, A.M. 1980. An assessment battery for assistive device systems recommendations, part I. Sacramento, CA: Assistive Device Center, California State University.

Newell, A.F. 1974. Morse Code and voice control for the disabled. In *Aids for the severely handicapped*, ed. K. Copeland. New York: Grune and Stratton, 54–58.

Nicholls, G.H. 1979. Cued Speech and the reception of spoken language. Unpublished Master's Thesis, McGill University, Montreal, Canada.

Nietupski, J., Stoll, A., Broome, D., and Brown, L. 1977. Curricular strategies for teaching selected problem solving skills to severely handicapped students. In *Curricular strategies for teaching functional object use, nonverbal communication, problem solving, and mealtime skills to severely handicapped students*, vol. VII, part 1, eds. L. Brown, J. Nietupski, S. Lyon, S. Hamre-Nietupski, T. Crowner, and L. Gruenewald. Madison, WI: Department of Specialized Educational Services.

Nietupski, J. and Williams, W. 1974. Teaching severely handicapped students to use the telephone to initiate selected recreational activities and to respond to telephone requests to engage in selected recreational activities. In *A collection of papers and programs related to publish school services for severely handicapped students*, vol. IV, eds. L. Brown, W. Williams and T. Crowner. Madison, WI: Madison Public Schools, 507–60.

Nietupski, J., Williams, W., and York, R. Teaching selected phonic word analysis reading skills to TMR labeled students. Unpublished manuscript.

Nietupski, J., Williams, W., York, R., Johnson, F., and Brown, L. A review of instructional programs designed to teach selected reading and spelling skills to severely handicapped students. Unpublished manuscript.

Norton, S.J., Schultz, M.C., Reed, C.M., Braida, L.D., Durlach, N.I., Rabinowitz, W.M., and Chomsky, C. 1977. Analytic study of the Tadoma Method: Background and preliminary results. *J. Speech Hear. Res.* 20: 574–95.

O'Rourke, T.J. 1971. *A basic course in Manual Communication.* Silver Spring, MD: National Association of the Deaf.

Overton, W.F. and Jackson, J.P. 1973. The representation of imagined objects in action sequences: A developmental study. *Child Develop.* 44: 309–14.

Paget, R. 1951. *The new Sign Language.* London, England: The Welcome Foundation.

Pennsylvania Association for Retarded Children v. Commonwealth of Pennsylvania, 1972. 343-F. Supp. 279.

Piaget, J. 1954. *The construction of reality in the child.* New York: Ballantine.

Piaget, J. 1963. *The origins of intelligence in children.* New York: W. W. Norton.

Piaget, J. and Inhelder, B. 1969. *The psychology fo the child.* New York: Basic Books.

Popovich, D. 1977. *A prescriptive behavioral checklist for the severely and profoundly retarded.* Baltimore: University Park Press.

Porch, B. 1971. *Porch index of communicative ability.* Palo Alto, CA: Consulting Psychologists.

Premack, D. 1970. A functional analysis of language. *J. Exp. Anal. Beh.* 14: 107-25.

Rees, N.S. 1975. Imitation and language development: Issues and clinical implications. *J. Speech Hear. Dis.* 40: 339-50.

Reich, R. 1978. Gestural facilitation of expressive language in moderately/severely retarded preschoolers. *Ment. Retard.* 16: 113-17.

Reichle, J.E. and Yoder, D.E. 1979. Assessment and early stimulation of communication in the severely and profoundly mentally retarded. In *Teaching the severely handicapped,* vol. IV, eds. R.L. York and E. Edgar. Columbus, OH: Special Press, 155-79.

Reid, B.A. and Reid, W.R. 1974. Role expectations of paraprofessional staff in special education. *Focus on Except. Child.* 6: 1-14.

Reike, J.A., Lynch, L.L., and Soltman, S.F. 1977. *Teaching strategies for language development.* New York: Grune & Stratton.

Reikehof, L.L. 1978. *The joy of signing.* Springfield, MO: Gospel Publishing House.

Rinard, G.A. and Rugg, D.E. 1977. Current state of development and testing of an ocular control device. A paper presented at the Conference on Systems and Devices for the Disabled, Seattle, WA.

Rinard, G.A. and Rugg, D.E. 1978. Application of the ocular transducer to the ETRAN Communicator. A paper presented at the Fifth Conference on Systems and Devices for the Disabled, Houston, TX.

Risley, T., Hart, B., and Doke, L. 1972. Operant language development: The outline of a therapeutic technology. In *Language of the mentally retarded,* ed. R. Schiefelbusch. Baltimore, MD: University Park Press, 107-23.

Robbins, N. 1978. *Sign Language curricula.* Watertown, MA: Perkins School for the Blind.

Robinson, C.C. and Robinson, J.H. 1978. Sensorimotor functions and cognitive development. In *Systematic instruction of the moderately and severely handicapped,* ed. M.E. Snell. Columbus, OH: Charles E. Merrill Publishing Co., 102-53.

Roos, P. 1977. A parent's view of what public education should accomplish. In *Educational programming for the severely and profoundly handicapped,* ed. E. Sontag. Reston, VA: Division on Mental Retardation, Council for Exceptional Children, 72-83.

Rubin. I., Plovnick, M. and Fry, R. 1975. *Improving the coordination of care: A program for health team development.* Cambridge, MA: Ballinger Publishing House.

Ruder, K. and Smith, M. 1974. Issues in language training. In *Language perspectives— Acquisition, retardation and intervention,* eds. R. Schiefelbusch, and L. Lloyd. Baltimore, MD: University Park Press.

Rumbaugh, D.M., ed. 1977. *Language learning by a chimpanzee: The Lana project.* New York: Academic Press.

Rumbaugh, D.M. 1978. LANA Project helps retarded children learn language. *Yerkes Newsletter* 15: 20-23.

Rumbaugh, D.M. and Savage-Rumbaugh, S. 1978. Chimpanzee language research: Status and potential. *Beh. Res. Meth. Instrumen.* 10: 119-31.

Rupert, J. 1969. Kindergarten program using cued speech at the Idaho State School for the Deaf. Report of the Proceedings of the 44th Meeting of the American Instructors of the Deaf, Berkeley, CA.

St. Louis, K.O. and Ruscello, D.M. *Oral Speech Mechanism Screening Examination.* Baltimore, MD: University Park Press.

St. Louis, K.W., Mattingly, S., Esposito, A., and Cone, J.D. 1980. *Receptive language curriculum for the moderately, severely and profoundly handicapped.* Morgantown, WV: The West Virginia System, West Virginia University.

St. Louis, K.W., Rejzer, R., and Cone, J.D. 1980. *Expressive language curriculum for the moderately, severely and profoundly handicapped.* Morgantown, WV: The West Virginia System, West Virginia University.

Sapon, S.M., Kaczmarek, L.A., Welber, E.R., Rouzer, R.M., and Sapon-Shevin, M.E. 1976. *Readings in the descriptive analysis of behavior: Teaching strategies.* Rochester, NY: University of Rochester Verbal Behavior Laboratory.

Savage-Rumbaugh, E.S., Rumbaugh, D.M., and Boysen, S. 1980. Do apes use language? *Am. Sci.* 68: 49–61.

Saya, M.J. 1979. Adult aphasics and the Bliss Symbol Language. A paper presented at the American Speech and Hearing Association Convention, Atlanta, GA.

Sayre, J.M. 1963. Communication for the non-verbal cerebral palsied. *Cereb. Palsy Rev.* 24: 3–8.

Schaeffer, B. 1980. Spontaneous language through signed speech. In *Nonspeech language and communication: Analysis and intervention,* ed. R. Schiefelbusch. Baltimore, MD: University Park Press, 421–46.

Scheuerman, N., Baumgart, D., Sipsma, K. and Brown, L. 1976. Toward the development of a curriculum for teaching nonverbal communication skills to severely handicapped students: Teaching basic tracking, scanning and selection skills. In *Madison's alternative for zero exclusion: Toward an integrated therapy model for teaching motor, tracking and scanning skills to severely handicapped students, vol. VI, part 3,* eds. L. Brown, N. Scheuerman, and T. Crowner. Madison, WI: Department of Specialized Educational Services.

Schienberg, S. 1980. PACE: An alternative approach to aphasia therapy. A mini-seminar presented at the Three Rivers Conference on Communicative Disorders, Pittsburgh, PA.

Schlanger, P.H. 1976. Training the adult aphasic to pantomime. A paper presented at the American Speech-Language-Hearing Association, Houston, TX.

Schlanger, P.H., Geffner, D.S., and DiCarrado, C. 1974. A comparison of gestural communication with aphasics. Pre and post therapy. A paper presented at the American Speech and Hearing Association Convention, Las Vegas, NV.

Schumaker, J.B. and Sherman, J.A. 1978. Parent as intervention agent: From birth onward. In *Language intervention strategies,* ed. R. Schiefelbusch. 237–315.

Schurman, J.A. 1974. Custom designing communication board frames: The role of the occupational therapist. In *Nonoral communication system project, 1964–1973,* ed. B. Vicker. Iowa City, IA: Campus Stores, Publishers, The University of Iowa.

Searcy, K.L., Opat, J., Welch, M.L. 1979. The Mercy approach to theraplay (MAT) facilitation of communication. A paper presented at the American Speech-Language-Hearing Association Convention, Atlanta, GA.

Shane, H.C. 1980. Approaches to assessing the communication of non-oral persons. In *Nonspeech language and communication: Analysis and intervention,* ed. R.L. Schiefelbusch. Baltimore, MD: University Park Press, 197–224.

Shane, H.C. Decision making in early augmentative communication system use. In R.L. Schiefelbusch and D. Bricker, *Early language intervention,* Baltimore, MD: University Park Press (in press).

Shane, H.C. and Bashir, A.S. 1978. Election criteria for determining candidacy for an argumentative communication system: Preliminary considerations. A paper presented at the American Speech-Language-Hearing Association Convention, San Francisco, CA.

Shane, H.C. and Bashir, A.S. 1980. Election criteria for the adoption of an augmentative communication system: Preliminary considerations. *J. Speech Hear. Dis.* 45: 408–14.

Shane, H.C. and Melrose, J. 1975. An electronic conversation board and an accompanying training program for aphonic expressive communication. A paper presented at the American Speech-Language-Hearing Association Convention, Washington, D. C.

Sheppard, J.J. 1964. Cranio-oropharyngeal motor patterns associated with cerebral palsy. *J. Speech Hear. Res.* 7: 373–80.

Siegel, G. and Spradlin, J. 1978. Programming for language and communication therapy. In *Language intervention strategies,* ed. R. Schiefelbusch. Baltimore, MD: University Park Press, 357–98.

Sigelman, D.K. and Bensberg, G.J. 1976. Supportive personnel for the developmentally disabled. In *Communication assessment and intervention strategies,* ed. L.L. Lloyd. Baltimore, MD: University Park Press, 653–90.

Silverman, F. 1980. *Communication for the speechless.* Englewood Cliffs, NJ: Prentice-Hall, Inc.

Silverman, H. and Kelso, D. 1977. The Bliss-Com. A portable symbol printing communication aid. Proceedings of the Fourth Annual Conference on Systems and Devices for the Disabled, Seattle, WA.

Silverman, H., McNaughton, S., and Kates, B. 1978. *Handbook of Blissymbolics for instructors, users, parents and administrators.* Toronto, Ontario: Blissymbolics Communication Institute.

Simmons, V. and Williams, I. 1976. *STEPS UP to language for the learning impaired.* Tucson, AZ: Communication Skill Builders, Inc.

Simpson, M.A. and McDade, H.L. 1979. A total communication approach in an interdisciplinary infant development program. A paper presented at the American Speech-Language-Hearing Association Convention, Atlanta, GA.

Siple, P. 1978. Linguistic and psychological properties of American Sign Language: An overview. In *Understanding language through sign language research,* ed. P. Siple. New York: Academic Press, 3–23.

Skelly, M. and Schinsky, L. 1979. *Amer-Ind gestural code based on universal American Indian Hand Talk.* New York: Elsevier North Holland, Inc.

Sklar, M. 1973. *Sklar aphasia scale.* Los Angeles, CA: Western Psychologial Service.

Sloane, H.N., Johnson, M.K., and Harris, F.R. 1968. Remedial procedures for teaching verbal behavior to speech deficient or defective young children. In *Operant procedures in remedial speech and language training,* eds. H.N. Sloane and B. McCauley. Boston, MA: Houghton-Mifflin Company, 77–101.

Smith, D.D. and Smith, J.O. 1978. Trends. In *Systematic instruction of the moderately and severely handicapped,* ed. M.E. Snell. Columbus, OH: Charles E. Merrill, 478–93.

Smith, L. 1972. Comprehension performance of oral deaf and normal hearing children at three stages of language development. Unpublished doctoral dissertation, University of Wisconsin, Madison, WI.

Snell, M.E. 1974. Sign language and total communication. In *Language acquisition program for the severely retarded,* ed. L. Kent. Champaign, IL: Research Press.

Snell, M.E. 1978. Functional reading. In *Systematic instruction of the moderately and severely handicapped,* ed. M.E. Snell. Columbus, OH: Charles E. Merrill Publishing Company, 324–85.

Snyder-McLean, L. 1978. Language training procedures for non-verbal severely retarded clients: Functional stimulus and response variables. A paper presented at the American Association for the Education of the Severely/Profoundly Handicapped, Baltimore, MD.

Soltman, S.F. and Rieke, J.A. 1977. Communication management for the nonresponsive child: A team approach. In *Educational programming for the severely and profoundly handicapped,* ed. E. Sontag. Reston, VA: The Council for Exceptional Children, 348–59.

Song, A.Y. 1979. Acquisition and use of Blissymbols by severely mentally retarded adolescents. *Ment. Retard.* 17: 253–55.

Sternat, J., Messina, R., Nietupski, J., Lyon, S., and Brown, L. 1977. Occupational and physical therapy services for severely handicapped students: Toward a naturalized public school service delivery model. In *Educational programming for the severely and profoundly handicapped*, ed. E. Sontag. Reston, VA: Division on Mental Retardation, The Council for Exceptional Children, 263-78.

Stokes, T. and Baer, D. 1977. An implicit technology of generalization. *J. Appl. Beh. Anal.* 10: 349-67.

Stokoe, W.C. 1980. The study and use of sign language. In *Nonspeech language and communication: Analysis and intervention*, ed. R.L. Schiefelbusch. Baltimore, MD: University Park Press, 123-55.

Stokoe, W.C., Casterline, D., and Croneberg, C. 1978. *Dictionary of American Sign Language*, rev. ed. Silver Spring, MD: Linstock Press.

Storm, R.H. and Willis, J.H. 1978. Small-group training as an alternative to individual programs for profoundly retarded persons. *Am. J. Ment. Deficiency* 83: 283-88.

Stremel, K. and Waryas, C. 1974. A behavioral-psycholinguistic approach to language training. In *Developing systematic procedures for training children's language*, ed. L.V. McReynolds. ASHA Monographs 18, 96-132.

Stremel-Campbell, K., Cantrell, D., and Halle, J. 1977. Manual signing as a language system and as a speech initiator for the nonverbal severely handicapped student. In *Educational programming for the severely and profoundly handicapped*, ed. E. Sontag. Reston, VA: Council for Exceptional Children, Division on Mental Retardation, 335-47.

Striefel, S. 1977. *Managing Behavior 7, Behavior modification: Teaching a child to imitate.* Lawrence, KS: H & H Enterprises.

Striefel, S., Wetherby, B., and Karlan, G.R. 1976. Establishing generalized verb-noun instruction-following skills in retarded children. *J. Exp. Child Psychol.* 22: 247-60.

Striefel, S., Wetherby, B., and Karlan, G.R. 1978. Developing generalized instruction-following behavior in the severely retarded. In *Quality of life in severely and profoundly mentally retarded people: Research foundation for improvement*, ed. C.E. Myers. Monograph, American Association of Mental Deficiency No. 3.

Struck, R. 1977. Santa Cruz Special Education Management System. *Behavioral characteristics progression (BCP).* Palo Alto, CA: VORT Corporation.

Stuckey, K.A., Kaehler, T., and Minihane, W.M. eds. 1977. *Deaf-blind bibliography* rev. ed. Watertown, MA: Perkins School for the Blind.

Sullivan, R.C. 1976. The role of the parent. In *Hey, don't forget about me*, ed. M.A. Thomas. Reston, VA: The Council for Exceptional Children, 36-45.

Supalla, T. and Newport, E.L. 1978. How many seats in a chair? The derivation of nouns and verbs in American Sign Language. In *Understanding language through Sign Language research*, ed. P. Siple. New York: Academic Press, 91-132.

Switzky, H., Rotator, A.F., Miller, T. and Freagon, S. 1979. The developmental model and its implications for assessment and instruction for the severely/profoundly handicapped. *Ment. Retard.* 17: 167-70.

Tawney, J.W., ed. 1979. *Programmed environments curriculum*, Columbus, OH: Charles E. Merrill Publishing Co.

Tilton, J.R., Liska, D.C., and Bourland, J.D., eds. 1977. *Guide to early developmental training: Wabash center for the mentally retarded*, Boston, MA: Allyn and Bacon, Inc.

Topper-Zweiban, S. 1977. Indicators of success in learning a manual communication mode. *Ment. Retard.* 15: 47-49.

Trantham, C. and Pedersen, J. 1976. *Normal language development: The key to diagnosis and therapy for language-disordered children.* Baltimore, MD: The Williams and Wilkins Company.

Traub, D. 1977. Training teachers to use communication boards with the mentally retarded. A paper presented at the American Speech and Hearing Association Convention, Chicago, IL.

Tucker, D.J. and Horner, R.D. 1977. Competency-based training of paraprofessional teaching associates for education of the severely and profoundly handicapped. In *Educational programming for the severely and profoundly handicapped*, ed. E. Sontag. Reston, VA: Division on Mental Retardation, Council for Exceptional Children, 405-17.

(Anon.) 1976. *Tune in the world with ham radio.* Newington, CT: The American Radio Relay League.

Turnbull, A.P. 1978. Parent-professional interactions. In *Systematic instruction of the moderately and severely handicapped,* ed. M.E. Snell. Columbus, OH: Charles E. Merrill Publishing Company, 458–76.

Utley, B.L., Holvoet, J.F., Barnes, K. 1977. Handling, positioning, and feeding the physically handicapped. In *Educational programming for the severely and profoundly handicapped,* ed. E. Sontag. Reston, VA: Division on Mental Retardation, Council for Exceptional Children, 279–99.

Uzgiris, J.C. and Hunt, J. 1975. *Assessment in infancy: Ordinal scales of psychological development.* Urbana, IL: University of Illinois Press.

Vanderheiden, G.C. 1976a. Providing the child with a means to indicate. In *Non-vocal communication technique and aids for the severely physically handicapped,* eds. G. Vanderheiden and K. Grilley. Baltimore, MD: University Park Press.

Vanderheiden, G.C. 1976b. Synthesized speech as a communication mode for non-verbal severely handicapped individuals. Madison, WI: Trace Research and Development Center.

Vanderheiden, G.C. 1977. Design and construction of a laptray: Preliminary notes. Madison, WI: The Trace Research and Development Center.

Vanderheiden, G.C., ed. 1978. *Non-vocal communication resource book.* Baltimore, MD: University Park Press.

Vanderheiden, G. and Grilley, K., eds. 1976. *Non-vocal communication techniques and aids for the severely physically handicapped.* Baltimore, MD: University Park Press.

Vanderheiden, G.C. and Harris-Vanderheiden, D. 1976. Communication techniques and aids for the non-vocal, severely handicapped. In *Communication assessment and intervention strategies,* ed. L.L. Lloyd. Baltimore, MD: University Park Press.

Velletri-Glass, A., Gazzaniga, M., and Premack, D. 1973. Artificial language training in global aphasics. *Neuropsychologia* 11: 95–104.

Vicker, B. 1974a. Advances in nonoral communication system programming: Project Summary #2, August 1973. In *Nonoral communication system project, 1964/1973,* ed. B. Vicker. Iowa City, IA: Campus Stores, Publishers, The University of Iowa, 105–75.

Vicker, B., ed. 1974b. *Nonoral communication system project, 1964/1973,* Iowa City, IA: Campus Stores, Publishers, The University of Iowa.

Von Glassersfeld, E. 1977. The Yerkish language and its automatic parser. In *Language learning by a chimpanzee: the Lana project,* ed. D.M. Rumbaugh. New York: Academic Press.

Warner, H., Bell, C.L., and Brown, J.V. 1977. The conversation board. In *Language learning by a chimpanzee: The Lana project,* ed. D.M. Rumbaugh. New York: Academic Press.

Waryas, C.L., and Stremel-Campbell, K. 1978. Grammatical training for the language-delayed child: A new perspective. In *Language intervention strategies,* ed. R.L. Schiefelbusch. Baltimore, MD: University Park Press, 145–92.

Washington State School for the Deaf 1972. *An introduction to Manual English.* Vancouver, WA: The Washington State School for the Deaf.

Waugh, M.M., and Gibson, P.K. 1979. Functional application of Bliss symbols with preschool cerebral palsied children. Evanston, IL: Institute for Continuing Professional Education.

Wepman, J.M. 1951. *Recovery from aphasia,* New York: The Ronald Press.

Wetherby, B. and Striefel, S. 1978. Application of miniature linguistic system of matrix-training procedures. In *Language intervention strategies,* ed. R.L. Schiefelbusch. Baltimore, MD: University Park Press, 317–56.

Whitman, T., Zakaras, M., and Chardos, S. 1971. Effects of reinforcement and guidance procedures or instruction-following behavior of severely retarded children. *J. Appl. Beh. Anal.* 4: 283–90.

Wilbur, R.B. 1976. The linguistics of manual language and manual systems. In

Communication assessment and intervention strategies, ed. L.L. Lloyd. Baltimore, MD: University Park Press, 423–500.

Wilbur, R.B. 1979. *American sign language and sign systems*. Baltimore, MD: University Park Press.

Wilcox, M.J., Davis, G.A., and Leonard, L.B. 1978. Diagnosis and treatment implications on analysis of an aphasic patient's contextual language comprehension. *Clinical aphasiology conference proceedings*. Minneapolis, MN: BRK Press.

Williams, W., Brown, L., and Certo, N. 1975. Basic components of instructional programs for severely handicapped students. *Theory Into Pract.* 14: 123–36.

Williams, W. and Fox, T., eds. 1977. Communication. In *Minimum objective system for pupils with severe handicaps: Working draft number one*, vol. 1. Burlington, VT: Center for Special Education, University of Vermont.

Wilson, P.S., Goodman, L., and Wood, R.K. 1975. *Manual language for the child without language: A behavioral approach for teaching the exceptional child*. Hartford, CT: Department of Mental Retardation Developmental Team.

(Anon.) 1978. *WISP parent program guide*. Laramie, WY: Project WISP/Outreach.

Woolman, D.H. 1980. A presymbolic training program. In *Nonspeech language and communication*, ed. R.L. Schiefelbusch. Baltimore, MD: University Park Press, 325–56.

Woodcock, R.W. 1968. Rebuses as a medium in beginning reading instruction. Nashville, TN: Institute on Mental Retardation and Intellectual Development.

Woodcock, R.W. 1970. The learning disabled and the Peabody Rebus Reading Program. A paper presented at the Council for Exceptional Children Convention, Chicago, IL.

Woodcock, R.W., Clark, C.R., and Davies, C.O. 1969. *The Peabody Rebus Reading Program*. Circle Pines, MN: American Guidance Service.

Woodward, J. 1976. Signs of change: Historical variation in American Sign Language. *Sign Lang. Studies* 10: 81–94.

Woodward, J. 1978. Historical bases of American Sign Language. In *Understanding language through sign language research*, ed. P. Siple. New York: Academic Press, 333–47.

Worthley, W.J. 1978. *Source book of language learning activities*. Boston, MA: Little, Brown and Company.

Wulz, S.V. and Hollis, J.J. 1980. Word identification and comprehension training for exceptional children. In *Nonspeech language and communication: Analysis and intervention*, ed. R.L. Schiefelbusch. Baltimore, MD: University Park Press, 357–87.

Yoder, D.E. and Reichle, J.E. 1977. Functions of language in the communication process. In *Research to practice in mental retardation, vol. 2*, ed. P. Mittler. Baltimore, MD: University Park Press.

(Anon.) 1980. *Your medicare handbook*. Washington, D. C.: Superintendent of Documents, U. S. Government Printing Office.

Yule, W., and Berger, M. 1975. Communication, language, and behavior modification. In *Behavior modification with the severely retarded*, eds. C.C. Kiernan and F.P. Woodford. Amsterdam, Holland: Association Scientific Publishers, 33–65.